Geographies of Health

Geographies of Health

Editor: Caleb Coleman

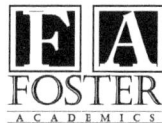

FA
FOSTER
ACADEMICS

www.fosteracademics.com

www.fosteracademics.com

FA
FOSTER
ACADEMICS

Cataloging-in-Publication Data

Geographies of health / edited by Caleb Coleman.
   p. cm.
Includes bibliographical references and index.
ISBN 978-1-63242-896-7
1. Medical geography. 2. Environmental health. 3. Health. 4. Medical care. I. Coleman, Caleb.
RA792 .G46 2020
614.42--dc23

Foster Academics,
118-35 Queens Blvd., Suite 400,
Forest Hills, NY 11375, USA

ISBN 978-1-63242-896-7 (Hardback)

Contents

Preface

An important dimension in the study of human health and healthcare is the adoption of a geographical perspective to the study of disease. Medical geography focuses on the analysis of spatial patterns of disease and the provision of healthcare. Medical geographic studies place diseases in the theoretical context of disease ecology. The study of health services and the spatial access to healthcare, health services planning and healthcare delivery are encompassed within this field. Health geography can be divided into two distinct segments. The first focuses on the geographies of disease and sickness, using disease statistics and distributions, and analytical research that strives to determine the factors that make individuals and a population susceptible to disease. The second component uses spatial analysis and behavioral economics to the study of health facility location, healthcare accessibility and utilization. This book aims to shed light on some of the unexplored aspects of the geographies of health and the recent researches in this field. Different approaches, evaluations, methodologies and advanced studies on medical and health geography have been included herein. It is a collective contribution of a renowned group of international experts.

This book is the end result of constructive efforts and intensive research done by experts in this field. The aim of this book is to enlighten the readers with recent information in this area of research. The information provided in this profound book would serve as a valuable reference to students and researchers in this field.

At the end, I would like to thank all the authors for devoting their precious time and providing their valuable contribution to this book. I would also like to express my gratitude to my fellow colleagues who encouraged me throughout the process.

Editor

Evaluating the risk for Usutu virus circulation in Europe: comparison of environmental niche models and epidemiological models

Yanchao Cheng[1]*[ID], Nils Benjamin Tjaden[1], Anja Jaeschke[1], Renke Lühken[2], Ute Ziegler[3], Stephanie Margarete Thomas[1] and Carl Beierkuhnlein[1,4]

Abstract

Background: Usutu virus (USUV) is a mosquito-borne *flavivirus*, reported in many countries of Africa and Europe, with an increasing spatial distribution and host range. Recent outbreaks leading to regional declines of European common blackbird (*Turdus merula*) populations and a rising number of human cases emphasize the need for increased awareness and spatial risk assessment.

Methods: Modelling approaches in ecology and epidemiology differ substantially in their algorithms, potentially resulting in diverging model outputs. Therefore, we implemented a parallel approach incorporating two commonly applied modelling techniques: (1) Maxent, a correlation-based environmental niche model and (2) a mechanistic epidemiological susceptible-exposed-infected-removed (SEIR) model. Across Europe, surveillance data of USUV-positive birds from 2003 to 2016 was acquired to train the environmental niche model and to serve as test cases for the SEIR model. The SEIR model is mainly driven by daily mean temperature and calculates the basic reproduction number R_0. The environmental niche model was run with long-term bio-climatic variables derived from the same source in order to estimate climatic suitability.

Results: Large areas across Europe are currently suitable for USUV transmission. Both models show patterns of high risk for USUV in parts of France, in the Pannonian Basin as well as northern Italy. The environmental niche model depicts the current situation better, but with USUV still being in an invasive stage there is a chance for under-estimation of risk. Areas where transmission occurred are mostly predicted correctly by the SEIR model, but it mostly fails to resolve the temporal dynamics of USUV events. High R_0 values predicted by the SEIR model in areas without evidence for real-life transmission suggest that it may tend towards over-estimation of risk.

Conclusions: The results from our parallel-model approach highlight that relying on a single model for assessing vector-borne disease risk may lead to incomplete conclusions. Utilizing different modelling approaches is thus crucial for risk-assessment of under-studied emerging pathogens like USUV.

Keywords: Usutu, Maxent, SEIR, Vector-borne disease, Risk map, Europe, Basic reproduction number, R_0, ENM

*Correspondence: yanchao1.cheng@uni-bayreuth.de
[1] Department of Biogeography, University of Bayreuth, Universitätsstr. 30, 95447 Bayreuth, Germany
Full list of author information is available at the end of the article

Background

Vector-borne diseases (VBDs) are of growing importance. Due to global transport, long-distance travel, population growth, environmental and climatic changes, VBDs are emerging all over the world [1–4]. In addition to human-mediated spread, mobile species such as migratory birds are promoting long-distance transport of pathogens [5]. If the local conditions at the introduction sites (e.g. hosts, vectors, and climate) are suitable, the pathogen can establish and evolve quickly, resulting in rapid local spread [6]. Usutu virus (USUV) is an example where both processes resulted in the recent arrival and spread of a zoonotic mosquito-borne virus in Europe [5].

USUV is a *flavivirus* [7] belonging to the Japanese encephalitis virus serocomplex [8]. As a member of the

family Flaviviridae, USUV is a single-stranded RNA virus closely related to Murray Valley encephalitis virus, Japanese encephalitis virus, and West Nile virus (WNV) [8]. It was first isolated in 1959 from *Culex neavei* mosquitoes in Swaziland and named after the Usutu river [7]. Its most important vectors are mosquito species of the genus *Culex* [9]. Since the first record, USUV has been reported for several African countries (e.g. Senegal, Central African Republic, Nigeria, Uganda) and detected in mosquitoes, birds, and humans [10]. In Europe USUV has been detected in 15 countries, with increasing spatial distribution and host range [9, 11–15] (Fig. 1). The earliest evidence of USUV in Europe came from a dead common blackbird (*Turdus merula*) found in Italy in 1996, although this case was not identified as such until 2013

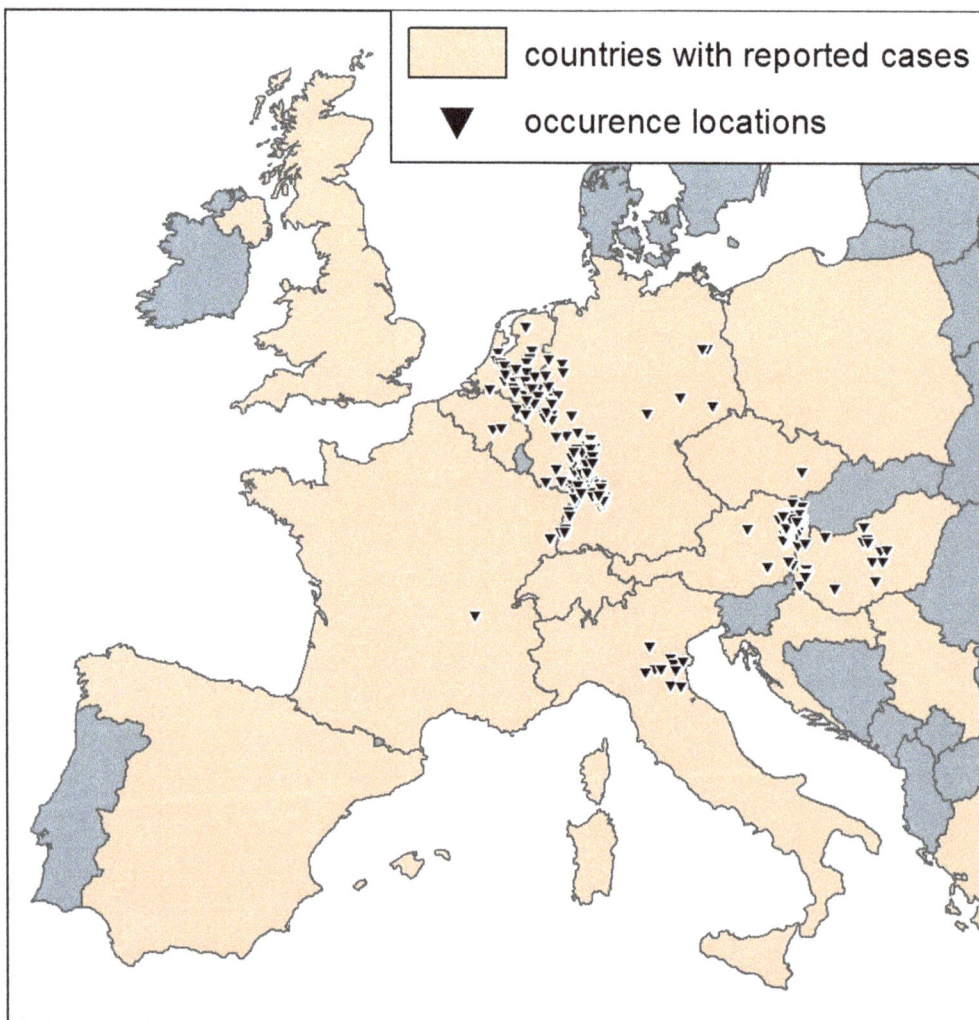

Fig. 1 USUV in Europe. Orange areas: European countries where cases of USUV have been reported, regardless of species and method of confirmation. Triangles: Spatially explicit records of USUV occurrence 2003—2016 before spatial rarefication. These are locations where individual USUV-positive dead birds have been found, confirmed by reverse transcription polymerase chain reaction (RT-PCR)

[16]. The first USUV epidemic in Europe was a series of dead common blackbirds reported from Austria in 2001 [17]. In the subsequent years, USUV was reported in further European countries. USUV or corresponding antibodies were detected in horses, bats, dogs [11, 18, 19], and at least 58 bird species, with common blackbirds as dominant avian host [14].

In 2009, the first human case of USUV infection in Europe was reported in Italy [20], followed by further human cases in Germany [21, 22], Croatia [23], Austria [24], and France [25]. Human cases are commonly characterized by mild symptoms including fever, rash, jaundice, headache, nuchal rigidity, hand tremor and hyperreflexia [20, 23, 26, 27]. However, at least in immunosuppressed patients USUV can cause a neuro-invasive infection [20], and it has recently been suspected to have caused idiopathic facial paralysis [25]. In addition to that, USUV infections were also detected from blood donors and healthy forestry workers in Germany and Italy [21, 22, 28], suggesting that asymptomatic infections can occur among humans. Recent data from Italy indicate that human USUV infections may not be a sporadic event and can even be more frequent than WNV infections in areas where both viruses co-circulate [9, 29, 30]. Furthermore, due to cross reactions in antibody tests, the number of human USUV cases may be underestimated through confusion with other flaviviruses [26]. As a consequence, the actual distribution of USUV and associated number of cases is likely to be larger than currently known [31].

The transmission cycle with birds as enzootic hosts creates a complex setting related to the risk for human health. First, migratory birds may transport the pathogen over large distances and can cause repeated re-introduction of the virus into a specific region that is not appropriate to maintain an outlasting population of the pathogen [5]. Second, common blackbirds are the predominant host [9, 14]. This species is very common across Europe and has grown accustomed to urban habitats, exhibiting high population densities in human settlements [32]. This means that vectors only need to cover short spatial distances between infected birds and humans—and the widespread mosquito species *Cx. pipiens* is a known bridge vector between mammals, birds and humans [33, 34]. In consequence, USUV is becoming an increasing threat for Europe as a mosquito-borne and zoonotic disease. Measures should be undertaken to improve or even create awareness towards zoonotic VBDs. For this purpose, spatial representations of risk are needed.

Models for vector borne viral diseases can be generated at various spatial and temporal scales [35]. Maps of vector occurrence or disease transmission risk derived from them can be used to direct vector surveillance and control programs as well as to inform public health officials, medicine practitioners and the general public about potential risks. Current approaches can be divided into two basic groups: correlative models (e.g. environmental niche models) and process-based models (e.g. epidemiological models). Both types of models have their own strengths and weaknesses [35]. Correlative environmental niche models, on the one hand, typically utilize species occurrence records and environmental predictor variables to estimate the current and future potential spatial distribution of a target species [36] or disease [37–42]. They do not require a priori knowledge about the specific effects single variables have, and are typically used on coarser spatio-temporal scales [35]. Process-based epidemiological models, on the other hand, aim to simulate the entire transmission process. Using knowledge gained from laboratory experiments or field observations, they require a deeper understanding of disease dynamics. As all models for VBD have their individual strengths and weaknesses, it is best practice not to rely on a single approach, but draw a conclusion from a consensus of multiple different models [35]. Although both model categories are widely used when modeling VBDs [35], comparisons of different models' outputs are typically made within those categories (e.g. [43]), and a comparison across categories is still missing.

To date only a limited number of USUV models for spatially confined areas exist. Based on an epidemiological model for WNV, Rubel et al. [44] developed a mechanistic susceptible-exposed-infected-removed (SEIR) model for USUV in Vienna (Austria) [44–46], which was later successfully applied to Germany and neighboring countries [47]. This model is mainly driven by daily mean temperature, and to enable the comparison of modeled bird deaths and observed bird deaths, it was originally carried out with interpolated monthly mean temperature values so as to achieve the same temporal resolution as the available bird death data [44]. A different, environmental niche model-based approach was followed by Lühken et al. [31], who adopted boosted regression trees to assess the spatio-temporal risk for USUV in Germany by estimating the risk in each grid cell.

Here we present, for the first time, USUV risk maps covering the entirety of the European mainland. Using two models in parallel, we utilize the mechanistic SEIR model by Rubel et al. [44] as well as a newly developed environmental niche model based on the machine-learning technique Maxent. Instead of using interpolated monthly mean temperature values for a single location, rasterized daily mean temperature was used to run the SEIR model. In order to increase comparability between the models, the same data source was also applied for the use of Maxent. Spatial risk maps were generated by both models. By using models from these two different groups, we are aiming at (1) estimating the potential risk for USUV transmission under current climate conditions in Europe and (2) investigating the differences between the outputs of two widely-used modelling approaches, which could be a first step towards interdisciplinary model comparison.

Methods
Study area and USUV occurrence records
In this study, we focus on current European occurrence records of USUV in the years of 2003–2016, from the earliest to the latest USUV cases available. The investigation area is limited by the natural coastlines, as well as through the reported USUV locations in Eastern Europe (Fig. 1).

To achieve a good data quality, only locations of USUV-positive birds confirmed by reverse transcription polymerase chain reaction (RT- PCR) were taken into account. This was done because (1) data from USUV-positive mammals or mosquitoes are collected quite unsystematic, i.e. data on USUV-positive birds are most consistent and comparable between the different European countries, and (2) other methods such as antibody analysis may not be able to distinguish USUV from other closely related flaviviruses such as WNV [48]. According to this rule, a total number of 376 USUV records was collected. USUV-positive data in Germany were collected by the German Mosquito Control Association (KABS), the Nature and Biodiversity Conservation Union (NABU), the local veterinary authorities and/or by the local state veterinary laboratories [47, 49–51]. Records for other European countries were derived from the literature (Additional file 1): Geographical coordinates published in the literature were directly entered into the database, precise site descriptions were digitized using Google Earth Pro, and high-quality occurrence maps were georeferenced using ESRI ArcGIS 10.2.2.

Climate data
Time series of daily mean temperature data, required by the SEIR model, were acquired from the E-OBS dataset version 15.0 [52] on a regular latitude–longitude grid with a spatial resolution of 0.25° (about 20 km). E-OBS provides gridded daily temperature and precipitation data for Europe based on data from weather stations. To compare the results from the SEIR model and the environmental niche model properly, bio-climatic variables, which are required by the environmental niche model, were generated from the E-OBS dataset as well. Therefore, time series of daily minimum, maximum

temperature and daily precipitation sums were acquired in addition to daily mean temperature.

Since the occurrence records for USUV cover the years of 2003–2016, these time series were trimmed accordingly. Considering that the spatial coverage of the E-OBS time series varies over time, grid cells with more than 10% missing data were excluded from our analyses. Monthly mean values were derived using the "raster" package [53] for R 3.2.1 [54] and 19 bio-climatic variables were calculated in SAGA-GIS version 2.1.4 [55] for use with the environmental niche model.

Environmental niche model: Maxent
For the environmental niche model, we used Maxent 3.3.3k [56]. Maxent is a powerful machine-learning technique that is widely used [35] to model the potential distribution of species, especially when the occurrence data are sparse [57]. Using occurrence records and environmental predictor variables as input data, Maxent generates maps of environmental suitability for transmission of USUV. Ranging between 0 for the lowest and 1 for the highest suitability, these maps can optionally be converted into presence/absence maps by applying a threshold value.

Maxent models are fitted assuming that all locations in the landscape are equally likely to be sampled. However, when the occurrence records are collected with different methods, sampling bias is inevitable. Compared to other methods, systematic sampling, also called spatial filtering of biased records [58], has a good performance regardless of species and bias type [58, 59]. It was applied by using the *SDM tool box* [60], an addon for ESRI ArcGIS that provides advanced tools and convenience functions for the Maxent workflow. To determine an appropriate spatial filtering resolution (the minimum distance between any two locations), the following rules were taken into consideration: (1) The spatial filtering process should decrease the bias distribution, but the remaining records should still represent the observed spatial patterns well. (2) There should be enough records left to run Maxent after spatial filtering. Consequently, the spatial filtering resolution was set to 20 km (about 0.25°), and 92 USUV records left after filtering in order to achieve optimum results and to avoid artefacts (Fig. 2).

Selection of the environmental predictors for the model followed a two-step approach (Table 1). First, 8 out of the 19 bio-climatic variables that were deemed unsuitable for the task were excluded due to the following ecological reasons: BIO2 and 3 ("mean diurnal range" and "isothermality") were excluded because while daily fluctuations in temperature are important for the mosquito life cycle and transmission dynamics, the monthly averages available here were considered unsuitable for capturing such

Table 1 Excluded and selected environmental predictor variables for the environmental niche model

Abbreviation	Variables
Excluded—monthly minima and maxima are not suitable to estimate daily fluctuations	
BIO2	Mean diurnal range (mean of monthly (max temp − min temp))
BIO3	Isothermality (BIO2/BIO7) × 100
Excluded—summer and winter precipitation are important to distinguish for mosquitoes and disease transmission dynamics	
BIO12	Annual precipitation
Excluded—wettest/driest time of the year can be in different seasons across Europe	
BIO8	Mean temperature of wettest quarter
BIO9	Mean temperature of driest quarter
BIO13	Precipitation of wettest month
BIO14	Precipitation of driest month
BIO16	Precipitation of wettest quarter
BIO17	Precipitation of driest quarter
Excluded by Jackknife	
BIO4	Temperature seasonality (standard deviation × 100)
BIO5	Maximum temperature of warmest month
BIO7	Temperature annual range (BIO5–BIO6)
BIO10	Mean temperature of warmest quarter
BIO19	Precipitation of coldest quarter
Model input	
BIO1	Annual mean temperature
BIO6	Minimum temperature of coldest month
BIO11	Mean temperature of coldest quarter
BIO15	Precipitation seasonality (coefficient of variation)
BIO18	Precipitation of warmest quarter

short-term fluctuations. BIO12 ("annual precipitation") was excluded because summer and winter precipitation play very different roles in this context and should be considered separately. All variables referring to the wettest/driest quarter or month of the year (BIO8, 9, 13, 14, 16, and 17) were excluded because seasonal precipitation patterns vary largely across Europe. As such, the wettest time of the year can be summer in some regions and winter in others, making this kind of variable unsuitable for larger scale analyses. The remaining eleven variables were further reduced through the built-in Jackknife feature in Maxent with a ten-fold cross-validation run, following the recommendations of Elith et al. [61]. In the end, a combination of five variables was chosen, consisting of annual mean temperature, minimum temperature of coldest month, mean temperature of coldest quarter, precipitation seasonality, and precipitation of warmest quarter. We used default settings for Maxent (10,000 background locations, 500 iterations), but disabled the use of "threshold" and "hinge" features, that would have led to over-fitting due to an inappropriate amount of model complexity.

Maxent, like many other environmental niche model approaches, generates pseudo-absence ("background")

locations to make up for the lack of field records of true absence of the target species. Careful selection of the area from which these background locations are allowed to be drawn from is an important part of model creation, as it can affect model performance and results. According to Barve et al. [62], this should be done by requiring the background locations to be within the area the species could realistically disperse to. We followed a buffer-based method [63] by setting a series of buffer radii from 0.5° to 24° (see Additional file 2), given the grid cell size of 0.25°. It is suggested to take the radius when the model performance stops increasing [63]. In addition to the built-in AUC (area under the receiver operator characteristic curve), true skill statistic (TSS) was also calculated as an indicator of model performance (Additional file 2). A radius of 12° was chosen as suggested, with the final model reaching an AUC of 0.92 and a TSS score of 0.78, both suggesting good model performance. In this model, the minimum temperature of the coldest month had the strongest contribution to the model (58%), followed by precipitation of the warmest quarter (21%) and annual mean temperature (13%). The threshold for distinguishing predicted presence and absence was based on the receiver operator characteristic (ROC), choosing the point along the ROC curve that maximized the sum of sensitivity and specificity. We chose this criterion also known as "maxSSS" because it is objective [64], widely used, performs consistently well with presence-only data [65, 66] and delivers threshold values that are relatively low [66], facilitating the high sensitivity desired in risk assessment studies.

Epidemiological model: SEIR

The SEIR model used in this study was developed by Rubel et al. [44] for Vienna (Austria) and surrounding areas based on data from different parts of the world. The model simulates the seasonal life cycles and inter-species USUV infections of the main vector and host species, *Cx. pipiens* and *T. merula* respectively. Health states of birds and mosquitoes are classified into nine compartments (larvae state of mosquitoes, health states susceptible/latent infected/infectious of mosquitoes and birds as well as recovered and dead birds, see [44]), and described by ordinary differential equations (see Additional file 3). The basic reproduction number R_0 is then calculated as the dominant eigenvalue of the next-generation matrix as described in [67], resulting in (see Table 2 for model parameters and Additional file 3 for details):

$$R_0 = \sqrt{\left[\frac{\delta_M \gamma_M \beta_M}{(\gamma_M + m_M) m_M} \frac{S_B}{K_B}\right]\left[\frac{\delta_M \gamma_B \beta_B}{(\gamma_B + m_B)(\alpha_B + m_B)} \frac{S_M}{K_B}\right]}$$

The SEIR model is mainly driven by variables responding to temperature. Further drivers are latitude, calendar day, and parameters with constant values [44].

The original SEIR R-code of the model was upgraded to work on a spatial grid rather than a single point location, and daytime length was calculated for each grid cell based on the geographical latitude of its center. Instead of interpolating daily data from monthly mean temperature, the model was run with true daily temperature data from the E-OBS dataset [52]. As an extensive literature review did not yield any new information, all other variables and parameters originally used by Rubel et al. were maintained in this study.

As the SEIR model for USUV was created for and calibrated within a temperate climate, water availability or precipitation were not considered a limiting factor by the developers. However, this assumption is not applicable for the entire study area, as the dry summers of Mediterranean climates can lead to a different, two peaked activity pattern of *Cx. pipiens* mosquitoes [68]. Consequently, the model was applied only to regions with a climate that is classified as cold or temperate with warm to hot summers but no dry season (Cfa, Cfb, Dfa and Dfb in the Köppen-Geiger system [69, 70]) (Fig. 2b).

The basic reproduction number R_0 (the number of secondary cases arising from a single infection in an

Table 2 Variables and parameters in the R_0 equation, following [44]

Parameter		Value
Mosquitoes		
Mortality rate	m_M	$m_M(T) = 0.00025T^2 - 0.0094T + 0.10257$
		T: daily mean temperature
Biting rate	κ	$\kappa(T) = \frac{0.344}{1+1.231\exp(-0.184(T-20))}$
Product of biting rate (κ) and transmission possibility from mosquitoes to birds (P_M)	β_M	$\beta_M(T) = P_M\kappa(T)$
		$P_M = 1$
Percentage of non-hibernating mosquitoes	δ_M	$\delta_M = 1 - \frac{1}{1+1775.7\exp[1.559(D-18.177)]}$
		$D = 7.639arcsin\left[\tan(\epsilon)\tan(\varphi) + \frac{0.0146}{\cos(\epsilon)\cos(\varphi)}\right] + 12$
		$\epsilon = 0.409sin\left(\frac{2\pi(d-80)}{365}\right)$
		D: daytime length, ϵ: declination, φ: geographic latitude
Exposed—infected/infectious rate	γ_M	$\gamma_M(T) = 0.0093T - 0.1352, T \geq 15°$
		$\gamma_M(T) = 0, T < 15°$
Susceptible mosquito population	S_M	Dynamic value, see Additional file 3
Birds		
Mortality rate	m_B	0.0012
Removal rate: fraction of infected birds either recovering or dying	α_B	0.182
Exposed—infected/infectious rate	γ_B	0.667
Product of biting rate (κ) and transmission possibility from birds to mosquitoes (P_B)	β_B	$\beta_B(T) = P_B\kappa(T)$
		$P_B = 0.125$
Susceptible black bird population	S_B	Dynamic value, see Additional file 3
Environmental capacity	K_B	see Additional file 3

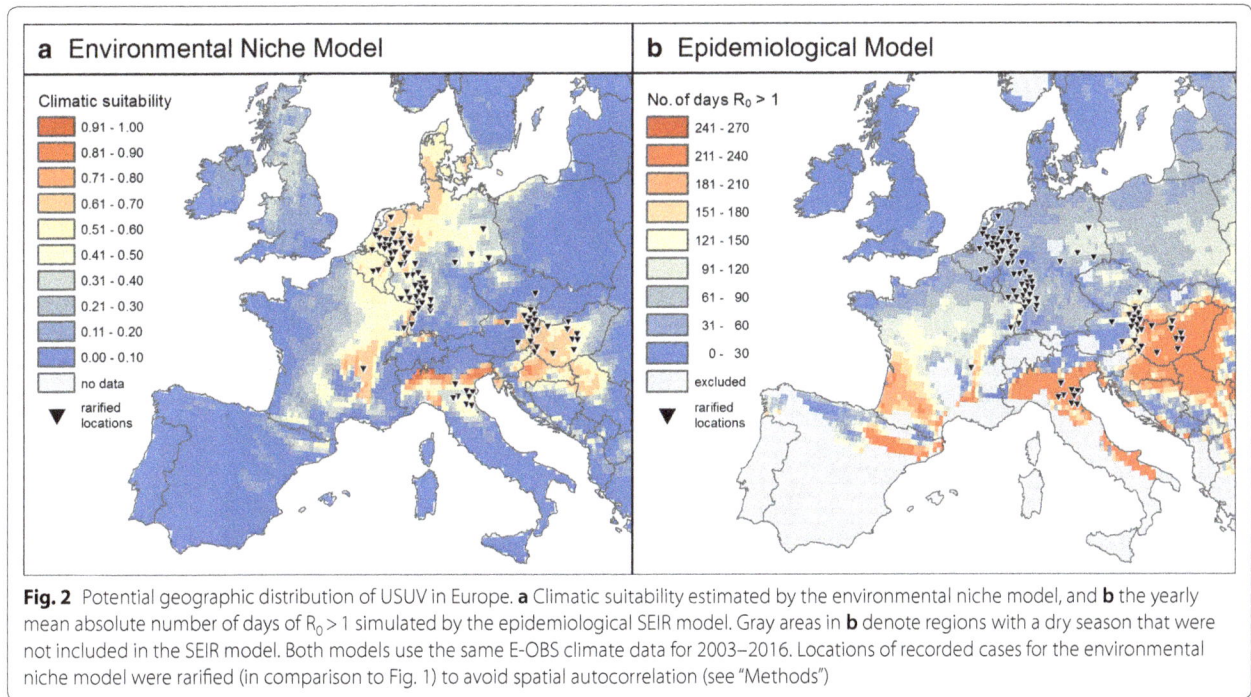

Fig. 2 Potential geographic distribution of USUV in Europe. **a** Climatic suitability estimated by the environmental niche model, and **b** the yearly mean absolute number of days of $R_0 > 1$ simulated by the epidemiological SEIR model. Gray areas in **b** denote regions with a dry season that were not included in the SEIR model. Both models use the same E-OBS climate data for 2003–2016. Locations of recorded cases for the environmental niche model were rarified (in comparison to Fig. 1) to avoid spatial autocorrelation (see "Methods")

otherwise uninfected population) of USUV calculated by the SEIR model is a threshold value: if $R_0 > 1$, an outbreak is possible after a single introduction of the pathogen; whereas if $R_0 < 1$, the introduced virus population will die out [67]. The daily R_0 value of each cell within the spatial raster was calculated within the time span of 2003-01-01 to 2016-12-31. From this, the average yearly number of days with $R_0 > 1$ was calculated for each raster cell and the maxSSS threshold was calculated for direct comparison with the environmental niche model based on the same presence and background locations that were used in the Maxent model. In addition to that, the average daily R_0 value of the main transmission season (June–September) was calculated for each year and raster cell.

Results

The potential geographic distribution of USUV predicted by both models on the continental European scale are shown in continuous form in Fig. 2, and as a direct comparison based on the maxSSS thresholds (environmental niche model: 0.35 in Maxent's logistic output format, epidemiological model: 40 days of $R_0 > 1$) in Fig. 3. While there are differences between the two models in parts of the study area, 15% of the study area are projected to be suitable by both approaches. The northern Italian outbreak region in and around the Po Valley is identified as a highly suitable area for USUV by both models. The same is true for eastern Austria, the Pannonian Basin and adjoining areas, as well as a narrow strip along the Rhône

river in France. Large parts of north-eastern France, the Benelux states and western and northern Germany are predicted to be at least somewhat suitable by both models. On the other hand, environmental niche model and SEIR agree on low risk being present in northern and mountainous regions (such as Sweden, Norway and the British Isles), where relatively low average and minimum temperatures keep the probability of transmission low.

In general, the environmental niche model accurately determines the occurrences of birds found positive with USUV. Compared to the SEIR, it suggests elevated climatic suitability for USUV to the north and west of the Jura Mountains as well as northwards along the Rhine and the North Sea coast until southern Denmark (Fig. 2a). Following the maxSSS threshold, the environmental niche model predicts a total of 17% of the study area to be suitable for transmission (sensitivity: 0.946, specificity: 0.852). 2% of the entire area are considered suitable only by the environmental niche model and not by the SEIR, including most parts of Denmark and adjoining parts of northern Germany, northern Netherlands, southern Belgium and a few areas in northern Britain (Fig. 3).

In contrast, the average yearly number of days with $R_0 > 1$ derived from the SEIR suggests a high risk for USUV in southwestern France and southeastern Italy, but shows relatively low risk in the northern Germany-Netherlands-Belgium region (Fig. 2b). North of the Pyrenees, the former French regions of Aquitaine and

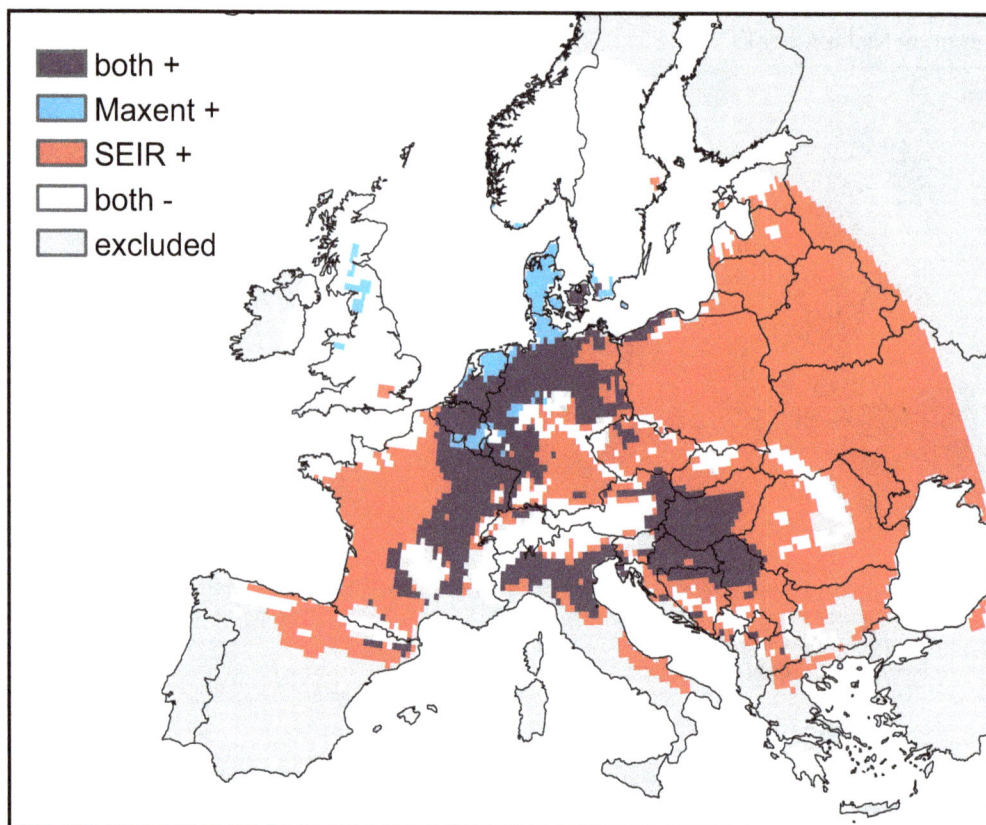

Fig. 3 Areas of agreement and disagreement of both models. Dark purple areas denote regions where both models predict suitable conditions for USUV-transmission based on the maxSSS threshold. In the blue and red areas, only the environmental niche model and SEIR predict suitable conditions, respectively. In white areas none of the models predicts suitable environmental conditions, while gray areas were excluded from further analyses because they are outside the climatic zones the SEIR model was developed for, or outside the buffer applied to the Maxent model

Midi-Pyrénées show a high transmission potential as well. Medium values mainly occur in Poland and northeastern Germany, along the Upper Rhine Valley and in central France. For the outbreak area in the Netherlands and northern Germany, the SEIR in this form suggests relatively low risk of transmission. However, following the maxSSS threshold, most of this region can still be classified as suitable for USUV transmission (Fig. 3). A total of 67% of the whole study area lies above the threshold for this model, resulting in a sensitivity that is slightly higher (0.989) than that of the environmental niche model but a very low specificity (0.274).

Zooming in towards the main areas of observed USUV transmission allows a closer inspection of the models. In the Austrian-Hungarian outbreak area, Maxent predicts climatic suitability values sufficient for USUV transmission at all observed occurrences (Fig. 4a1). The SEIR model predicts the highest R_0 values for the largest USUV event in 2003 (Fig. 4a2) and considerably lower values for the following 2 years with less observed cases (Fig. 4a). Relatively high R_0 values are observed again for the last USUV event in 2016. Interestingly, though, values for the USUV-free years of 2006–2015 are higher than those of 2004/5 (Fig. 4a2).

(See figure on next page.)

Fig. 4 Temporal patterns of the average R_0 values for three selected regions of Europe. **a** Austria and the Pannonian Basin, **b** northern Italy, and **c** Germany and the Netherlands. (1) Spatial representation of both models for years with USUV events. Color coding in the maps shows the average daily R_0 values throughout June to September for the given years. Gray areas denote climate types with dry seasons, thus the SEIR model was not applied there. Cross-hatching indicates areas where the environmental niche model suggests absence of USUV, based on climate data for the whole time period from 2003 to 2016. (2) Time series curves illustrate the daily R_0 value, averaged over all occurrence records of the respective region for each given year

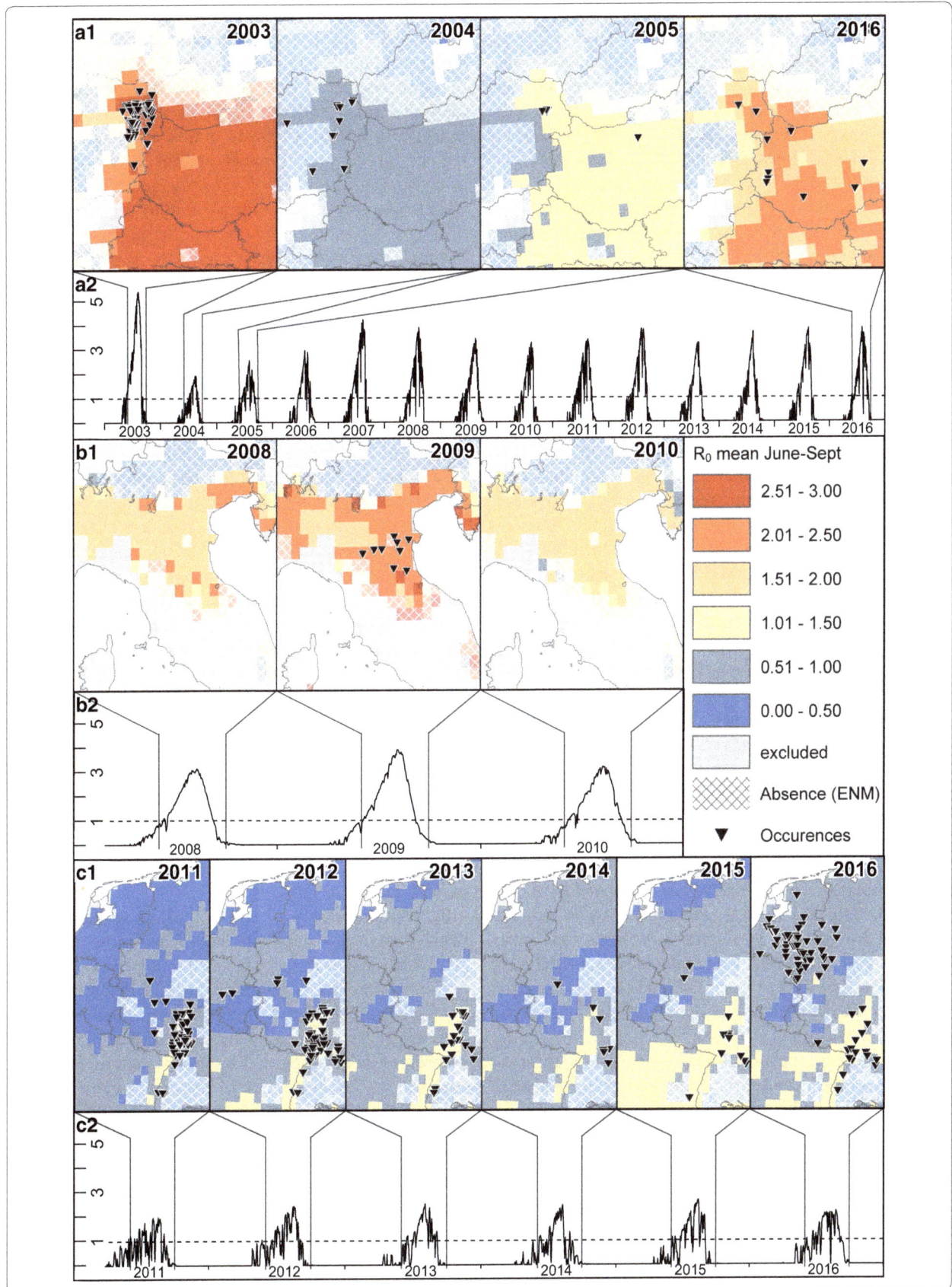

In Italy, Maxent is able to predict the general outbreak area (Fig. 4b1). The SEIR model predicts elevated R_0 values for the year of 2009 where USUV occurred, but similarly high values for the USUV-free years before and after (Fig. 4b2).

In the largest outbreak area in western Germany and the Benelux states, Maxent closely resembles the observed pattern of USUV occurrence (Fig. 4c1). Compared to the other two regions, the SEIR model in these areas shows much lower average and absolute R_0 values as well as higher temporal variability throughout the transmission season (Fig. 4c2). Average R_0 values for the transmission season rise above 1 and match the occurrence records well in the Rhine Valley but stay below 1 in the northern parts of the area, i.e. the Netherlands and northwestern Germany.

Discussion

In face of emerging VBDs and rapid spread into new regions with suitable climatic conditions, models that show the current geographic regions at risk are required to allow local health authorities to be prepared. However, modelling approaches can differ substantially in philosophy, structure, and algorithms. Pros and cons of different approaches are evident and, obviously, there is not one single approach to be preferred for every pathogen, area or timespan.

In this study, two fundamentally different models were applied to describe the current emergence of USUV in Europe. This disease exhibits a series of complex interactions between the virus, vectors and host species [9]. Process-based models offer direct links between model outcome and underlying mechanisms, which makes interpretation of the observed spatial patterns relatively straightforward. However, exact knowledge on the parameters of USUV transmission is still scarce. With large numbers of USUV-positive birds reported from distinct geographical hot spots, the application of biogeographical distribution models may be a viable alternative. In order to identify coinciding and deviating model output, we ran the analyses based on the same climate data and following standard processes to detect regions at risk for the transmission of USUV.

The large-scale spatial patterns predicted by the two models (Figs. 2, 3) are quite similar close to the observed USUV events—with the notable exception of northern Germany and the Netherlands. Here, the environmental niche model favors higher latitudes as far north as Denmark, while the epidemiological model suggests good conditions for transmission in southwestern France and northeastern Spain (Fig. 2b) and at least suitable conditions for most parts of Eastern Europe (Fig. 3). Given the observed recent increase in temperatures across Europe

and the projected further increase during the upcoming century [IPCC] [71], it can be expected that both models under-estimate future potential for USUV transmission to some degree. If precipitation patterns change dramatically so as to affect mosquito populations, the SEIR model may not be a reliable option any more in some regions. Similarly, both models are not suitable to predict today's potential for USUV transmission in areas that are climatically very different from the study region.

Environmental niche model

As the environmental niche model is strongly driven by existing spatial records, it is not surprising that it reflects the current distribution of USUV records better. However, it has to be kept in mind that there is no consistent monitoring of USUV across Europe, leading to biases in the occurrence records. For instance, many USUV events were reported in Italy, Austria, Hungary, and Croatia (though no RT-PCR positive birds), but to date no USUV case was reported in their neighbor countries—Slovenia and Slovakia. Due to the same reason, only bird cases were included in our approach, as it is the least biased dataset in Europe, compared to USUV cases from wild mammals (e.g. bats and wild boars) or humans. Furthermore, we restricted our USUV dataset to USUV cases confirmed by RT-PCR counts, as other methods bear the possibility of false positives that would lead to over-estimation of risk. Given the high activity of West Nile Virus in the area that could easily be mistaken for USUV in antibody tests, the gain from avoiding false positives should outweigh the loss from potentially excluding some true positives. Even though Maxent is relatively insensitive to sampling bias compared to other environmental niche models [57] and records were spatially rarified in this study, the modelling output would still be inevitably affected, e.g. in Italy, where occurrence records are comparably sparse.

In addition, USUV is still spreading in Europe and likely does not occupy its entire environmental niche yet, which may lead to under-estimation of risk through the environmental niche model in areas that may be climatically suitable, but have not been reached yet (compare e.g. [72]). The quality and accessibility of observed records of occurrence of vectors, hosts and especially pathogens is a major practical obstacle for the development of models of the environmental niche model family. Only a consistent and advanced monitoring system covering a selection of representative areas across Europe could give more accurate and reliable occurrence records to produce risk maps. Consequently, the environmental niche model performance can be improved as more occurrence data with high quality are available and the sampling bias is minimized. Ideally, such a monitoring system is centralized, open access and would not only focus on birds or mosquitoes but also include mammalian hosts such as rodents or bats to cover different types of potentially circulating pathogens. Especially the latter have been suspected to be under-estimated but important hosts for other viral zoonotic diseases [73]. As USUV outbreaks typically cease with the arrival of winter, hibernating bats could enable overwintering of the virus. However, coordinated efforts are also needed for centralized and open access to the occurrence records resulting from these improved measures [35].

Epidemiological model

As an absence of records does not necessarily indicate an absence of risk, it makes sense to use a mechanistic model to point out regions such as southwestern France, where transmission appears to be possible. The SEIR model captured the USUV events in the Pannonian Basin and Po Valley regions well, though the events in Germany and the Netherlands were not represented correctly. Hence, it must be questioned whether the current knowledge on processes, mechanisms and underlying parameters is sufficient to explain USUV transmission patterns and outbreaks. Although an extensive literature review was conducted with the aim of improving and updating the parameters for the SEIR model, no information supporting the integration of additional processes, drivers or variables was found. Therefore, all the parameters and variables used already in the 2008 study of Rubel et al. [44] were kept unchanged, even though some of them are probably not suitable for the whole study area. For instance, population density as well as birth and mortality rates of common blackbirds are unlikely to be constant across the whole study area. An advanced, open-access monitoring system as discussed above could also be of great use for this.

Furthermore, although precipitation is known to affect mosquito life cycles and disease transmission dynamics [74, 75], the applied SEIR model does not take this into account. The SEIR model for USUV was originally developed and calibrated for temperate climates. It is thus possible that certain ecological factors (e.g. precipitation), which are not limiting in the calibration area but could be limiting elsewhere, are not included in the model. In our study we restrained the extent for the SEIR model by excluding climate types with dry seasons in order to avoid making predictions for regions the model is not suitable for. Future models should aim to improve the population model components for vectors and hosts, leading to a more universally useful model. In addition, explicit parameters for USUV are not available yet and had to be substituted by data for the related WNV. For instance, no information about the extrinsic incubation period and

its relation to ambient temperature is currently available. Data from a single experiment on a single strain of another virus (i.e. West-Nile virus) [76] is far from optimal, as it has been shown that these experiments are subject to large uncertainty for various reasons [77]. This is a common problem, though, since updated and realistic experiments are sorely needed for many VBDs [35]. Future models could account for some of this uncertainty by incorporating stochastic variations instead of relying on fixed values, as it has already been done e.g. for Chikungunya [78].

Another point worth considering is that so far there is no standardized way of converting the daily values of R_0 calculated by the SEIR model for each grid cell into interpretable maps. Obviously, some amount of temporal aggregation needs to be applied in order to gain low dimensional, printable maps. In practice, this ranges from R_0 being displayed as averages for single months (e.g. [79]) up to R_0 values being averaged over 30-year periods (e.g. [80]). Here, we chose to display average R_0 values for single transmission seasons, which apparently failed to predict the 2016 USUV event in Northwest Europe (Fig. 4c). However, R_0 is a threshold value. Thus, while a value of $R_0 > 1$ indicates high risk of disease spread, an average $R_0 < 1$ for the same period does not necessarily mean no or even low risk, depending on how the length of that period was chosen and how often the threshold was exceeded. This is a serious drawback of SEIR model results to visualize the spatial-explicit risk of pathogen transmission. Hence, an alternative way of illustrating these models is concentrating on the duration of time where $R_0 > 1$. Here, we chose to count the (average) number of days per year where $R_0 > 1$, but this can also be done on other temporal scales (e.g. months [81]). In our case, this value apparently fails to capture the outbreak area in Germany and the Netherlands (Fig. 2b). However, a closer look reveals that this again is a lack of knowledge about the details of the disease that prevents a meaningful interpretation of these maps, i.e., how many days of $R_0 > 1$ are actually needed for an USUV event to occur. When this threshold would be known, the average yearly number of days of $R_0 > 1$ map can be converted to a categorized risk map showing whether there is a risk and how severe it is. Furthermore, it has to be questioned, if higher absolute R_0 values during the transmission season would reduce the number of days of $R_0 > 1$ days required for an USUV outbreak. Only when these primary questions are addressed, a more reasonable risk map can be generated.

Outlook

Further efforts should strive towards the unification of the two streams of modeling. As shown in this study, the ecological niche model reflects spatial distribution better, while the epidemiological model has the advantage of capturing short term variabilities, as it uses daily temperature data. Ecological niche models are run with climate data which typically covers decades, and as a consequence, extreme weather events such as heat waves would not be captured. An integrated model could benefit from both models' advantages. For example, in a hierarchical approach, spatial distribution of risk could first be estimated by an environmental niche model, followed by a zoom into a finer scale for the investigation of temporal risk patterns in high risk areas through an epidemiological model with well-updated parameters and variables. In this case, the finer temporal scale epidemiological model, using daily weather data or even weather forecast data, can work as a live early warning forecast. Instead of projecting where climate is suitable, ecological niche models can also be applied to exclude unsuitable regions. In addition, in an integrated approach, environmental niche models that estimate the abundance of vectors and hosts could be nested in an epidemiological model as well, in order to gain more precise information on the required vector-to-host ratio.

Conclusion

In conclusion, this study highlights the necessity to consider different approaches to detect the current and future areas under risk of VBDs. Environmental niche models and epidemiological models examine rather complementary aspects, especially in terms of short-term weather conditions versus long-term climatic conditions. Environmental niche models are typically built upon long-term climate data and thus can be used to gain a general overview of the areas at risk and estimate potential effects of climate change. Given enough spatially explicit occurrence records are available, these models are particularly useful for a rapid risk assessment of emerging VBDs, while more detailed data about the transmission mechanisms is gathered. Once this data is available, elaborate mechanistic models can offer more fine-grained insights on the progression of outbreaks, with the potential for short-term forecasts based on weather models. At this point, environmental niche models for host or vector populations can provide valuable input data for advanced epidemiological models. Thus, using both approaches complementing each other is key for a comprehensive and effective risk evaluation.

Wide parts of Europe are currently at risk of USUV circulation, and its status of a mostly neglected emerging disease makes estimation of its potential future range difficult. Evidence suggests that USUV event s may be

more likely to occur in climatically favored regions within Europe such as the Po Valley in northern Italy [82] and the Rhine Valley [48, 50]. At the same time, these areas have a high human population density and exhibit large urban areas and cities. Remnant wetland habitats along rivers serve as habitats for migratory bird stops result‐ ing in a combined setting with humans being exposed to high risk. The detected spatial patterns can be used to indicate regions where surveillance activities should be focused and intensified.

Additional files

Additional file 1. Records of USUV-infected bird locations confirmed by RT PCR collected from the literature.

Additional file 2. Buffer radii versus model performance.

Additional file 3. Detailed description of the SEIR model.

Authors' contributions
YC, NT, ST, AJ, RL, and CB developed the concept of the study. YC, UZ and RL complied the occurrence records. NT and YC processed the climate data and adapted the SEIR model. YC and NT ran the Maxent models. CB, ST and AJ supervised the modelling process. YC prepared the figures. All authors discussed the preliminary results and figures at various stages of the modelling process. YC and NT wrote the original draft of the manuscript. All authors discussed and revised the manuscript. All authors read and approved the final version of the manuscript.

Author details
[1] Department of Biogeography, University of Bayreuth, Universitätsstr. 30, 95447 Bayreuth, Germany. [2] Bernhard Nocht Institute for Tropical Medicine, World Health Organization Collaborating Centre for Arbovirus and Hemorrhagic Fever Reference and Research, Hamburg, Germany. [3] Friedrich-Loeffler-Institut, Institute of Novel and Emerging Infectious Diseases, Südufer 10, 17493 Greifswald – Insel Riems, Germany. [4] BayCEER, Bayreuth Center for Ecology and Environmental Research, Bayreuth, Germany.

Acknowledgements
We would like to thank Reinhold Stahlmann for his work on the figures. We acknowledge the E-OBS dataset from the EU-FP6 project ENSEMBLES (http://ensembles-eu.metoffice.com) and the data providers in the ECA&D project (http://www.ecad.eu). This publication was funded by the German Research Foundation (DFG) and the University of Bayreuth in the funding programme Open Access Publishing.

Competing interests
The authors declare that they have no competing interests.

Funding
This work was partly funded by the Federal Ministry of Education and Research of Germany (BMBF), Grant Nos. 01EI1702A and 01KL1601. Yanchao Cheng is funded by China Scholarship Council, No. 201506040059. This publication was funded by the German Research Foundation (DFG) and the University of Bayreuth in the funding programme Open Access Publishing.

References

1. Mangili A, Gendreau MA. Transmission of infectious diseases during commercial air travel. Lancet. 2005;365(9463):989–96.

2. Tatem AJ, Rogers DJ, Hay SI. Global transport networks and infectious disease spread. Adv Parasitol. 2006;62:293–343.

3. Gage KL, Burkot TR, Eisen RJ, Hayes EB. Climate and vectorborne diseases. Am J Prev Med. 2008;35(5):436–50.

4. Wu T, Perrings C, Kinzig A, Collins JP, Minteer BA, Daszak P. Economic growth, urbanization, globalization, and the risks of emerging infectious diseases in China: a review. Ambio. 2017;46(1):18–29.

5. Engel D, Jöst H, Wink M, Börstler J, Bosch S, Garigliany MM, et al. Reconstruction of the evolutionary history and dispersal of Usutu virus, a neglected emerging arbovirus in Europe and Africa. MBio. 2016;7(1):e01938-01915.

6. Kilpatrick AM, Randolph SE. Drivers, dynamics, and control of emerging vector-borne zoonotic diseases. Lancet. 2012;380(9857):1946–55.

7. Williams MC, Knight EM, Haddow AJ, Simpson DIH. Isolation of West Nile virus from man and of Usutu virus from the bird-biting mosquito *Mansonia aurites* (Theobald) in Entebbe area of Uganda. Ann Trop Med Parasitol. 1964;58(3):367–74.

8. Poidinger M, Hall RA, Mackenzie JS. Molecular characterization of the Japanese encephalitis serocomplex of the *flavivirus* genus. Virology. 1996;218(2):417–21.

9. Nikolay B. A review of West Nile and Usutu virus co-circulation in Europe: how much do transmission cycles overlap? Trans R Soc Trop Med Hyg. 2015;109(10):609–18.

10. Nikolay B, Diallo M, Boye CSB, Sall AA. Usutu virus in Africa. Vector Borne Zoonotic Dis. 2011;11(11):1417–23.

11. Barbic L, Vilibic-Cavlek T, Listes E, Stevanovic V, Gjenero-Margan I, Ljubin-Sternak S, et al. Demonstration of Usutu virus antibodies in horses, Croatia. Vector Borne Zoonotic Dis. 2013;13(10):772–4.

12. Vittecoq M, Lecollinet S, Jourdain E, Thomas F, Blanchon T, Arnal A, et al. Recent circulation of West Nile virus and potentially other closely related flaviviruses in southern France. Vector Borne Zoonotic Dis. 2013;13(8):610–3.

13. Escribano-Romero E, Lupulović D, Merino-Ramos T, Blázquez AB, Lazić G, Lazić S, et al. West Nile virus serosurveillance in pigs, wild boars, and roe deer in Serbia. Vet Microbiol. 2015;176(3–4):365–9.

14. Ashraf U, Ye J, Ruan XD, Wan SF, Zhu BB, Cao SB. Usutu virus: an emerging *flavivirus* in Europe. Viruses. 2015;7(1):219–38.

15. Rijks J, Kik M, Slaterus R, Foppen R, Stroo A, Ijzer J, et al. Widespread Usutu virus outbreak in birds in the Netherlands, 2016. Eurosurveillance. 2016;21(45):30391.

16. Weissenböck H, Bakonyi T, Rossi G, Mani P, Nowotny N. Usutu virus, Italy, 1996. Emerg Infect Dis. 2013;19(2):274–7.

17. Weissenböck H, Kolodziejek J, Url A, Lussy H, Rebel-Bauder B, Nowotny N. Emergence of Usutu virus, an African mosquito-borne *flavivirus* of the Japanese encephalitis virus group, central Europe. Emerg Infect Dis. 2002;8(7):652–6.

18. Durand B, Haskouri H, Lowenski S, Vachiery N, Beck C, Lecollinet S. Seroprevalence of West Nile and Usutu viruses in military working horses and dogs, Morocco, 2012: dog as an alternative WNV sentinel species? Epidemiol Infect. 2016;144(9):1857–64.

19. Cadar D, Becker N, Campos RDM, Börstler J, Jöst H, Schmidt-Chanasit J. Usutu virus in bats, Germany, 2013. Emerg Infect Dis. 2014;20(10):1771–3.

20. Pecorari M, Longo G, Gennari W, Grottola A, Sabbatini AM, Tagliazucchi S, et al. First human case of Usutu virus neuroinvasive infection, Italy, August–September 2009. Eurosurveillance. 2009;14(50):19446.

21. Cadar D, Maier P, Müller S, Kress J, Chudy M, Bialonski A, et al. Blood donor screening for West Nile virus (WNV) revealed acute Usutu virus (USUV) infection, Germany, September 2016. Eurosurveillance. 2017;22(14):30501.

22. Allering L, Jöst H, Emmerich P, Günther S, Lattwein E, Schmidt M, et al. Detection of Usutu virus infection in a healthy blood donor from south-west Germany, 2012. Eurosurveillance. 2012;17(50):20341.

23. Vilibic-Cavlek T, Kaic B, Barbic L, Pem-Novosel I, Slavic-Vrzic V, Lesnikar V, et al. First evidence of simultaneous occurrence of West Nile virus and Usutu virus neuroinvasive disease in humans during the 2013 outbreak. Infection. 2014;42(4):689–95.

24. Bakonyi T, Erdélyi K, Brunthaler R, Dán Á, Weissenböck H, Nowotny N. Usutu virus, Austria and Hungary, 2010-2016. Emerg Microbes Infect. 2017;6(10):e85.

25. Simonin Y, Sillam O, Carles MJ, Gutierrez S, Gil P, Constant O, et al. Human Usutu virus infection with atypical neurologic presentation, Montpellier, France, 2016. Emerg Infect Dis. 2018;24(5):875–8.

26. Santini M, Vilibic-Cavlek T, Barsic B, Barbic L, Savic V, Stevanovic V, et al. First cases of human Usutu virus neuroinvasive infection in Croatia, August–September 2013: clinical and laboratory features. J Neurovirol. 2015;21(1):92–7.

27. Cavrini F, Gaibani P, Longo G, Pierro AM, Rossini G, Bonilauri P, et al. Usutu virus infection in a patient who underwent orthotropic liver transplantation, Italy, August–September 2009. Eurosurveillance. 2009;14(50):19448.

28. Percivalle E, Sassera D, Rovida F, Isernia P, Fabbi M, Baldanti F, et al. Usutu virus antibodies in blood donors and healthy forestry workers in the Lombardy region, northern Italy. Vector Borne Zoonotic Dis. 2017;17(9):658–61.

29. Calzolari M, Gaibani P, Bellini R, Defilippo F, Pierro A, Albieri A, et al. Mosquito, bird and human surveillance of West Nile and Usutu viruses in Emilia-Romagna region (Italy) in 2010. PLoS One. 2012;7(5):e38058.

30. Grottola A, Marcacci M, Tagliazucchi S, Gennari W, Di Gennaro A, Orsini M, et al. Usutu virus infections in humans: a retrospective analysis in the municipality of Modena, Italy. Clin Microbiol Infect. 2017;23(1):33–7.

31. Lühken R, Jöst H, Cadar D, Thomas SM, Bosch S, Tannich E, et al. Distribution of Usutu virus in Germany and its effect on breeding bird populations. Emerg Infect Dis. 2017;23(12):1991–8.

32. Møller AP, Jokimäki J, Skorka P, Tryjanowski P. Loss of migration and urbanization in birds: a case study of the blackbird (*Turdus merula*). Oecologia. 2014;175(3):1019–27.

33. Muñoz J, Eritja R, Alcaide M, Montalvo T, Soriguer RC, Figuerola J. Host-feeding patterns of native *Culex pipiens* and invasive *Aedes albopictus* mosquitoes (Diptera: Culicidae) in urban zones from Barcelona, Spain. J Med Entomol. 2011;48(4):956–60.

34. Börstler J, Jöst H, Garms R, Krüger A, Tannich E, Becker N, et al. Host-feeding patterns of mosquito species in Germany. Parasit Vectors. 2016;9:318.

35. Tjaden NB, Caminade C, Beierkuhnlein C, Thomas SM. Mosquito-borne diseases: advances in modelling climate-change impacts. Trends Parasitol. 2018;34(3):227–45.

36. Elith J, Graham CH, Anderson RP, Dudík M, Ferrier S, Guisan A, et al. Novel methods improve prediction of species' distributions from occurrence data. Ecography. 2006;29(2):129–51.

37. Tjaden NB, Suk JE, Fischer D, Thomas SM, Beierkuhnlein C, Semenza JC. Modelling the effects of global climate change on Chikungunya transmission in the 21st century. Sci Rep. 2017;7(1):3813.

38. Bhatt S, Gething PW, Brady OJ, Messina JP, Farlow AW, Moyes CL, et al. The global distribution and burden of Dengue. Nature. 2013;496(7446):504–7.

39. Nsoesie EO, Kraemer MU, Golding N, Pigott DM, Brady OJ, Moyes CL, et al. Global distribution and environmental suitability for Chikungunya virus, 1952 to 2015. Eurosurveillance. 2016;21(20):30234.

40. Samy AM, Thomas SM, Abd El Wahed A, Cohoon KP, Peterson AT. Mapping the global geographic potential of Zika virus spread. Mem Inst Oswaldo Cruz. 2016;111(9):559–60.

41. Samy AM, van de Sande WWJ, Fahal AH, Peterson AT. Mapping the potential risk of Mycetoma infection in Sudan and South Sudan using ecological niche modeling. PLoS Negl Trop Dis. 2014;8(10):e3250.

42. Peterson AT. Mapping disease transmission risk: enriching models using biogeography and ecology. Baltimore: Johns Hopkins University Press; 2014.

43. Cianci D, Hartemink N, Ibanez-Justicia A. Modelling the potential spatial distribution of mosquito species using three different techniques. Int J Health Geogr. 2015;14:10.

44. Rubel F, Brugger K, Hantel M, Chvala-Mannsberger S, Bakonyi T, Weissenböck H, et al. Explaining Usutu virus dynamics in Austria: model development and calibration. Prev Vet Med. 2008;85(3–4):166–86.

45. Brugger K, Rubel F. Simulation of climate-change scenarios to explain Usutu-virus dynamics in Austria. Prev Vet Med. 2009;88(1):24–31.

46. Reiczigel J, Brugger K, Rubel F, Solymosi N, Lang Z. Bayesian analysis of a dynamical model for the spread of the Usutu virus. Stoch Environ Res Risk Assess. 2010;24(3):455–62.

47. Cadar D, Lühken R, van der Jeugd H, Garigliany M, Ziegler U, Keller M, et al. Widespread activity of multiple lineages of Usutu virus, western Europe, 2016. Eurosurveillance. 2017;22(4):30452.

48. Jöst H, Bialonski A, Maus D, Sambri V, Eiden M, Groschup MH, et al. Short report: isolation of Usutu virus in Germany. Am J Trop Med Hyg. 2011;85(3):551–3.

49. Becker N, Jöst H, Ziegler U, Eiden M, Hoper D, Emmerich P, et al. Epizootic emergence of usutu virus in wild and captive birds in Germany. PLoS One. 2012;7(2):e32604.

50. Ziegler U, Jöst H, Müller K, Fischer D, Rinder M, Tietze DT, et al. Epidemic spread of Usutu virus in southwest Germany in 2011 to 2013 and monitoring of wild birds for Usutu and West Nile viruses. Vector Borne Zoonotic Dis. 2015;15(8):481–8.

51. Ziegler U, Fast C, Eiden M, Bock S, Schulze C, Hoeper D, et al. Evidence for an independent third Usutu virus introduction into Germany. Vet Microbiol. 2016;192:60–6.

52. Haylock MR, Hofstra N, Klein Tank A, Klok EJ, Jones PD, New M. A European daily high-resolution gridded data set of surface temperature and precipitation for 1950–2006. J Geophys Res. 2008;113:D20119.

53. Hijmans RJ. Raster: geographic data analysis and modeling. R package version 2.5-8. 2016. http://CRAN.R-project.org/package=raster.

54. R Core Team. R:A language and environment for statistical computing. R Foundation for Statistical Computing, Vienna, Austria. 2015. http://www.R-project.org/.

55. Conrad O, Bechtel B, Bock M, Dietrich H, Fischer E, Gerlitz L, et al. System for automated geoscientific analyses (SAGA). Geosci Model Dev. 2015;8:1991–2007.

56. Phillips SJ, Anderson RP, Schapire RE. Maximum entropy modeling of species geographic distributions. Ecol Model. 2006;190(3–4):231–59.

57. Baldwin RA. Use of maximum entropy modeling in wildlife research. Entropy. 2009;11(4):854–66.

58. Kramer-Schadt S, Niedballa J, Pilgrim JD, Schröder B, Lindenborn J, Reinfelder V, et al. The importance of correcting for sampling bias in MaxEnt species distribution models. Divers Distrib. 2013;19(11):1366–79.

59. Fourcade Y, Engler JO, Rödder D, Secondi J. Mapping species distributions with MAXENT Using a geographically biased sample of presence data: a performance assessment of methods for correcting sampling bias. PLoS One. 2014;9(5):e97122.

60. Brown JL. SDMtoolbox: a python-based GIS toolkit for landscape genetic, biogeographic and species distribution model analyses. Methods Ecol Evol. 2014;5(7):694–700.

61. Elith J, Phillips SJ, Hastie T, Dudík M, Chee YE, Yates CJ. A statistical explanation of MaxEnt for ecologists. Divers Distrib. 2011;17(1):43–57.

62. Barve N, Barve V, Jiménez-Valverde A, Lira-Noriega A, Maher SP, Peterson AT, et al. The crucial role of the accessible area in ecological niche modeling and species distribution modeling. Ecol Model. 2011;222(11):1810–9.

63. VanDerWal J, Shoo LP, Graham C, William SE. Selecting pseudo-absence data for presence-only distribution modeling: how far should you stray from what you know? Ecol Model. 2009;220(4):589–94.

64. Liu CR, Barry PM, Dawson TP, Pearson RG. Selecting thresholds of occurrence in the prediction of species distributions. Ecography. 2005;28:385–93.

65. Liu CR, White M, Newell G. Selecting thresholds for the prediction of species occurrence with presence-only data. J Biogeogr. 2013;40:778–89.

66. Liu CR, Newell G, White M. On the selection of thresholds for predicting species occurrence with presence-only data. Ecol Evol. 2015;6:337–48.

67. Diekmann O, Heesterbeek JAP, Metz JAJ. On the definition and computation of the basic reproduction ratio R_0 in models for infectious-diseases in heterogeneous populations. J Math Biol. 1990;28(4):365–82.

68. Roiz D, Ruiz S, Soriguer R, Figuerola J. Climatic effects on mosquito abundance in Mediterranean wetlands. Parasit Vectors. 2014;7:333.

69. Peel MC, Finlayson BL, McMahon TA. Updated world map of the Köppen-Geiger climate classification. Hydrol Earth Syst Sci. 2007;11(5):1633–44.

70. Kottek M, Grieser J, Beck C, Rudolf B, Rubel F. World map of the Köppen-Geiger climate classification updated. Meteorol Z. 2006;15(3):259–63.

71. Cramer W, Holten JI, Kaczmarek Z, Martens P, Nicholls RJ, Öquist M et al. Europe. In: McCarthy JJ, Canziani OF, A. LN, Dokken DJ, White KS, editors. Climate change 2001: impacts, adaptation, and vulnerability—Contribution of Working Group II to the 3rd Assessment Report of the Intergovernmental Panel on Climate Change. Cambridge: Cambridge University Press; 2001.

72. Elith J, Kearney M, Phillips S. The art of modelling range-shifting species. Methods Ecol Evol. 2010;1(4):330–42.

73. Calisher CH, Childs JE, Field HE, Holmes KV, Schountz T. Bats: important reservoir hosts of emerging viruses. Clin Microbiol Rev. 2006;19(3):531–45.

74. Morin CW, Comrie AC, Ernst K. Climate and dengue transmission: evidence and implications. Environ Health Perspect. 2013;121(11–12):1264–72.

75. Kang DS, Tomas R, Sim C. The effects of temperature and precipitation on *Culex quinquefasciatus* (Diptera: Culicidae) abundance: a case study in the Greater Waco city, Texas. Vector Biol J. 2017;2(1):1000116.

76. Reisen WK, Fang Y, Martinez VM. Effects of temperature on the transmission of West Nile virus by *Culex tarsalis* (Diptera: Culicidae). J Med Entomol. 2006;43(2):309–17.

77. Tjaden NB, Thomas SM, Fischer D, Beierkuhnlein C. Extrinsic incubation period of dengue: knowledge, backlog, and applications of temperature dependence. PLoS Negl Trop Dis. 2013;7(6):e2207.

78. Ng V, Fazil A, Gachon P, Deuymes G, Radojević M, Mascarenhas M, et al. Assessment of the probability of autochthonous transmission of Chikungunya virus in Canada under recent and projected climate change. Environ Health Perspect. 2017;125(6):067001.

79. Rocklöv J, Quam MB, Sudre B, German M, Kraemer MUG, Brady O, et al. Assessing seasonal risks for the introduction and mosquito-borne spread of Zika virus in Europe. Ebiomedicine. 2016;9:250–6.

80. Ogden NH, Radojevic M, Wu XT, Duvvuri VR, Leighton PA, Wu JH. Estimated effects of projected climate change on the basic reproductive number of the Lyme disease vector *Ixodes scapularis*. Environ Health Perspect. 2014;122(6):631–8.

81. Mordecai EA, Cohen JM, Evans MV, Gudapati P, Johnson LR, Lippi CA, et al. Detecting the impact of temperature on transmission of Zika, dengue, and chikungunya using mechanistic models. PLoS Negl Trop Dis. 2017;11(4):e0005568.

82. Pautasso A, Radaelli MC, Ballardini M, Francese DR, Verna F, Modesto P, et al. Detection of West Nile and Usutu viruses in Italian free areas: entomological surveillance in Piemonte and Liguria Regions, 2014. Vector Borne Zoonotic Dis. 2016;16(4):292–4.

2

A cross-sectional ecological analysis of international and sub-national health inequalities in commercial geospatial resource availability

Winfred Dotse-Gborgbortsi[1,2], Nicola Wardrop[2], Ademola Adewole[2], Mair L. H. Thomas[2] and Jim Wright[2*]

Abstract

Background: Commercial geospatial data resources are frequently used to understand healthcare utilisation. Although there is widespread evidence of a digital divide for other digital resources and infra-structure, it is unclear how commercial geospatial data resources are distributed relative to health need.

Methods: To examine the distribution of commercial geospatial data resources relative to health needs, we assembled coverage and quality metrics for commercial geocoding, neighbourhood characterisation, and travel time calculation resources for 183 countries. We developed a country-level, composite index of commercial geospatial data quality/availability and examined its distribution relative to age-standardised all-cause and cause specific (for three main causes of death) mortality using two inequality metrics, the slope index of inequality and relative concentration index. In two sub-national case studies, we also examined geocoding success rates versus area deprivation by district in Eastern Region, Ghana and Lagos State, Nigeria.

Results: Internationally, commercial geospatial data resources were inversely related to all-cause mortality. This relationship was more pronounced when examining mortality due to communicable diseases. Commercial geospatial data resources for calculating patient travel times were more equitably distributed relative to health need than resources for characterising neighbourhoods or geocoding patient addresses. Countries such as South Africa have comparatively high commercial geospatial data availability despite high mortality, whilst countries such as South Korea have comparatively low data availability and low mortality. Sub-nationally, evidence was mixed as to whether geocoding success was lowest in more deprived districts.

Conclusions: To our knowledge, this is the first global analysis of commercial geospatial data resources in relation to health outcomes. In countries such as South Africa where there is high mortality but also comparatively rich commercial geospatial data, these data resources are a potential resource for examining healthcare utilisation that requires further evaluation. In countries such as Sierra Leone where there is high mortality but minimal commercial geospatial data, alternative approaches such as open data use are needed in quantifying patient travel times, geocoding patient addresses, and characterising patients' neighbourhoods.

Keywords: Geocoding, Drive-times, Patient travel, Neighbourhood statistics, Digital divide, Geospatial data, Health inequalities, Inverse care law, GIS

*Correspondence: j.a.wright@soton.ac.uk
[2] Geography and Environment, University of Southampton, Highfield, Southampton SO17 1BJ, UK
Full list of author information is available at the end of the article

Background

Sustainable Development Goal (SDG) 3, Target 3.8 seeks to 'achieve universal health coverage, including financial risk protection, access to quality essential health-care services...for all' [1], with a similar target 3.7 seeking to deliver universal maternal healthcare coverage. GIS has been proposed as an integrative information and communication technology tool for accelerating progress towards universal health coverage (UHC) [2]. Informed decision-making is central to achieving UHC and spatial analysis enables precise identification of health needs to inform system strengthening interventions and can help to identify localised gaps in service provision, masked by national or provincial averages [2]. Supporting UHC has been proposed as a means of reducing mortality. For example, increasing the proportion of births attended by a skilled birth attendant at primary healthcare facilities can contribute to reduced maternal mortality [3].

To realise the potential of GIS, it has been argued that the health sector has to 'geoenable' its health information systems [2]. 'Geoenabling' entails putting in place the necessary governance structures, technical capacity, guidelines, standards, protocols, technology and core data to harness GIS' potential. Thus, a management structure that provides sufficient funding to underpin GIS adoption, resources for creating and maintaining health information systems, and an underlying national spatial data infrastructure are all prerequisites for GIS uptake in the health sector. Awareness of GIS use in healthcare planning remains low even in developed countries [4], where within the UK National Health Service its use remains largely restricted to mapping.

Here, we focus on one such potential barrier to GIS uptake in the health sector, namely the availability of core data. In representing population demand for healthcare and examining patient interactions with healthcare facilities, the use of several key commercial geospatial resources has become widespread in many developed countries. These geospatial resources include reference data sets and tools for geocoding the residential addresses of patients presenting at healthcare facilities [5, 6], and transportation data that enable patient travel times to be computed from place of residence to facility [7, 8]. They also include area statistics and geodemographic data sets, which provide insights into neighbourhood characteristics that may be associated with healthcare demand and utilisation [9–11].

Although such data resources are generally available in high income countries, in many low and middle income countries (LMICs), such data may be patchy in coverage, imprecise, or lacking altogether. Furthermore, in developed countries, national spatial data infra-structures (SDIs) typically enable national mapping and statistical agencies to maintain address databases or dwelling frameworks, and thereby construct small area statistics. In LMICs, however, barriers relating to the global digital divide such as lack of financial resources, insufficient leadership and governance, poor internet bandwidth [12], lack of trained personnel, lack of vendor support, and power dynamics over information release all inhibit SDI development [13]. Even where open data initiatives exist as in the example of Kenya, such resources may still remain limited [14], although there is evidence [15, 16] that coverage of the world's largest open geospatial database, OpenStreetMap (OSM), is rapidly expanding in many LMICs.

Over 30 years ago, an 'inverse care law' was first identified by Hart [17], which highlighted the frequently encountered perverse relationship between healthcare provision and need. Since then, there have been numerous studies that have quantified greater healthcare provision among areas of low need and lower healthcare provision in areas of high need [18–21], confirming this phenomenon in many settings. It is unclear whether data for planning healthcare delivery follow a similar pattern.

Methods

Aims

In this paper, we aim to quantify the extent to which the same perverse relationship with health needs applies to geospatial data availability as with healthcare provision. We explore two scales through a cross-sectional, ecological study design. We firstly examine the relationship between geospatial data availability and health need as measured by all-cause mortality and mortality due to three groups of causes, globally at national level. We then consider the relationship between health need and geospatial data availability in two sub-national case studies from Ghana and Nigeria.

Data

At international level, we examine the availability, by country, of three sets of commercial data resources that are central to understanding population demand for healthcare and spatial patterns of healthcare utilisation. These are geocoding tools for locating patients' residences; transportation network resources for computing patient travel from place of residence to health facility; and area statistics for characterising the neighbourhoods where patients live. We excluded other commercial geospatial data resources not directly related to healthcare-seeking behaviour, such as remotely sensed imagery. To identify such resources, we used the search strategy in Additional file 1: Table S1. We included only geospatial data resources that met the following criteria:

- Related to more than five countries, thereby having an international rather than national or regional remit
- Were not derived exclusively from open data and were provided as a commercial service
- Did not duplicate data resources already included in our analysis (for example where there were several APIs based on the same underlying data resource)
- Provided published statements of data availability or quality by country.

Where necessary, we contacted data providers to request permission to use data availability or quality statements in our analysis, only including those where such permission was granted. The geospatial resources that met all these criteria were included in our analysis are shown in Table 1 (Additional file 1: Tables S2–S4 documents data resources that were excluded and reasons for this).

Alongside these resources, we used all-cause mortality by country for the most recent period (2000–2015) reported by the World Health Organisation (WHO)

[22], as a general health outcome measure and thereby metric of healthcare need. We also separately examined the major WHO categorization of mortality: non-communicable diseases; injuries; communicable diseases, maternal, perinatal, and nutritional conditions for 183 countries.

Analysis
International analysis
National mortality data from WHO were age-standardised to account for differences in population structure between countries. As dependent territories are not reported separately in WHO mortality data, these were excluded from our analysis.

We then generated commercial geospatial resource indicators by country as follows:

- *Geocoding resources* Since the published level of geocoding availability and quality via the Google Application Programming Interface (API) scarcely varied by country, we used the geocoding precision

Table 1 Commercial geospatial data resources for geocoding patient addresses, estimating travel times, and characterising patients' neighbourhoods

Geospatial resource	Description	Web link
Geocoding		
ESRI geocoding resources	Underpinning resources for geocoding via API, desktop and online software	https://developers.arcgis.com/rest/geocode/api-reference/geocode-coverage.htm
Pitney Bowes	Geocoding API	https://developer2.pitneybowes.com/docs/location-intelligence/v1/en/index.html#GeoCode/Geocode/LI_GGM_Geo_Geocoding.html#GGM_Geo_Geocoding__Geocoding_CountrySpecific
TomTom	Resources for geocoding API	https://developer.tomtom.com/market-coverage-1
MapBox	Resources for geocoding API	https://www.mapbox.com/geocoding/#data
Loqate	Resources for geocoding service	https://loqate.com/countries-covered/
Patient travel		
ESRI/HERE	Underpinning resources for travel time estimation via API, desktop and online software	https://doc.arcgis.com/en/arcgis-online/reference/network-coverage.htm
Google traffic/speed limits	Resources accessible via Google Maps API	https://developers.google.com/maps/coverage
iGeoloise TravelTime Platform	Resources for API for computing travel times via public transport and driving	http://docs.traveltimeplatform.com/overview/supported-countries/
TomTom	API resources for routing and drive-times	https://developer.tomtom.com/market-coverage-1
MapBox Directions API	Resources for travel time API	https://www.mapbox.com/api-documentation/pages/traffic-countries.html
Neighbourhood characterisation		
Michael Bauer	Area statistics covering topics such as population, age-sex structure, consumer lifestyles, unemployment and purchasing power	http://www.english.mb-research.de/market-data-overseas.html
Mosaic Global geodemographic resources	Area statistics based on consumer classification system	http://www.experian.co.uk/assets/business-strategies/brochures/Mosaic_Global_factsheet%5b1%5d.pdf
Cameo International	Area statistics based on consumer classification system	http://www.callcredit.co.uk/media/1287258/cameo%20global%20map.jpg
Maptitude	Spatially disaggregated demographic data that are more than headcounts	https://www.caliper.com/maptdata.htm

levels published by Pitney Bowes, TomTom, MapBox, Loqate, and the Environmental Systems Research Institute (ESRI).

- *Resources for computing patient travel times* To characterise availability and quality of resources for computing travel times via the Google API, we generated a composite index by summing reported data availability for cycling directions, walking directions, driving directions, speed limits and availability of a traffic layer. Each of these was scored as two for 'good quality and availability', one for 'approximate data quality and availability' and zero otherwise. ESRI/HERE data quality and availability was characterised by six levels, based on availability of traffic and speed limit data, and completeness of street network coverage, whilst TomTom resources were characterised by availability of traffic flows, traffic incidents, and online routing. We separately recorded the availability of a traffic layer via MapBox and availability of routing for car travel only or car travel and public transport via iGeoloise TravelTime.

- *Area statistics for characterising patients' neighbourhoods* To quantify availability of neighbourhood statistics by country, we computed three measures. Firstly, as a measure of spatial data disaggregation, we used the mean population per areal unit (lower mean populations indicate a higher level of spatial disaggregation) in Michael Bauer data sets. Where no data were available from this provider for a given country, we used the national 2015 population estimate from the WHO mortality database. Secondly, for the most detailed geography available in the Michael Bauer data, we counted the number of areal attributes available per country, setting this to zero where no data were available. Finally, for each country, we identified whether only one or both the geodemographic classifications (i.e. CAMEO Worldwide and Mosaic Global) were available, alongside availability of Maptitude demographic data.

To examine the availability of these geospatial resources relative to healthcare need, as measured by standardised all-cause mortality and cause-specific mortality, we computed relative concentration indices and slope indices of inequality [23] for each of these measures of geospatial data availability using a tool from Public Health England [24]. In this context, the slope index of inequality measured the change in mortality relative to ranked geospatial data availability/quality, whilst the relative concentration index measured the mortality gradient against relative geospatial data availability/quality.

We also created a composite index of commercial geospatial resource quality/availability (geospatial resource index) by combining these various indicators. For each of the three index domains (geocoding resources, patient travel, and neighbourhood characterisation), we ranked each country from highest to lowest based on each of the above indicators, then summed these ranks, dividing the total by the maximum possible summed rank to give an index for each domain between 0 and 1. To avoid the index being dominated by indicator availability at domain level, we then summed the three domain index values. We regressed logged standardised mortality against the geospatial resource index, identifying as outliers in terms of data availability those countries with studentised residuals greater than two. We also calculated the correlation of the geospatial resource index with the percentage of internet users and gross domestic product (GDP) per capita for 2016 in each country [25].

Sub-national case studies

To examine sub-national geospatial commercial resource availability and quality, two sub-national case studies were conducted, one in Eastern Region, Ghana and the other in Lagos State, Nigeria. Both focussed on success rates for geocoding facility locations (health facilities and schools respectively). In the absence of robust district-level mortality estimates, both studies examined geocoding success rates relative to area deprivation at administrative level 2 (districts in Ghana or local government areas in Nigeria). In this context, we consider area deprivation to reflect 'an area's potential for health risk from ecological concentration of poverty, unemployment, economic disinvestment, and social disorganisation' [26].

In Eastern Region, 984 health facility place-names from 25 districts were obtained from the Ghana Health Service routine data repository (DHIMS2) and geocoded via an interface to the Google Maps API Version 2 [27]. Geocoding success was measured as the proportion of facilities per district for which a location within Eastern Region was returned. District deprivation was assessed firstly via the 2017 UNICEF District League Table (DLT) [28], a composite index of district development based on indicators of education, sanitation, rural water, health, security and governance. Secondly, district deprivation was also assessed via a bespoke district deprivation index. The bespoke deprivation index was created from 12 indicators representing six domains: information access, education, energy, employment, water and sanitation, and living conditions, adapting an approach used in South Africa [29]. Indicators values were drawn from 2010 census data [30]. Within each domain, each indicator was standardised by conversion to a z-score, with z-scores averaged for each domain. The average scores for the six domains were then summed to give a composite deprivation score.

Similarly, in Lagos State 310 schools, both private and public, from 20 Local Government Areas (LGAs) were obtained from online news media [31]. These were then geocoded using the Google Maps API Version 2 via BatchGeo [32]. A deprivation index with the same six domains as Ghana was created for the LGAs, but with 9 indicators drawn from 2006 census data acquired from the National Population Commission. These were then standardised and combined using the same method as for Eastern Region. For both case studies, geocoding success per district/LGA was then plotted against deprivation. Relative concentration indices and slope indices of inequality were computed for district-level geocoding success rates versus the deprivation measures.

Results

Characteristics of commercial geospatial data resources

Table 2 summarises the availability and precision of commercial geospatial resources for the 183 countries for which data were available in the WHO mortality database. There is considerable international variation in each indicator's availability, with for example both predictive and live traffic data underpinning ESRI's drive-time calculations in 11 countries, but conversely only partial coverage of the major road network being available in 24 countries. Similarly, market and demographic statistics were available for areas with average populations of less than a thousand in some countries, but over ten million in others.

International inequality in access to commercial geospatial data resources

Table 3 shows two health inequality metrics, the relative concentration index and slope index of inequality, for national all-cause mortality versus international availability and quality of various commercial geospatial data resources. Slope index of inequality values indicate the effect on all-cause mortality of moving from the most data-poor country to the most data-rich. Negative concentration indices suggest mortality is concentrated among data-poor populations, whilst zero indicates no mortality gradient relative to geospatial data. Slope indices of inequality were significantly different from zero for most sources of commercial geospatial data considered, suggesting significant health inequalities for most resources. However, levels of inequality were lower for resources for computing patient travel times than for resources for geocoding patient addresses or characterising patients' areas of residence. For example, concentration indices for ESRI's geocoding service and population size of Michael Bauer's areal units were − 0.14 and − 0.12 respectively, whereas concentration indices for Google and ESRI's patient travel resources were less than − 0.07.

Table 4 shows the inequality metrics broken down by the WHO cause-specific mortality categorization. As indicated by the concentration index values differing from zero, measured inequalities were greatest for the communicable disease group and lowest for non-communicable diseases, both for the overall index and for the geocoding and neighbourhood characterisation domains. Concentration index values and therefore measured inequality were closer to zero for the patient travel domain, as with all-cause mortality.

International geospatial resource index

Figure 1 shows the international geospatial resource index (illustrating quality/availability of commercial geospatial data resources for healthcare planning). According to the composite index, the quality/availability is generally high in the Americas, Australasia and Europe, but low in Africa and south Asia. However, some data providers document potentially valuable geospatial resources for healthcare planning in countries with high mortality, particularly in west and southern Africa. For example, a traffic layer is available via Google and interpolated street address level geocoding is documented by Pitney Bowes for Nigeria, both potentially valuable in understanding patient travel.

The geospatial resource index was strongly correlated with the percentage of internet users per country in 2016 ($r = 0.77$, $p < 0.001$, $n = 183$) and to a lesser extent with GDP per capita ($r = 0.68$, $p < 0.001$, $n = 174$). Several African countries such as South Africa and Mozambique had comparatively high geospatial data availability/quality scores given GDP, whilst several of the Gulf States (e.g. Qatar, United Arab Emirates) and smaller island states (e.g. Iceland, the Seychelles) had comparatively low index values given their GDP per capita. Similar patterns were observable for index values versus internet use.

Figure 2 shows the distribution of standardised all-cause mortality in relation to the geospatial resource index. As anticipated from the deprivation indicators above, the pattern of all-cause mortality broadly follows geospatial resource quality/availability. Several outliers are labelled in Fig. 2. Countries with low all-cause mortality and low commercial geospatial data resources were typically either small island states such as Malta and the Maldives, or states with strict controls on international transfers of national data, such as South Korea and Cuba. South Africa was notable for its high all-cause mortality but comparatively high commercial geospatial resource availability, with similar outliers being in southern or west Africa.

Table 2 Geospatial resource availability and precision for 183 countries (portions of this table are modifications based on work created and shared by Google and used according to terms described in the Creative Commons 3.0 Attribution License. Used with permission. Copyright © 2017 Esri, ArcGIS Online, HERE, Increment P, GlobeTech and the GIS User Community. All rights reserved. © 2017 Michael Bauer Research GmbH, © TomTom 2018)

Availability and precision of geospatial data resources	No of countries (%)
Geocoding	
ESRI	
Level 1: address searches likely to result in either precise coordinates or interpolated location along street for address	42 (23.0%)
Level 2: address searches often result in precise coordinates or interpolated location along street, but sometimes street-level coordinates or coarser	16 (8.7%)
Level 3: address searches sometimes result in precise coordinates or interpolated location along street, but more often street-level coordinates or coarser	51 (27.9%)
Level 4: address searches result in imprecise locations, e.g. centroids of higher-level administrative boundaries	74 (40.4%)
Pitney Bowes Geocoding (highest precision available)	
Precise address point geocoding	20 (10.9%)
Address geocoding	39 (21.3%)
Street-level geocoding	60 (32.8%)
Post code	34 (18.6%)
Administrative boundaries or place-names	29 (15.8%)
Not specified	1 (0.5%)
TomTom geocoding (highest precision available)	
Address point	42 (23.0%)
Interpolated address	20 (10.9%)
Street-level	77 (42.1%)
Locality	44 (24.0%)
MapBox geocoding (highest precision available)	
Address geocoding	25 (13.7%)
Postcode	20 (10.9%)
Place-name	60 (32.8%)
No service	79 (42.6%)
Loqate geocoding	
Premises—point	52 (28.4%)
Premises	44 (24.0%)
Thoroughfare	68 (37.2%)
Locality	19 (10.4%)
Patient travel	
ESRI/HERE travel times	
Predictive traffic: comprehensive street data with live, historic, and predictive traffic	11 (6.0%)
Live traffic: comprehensive street data with live and historic traffic	40 (21.9%)
Historical traffic: comprehensive street data with historic traffic only	20 (10.9%)
Posted speed limits: comprehensive street data but with time-invariant travel times derived from speed limits	15 (8.2%)
Limited street coverage: partial street data for major roads only without minor or secondary roads; time-invariant travel times derived from speed limits	73 (39.9%)
Minimal street coverage: partial street data for some major roads only; no ground verification of network; no speed limit data	24 (13.1%)
Google travel times—traffic	
Traffic layer—available with good data quality and availability	91 (49.7%)
Traffic layer—available with approximate data quality or availability	1 (0.5%)
Traffic layer not available	91 (49.7%)
Google travel times—speed limits	
Speed limits—available with good data quality and availability	11 (6.0%)
Speed limits—available with approximate data quality or availability	166 (90.7%)
Speed limits not available	6 (3.3%)

Table 2 (continued)

Availability and precision of geospatial data resources	No of countries (%)
Google travel times—cycling	
Cycling directions available	21 (11.5%)
Cycling directions unavailable	162 (88.5%)
iGeolise TravelTime Platform	
Travel times for public transport and driving	23 (12.6%)
Travel times for driving only	3 (1.6%)
Travel times unavailable	157 (85.8%)
TomTom	
Online routing with traffic incidents and traffic flows	42 (23.0%)
Online routing with traffic flows only	15 (8.2%)
Online routing without traffic	57 (31.1%)
No online routing	69 (37.7%)
MapBox	
Traffic layer available	33 (18.0%)
Traffic layer unavailable	150 (82.0%)
Neighbourhood characterisation	
Michael Bauer neighbourhood statistics	
Number of areal attribute groups per country—global mean (5th centile; 95th centile)	4 (0; 9)
Mean population per areal unit by country—global median (5th centile; 95th centile)	130,000 (411; 23,801,400)
Mosaic Global	
Geodemographic classification available	24 (13.1%)
Geodemographic classification unavailable	159 (86.9%)
Cameo worldwide	
Geodemographic classification available	39 (21.3%)
Geodemographic classification unavailable	144 (78.7%)
Maptitude	
Demographic data (beyond population headcounts) available	13 (7.1%)
Demographic data (beyond population headcounts) unavailable	170 (92.9%)

Sub-national case studies

Figure 3 shows the relationship between geocoding success rate and deprivation, in Lagos State and Eastern Region, with no clear relationship emerging overall. Geocoding success rates were low for health facilities in Eastern Region, but much higher for schools in Lagos State. In Eastern Region, districts such as East Akim and Birim Central had high success rates although their deprivation score was close to the average. Further exploration revealed these two districts had the highest number of hospitals (4 each) in the region and hospitals had the highest geocoding success rate (70.6%) compared with other health facility types. Likewise, the regional capital of New Juaben with 3 hospitals, was least deprived and had a high geocoding success rate. In Nigeria, two LGAs containing a small number of schools, Badagry and Ibeju-Lekki, were more deprived and had lower geocoding success rates, particularly influencing the observed relationship between deprivation and geocoding success.

Table 5 shows inequality metrics for geocoding success rates versus area deprivation at the LGA or district level in Lagos State, Nigeria, and Eastern Region, Ghana. There was no evidence of inequality in geocoding success relative to area deprivation in Lagos State, as indicated by the concentration index of zero. In Ghana, evidence for lower geocoding success in more deprived areas was mixed. When the DLT was used to measure area deprivation, confidence intervals for the slope index of inequality straddled zero, indicating no significant inequality. When the bespoke area deprivation index was used, the slope index of inequality was significantly different from zero.

Discussion

To our knowledge, our analysis is the first to examine global patterns of commercial geospatial data availability in relation to health outcomes. As observed with healthcare services, both internationally and for two sub-national case studies, these data are inversely correlated with health need, as measured by mortality and

Table 3 Metrics of inequality in international availability of commercial geospatial data resources, relative to age-standardised all-cause mortality for 2015 in 183 countries (portions of this table are modifications based on work created and shared by Google and used according to terms described in the Creative Commons 3.0 Attribution License. Used with permission. Copyright © 2017 Esri, ArcGIS Online, HERE, Increment P, GlobeTech and the GIS User Community. All rights reserved. © 2017 Michael Bauer Research GmbH, © TomTom 2018)

Index domain	Commercial geospatial resource availability/quality measure	Relative concentration index	Slope index of inequality (95% confidence intervals)
Geocoding	ESRI	− 0.14	7.54 (6.47–8.61)
	Pitney Bowes	− 0.04	2.18 (0.66–3.69)
	TomTom	− 0.02	0.9 (− 0.70 to 2.49)
	MapBox	− 0.07	4.24 (2.77–5.71)
	Loqate	− 0.01	0.45 (− 1.12 to 2.03)
	Geocoding domain	− 0.07	3.21 (1.81–4.62)
Patient travel	ESRI / HERE	− 0.03	1.55 (0.05–3.06)
	Google Maps	− 0.06	3.24 (1.75–4.72)
	MapBox	− 0.07	7.79 (5.88–9.70)
	iGeolise TravelTime	− 0.05	7.25 (4.89–9.61)
	TomTom	− 0.01	0.32 (− 1.27 to 1.90)
	Patient travel domain	− 0.04	1.93 (0.47–3.39)
Neighbourhood characterisation	Michael Bauer—average population per areal unit	− 0.12	6.08 (4.89–7.27)
	Michael Bauer—no. of areal attribute groups	− 0.07	3.54 (2.14–4.94)
	Geodemographic classification/demographic data availability (Experian Global & Cameo Worldwide; Maptitude)	− 0.10	5.91 (4.56–7.25)
	Neighbourhood characterisation domain	− 0.13	6.39 (5.24–7.54)
Overall index	Overall commercial geospatial resource quality/availability index	− 0.08	4.01 (2.64–5.37)

Table 4 Metrics of inequality in international availability of commercial geospatial data resources, relative to age-standardised cause-specific mortality for 2015 in 183 countries

Commercial geospatial resource availability/quality measure	Relative concentration index	Slope index of inequality (95% confidence intervals)
Relative to mortality from communicable, maternal, perinatal and nutritional conditions		
Geocoding domain	− 0.121	3.05 (0.82–5.27)
Patient travel domain	− 0.020	0.52 (− 1.77 to 2.80)
Neighbourhood characterisation domain	− 0.335	8.44 (6.53–10.35)
Overall geospatial resource index	− 0.159	4.01 (1.81–6.20)
Relative to mortality from non-communicable diseases		
Geocoding domain	− 0.040	1.38 (0.84–1.91)
Patient travel domain	− 0.034	1.18 (0.63–1.73)
Neighbourhood characterisation domain	− 0.056	1.91 (1.41–2.41)
Overall geospatial index	− 0.045	1.54 (1.01–2.06)
Relative to mortality from injuries		
Geocoding domain	− 0.092	0.39 (0.22–0.56)
Patient travel domain	− 0.034	0.14 (− 0.03 to 0.32)
Neighbourhood characterisation domain	− 0.170	0.72 (0.58–0.87)
Overall geospatial index	− 0.103	0.44 (0.27–0.60)

deprivation respectively. This disparity in geospatial data availability is more pronounced for mortality due to communicable diseases. Such data are thus frequently unavailable for planning healthcare provision or geocoding cases for widespread communicable diseases such as malaria. The availability of commercial geospatial data resources broadly follows the same pattern as that identified in analyses of the global digital divide, with for

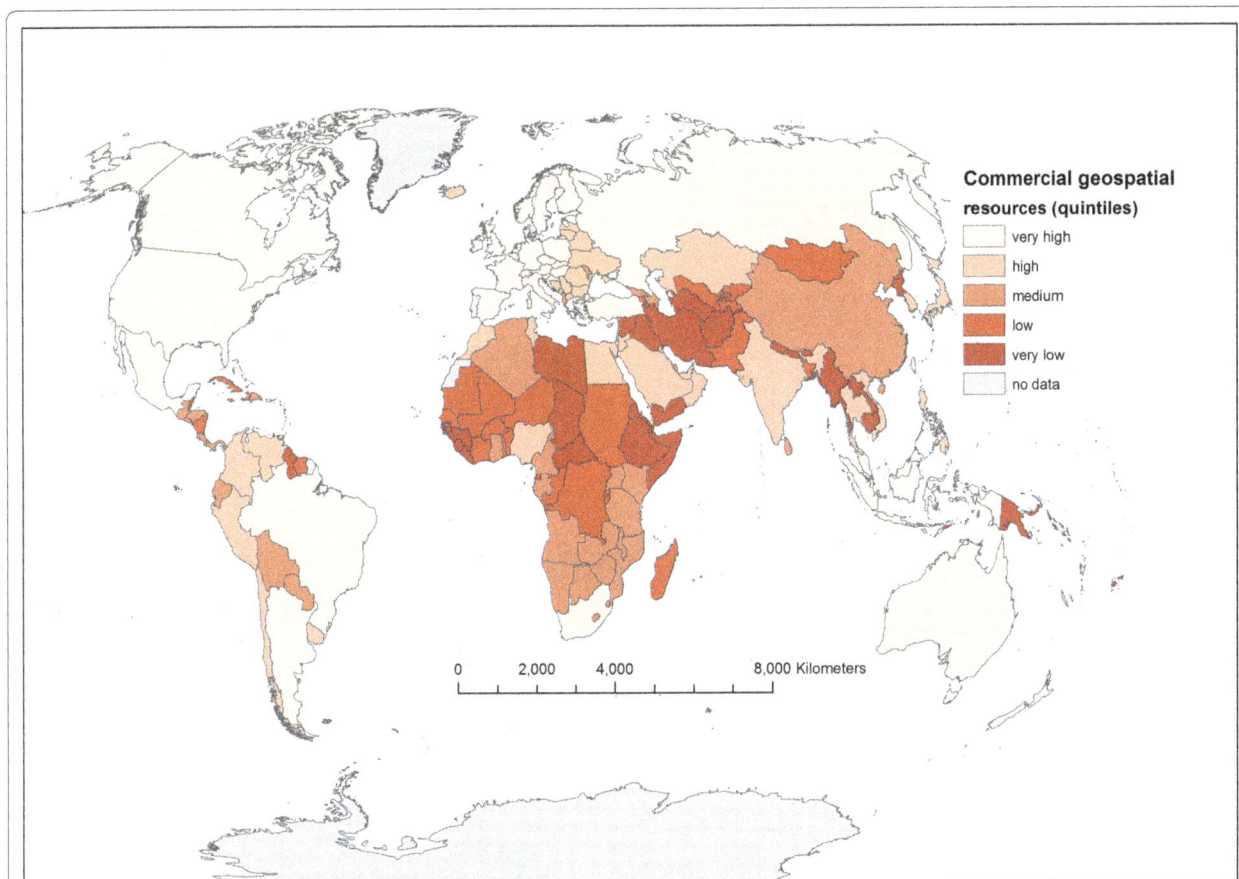

Fig. 1 An index of commercial geospatial resource quality/availability for healthcare planning by country (based on a Winkel-Tripel projection. Portions of this graphic are modifications based on work created and shared by Google and thematicmapping.org and used according to terms described in the Creative Commons 3.0 Attribution License. Used with permission. Copyright © 2017 Esri, ArcGIS Online, HERE, Increment P, GlobeTech and the GIS User Community. All rights reserved. © 2017 Michael Bauer Research GmbH, © TomTom 2018)

example sub-Saharan Africa being the world region lagging furthest behind North America in internet users [33] and Africa having the lowest Information and Communication Technology Development Index [34]. The pattern of outliers is somewhat different to these more general analyses of the global digital divide, however. For example, an assessment of digitalisation relative to GDP per capita [35] indicated lower than anticipated digitalisation in Oman and Kuwait but higher digitalisation in South Korea. We observed the same relationship for the Gulf States in relation to our commercial geospatial index but low international availability of commercial geospatial data in South Korea. However, because of restrictions on the export of mappable data out of the country, South Korea has previously been reported as lacking data from major providers such as Google [36].

In the absence of such commercial tools, and where sufficient capacity exists, researchers in LMICs have resorted to alternative strategies for geocoding data, computing drive-times, and characterising patients'

places of residence. Where the human resources, infrastructure, and tools exist, one geocoding strategy is to rely on open data, particularly OSM, as has been attempted in Thailand and Mozambique for healthcare management [37, 38]. Elsewhere, a study in Yemen, relied on direct measurement of drive-times taken on specific routes [39]. A Kenyan study explored participatory mapping and use of local landmarks as strategies for geocoding patient addresses [40], whilst in a Mexican study, a software application was developed that allowed patients to identify their place of residence through interpretation of Google Earth and StreetView imagery [41]. In Cote d'Ivoire, aggregated call record data from mobile phones have been used to develop a proxy for regional socio-economic indicators [42], whilst in Accra, vegetation metrics derived from QuickBird satellite imagery were correlated with a slum index [43]. Without such innovative geocoding or neighbourhood characterisation strategies, there is potential for misclassification of neighbourhood characteristics [44] and environmental exposures [45] when

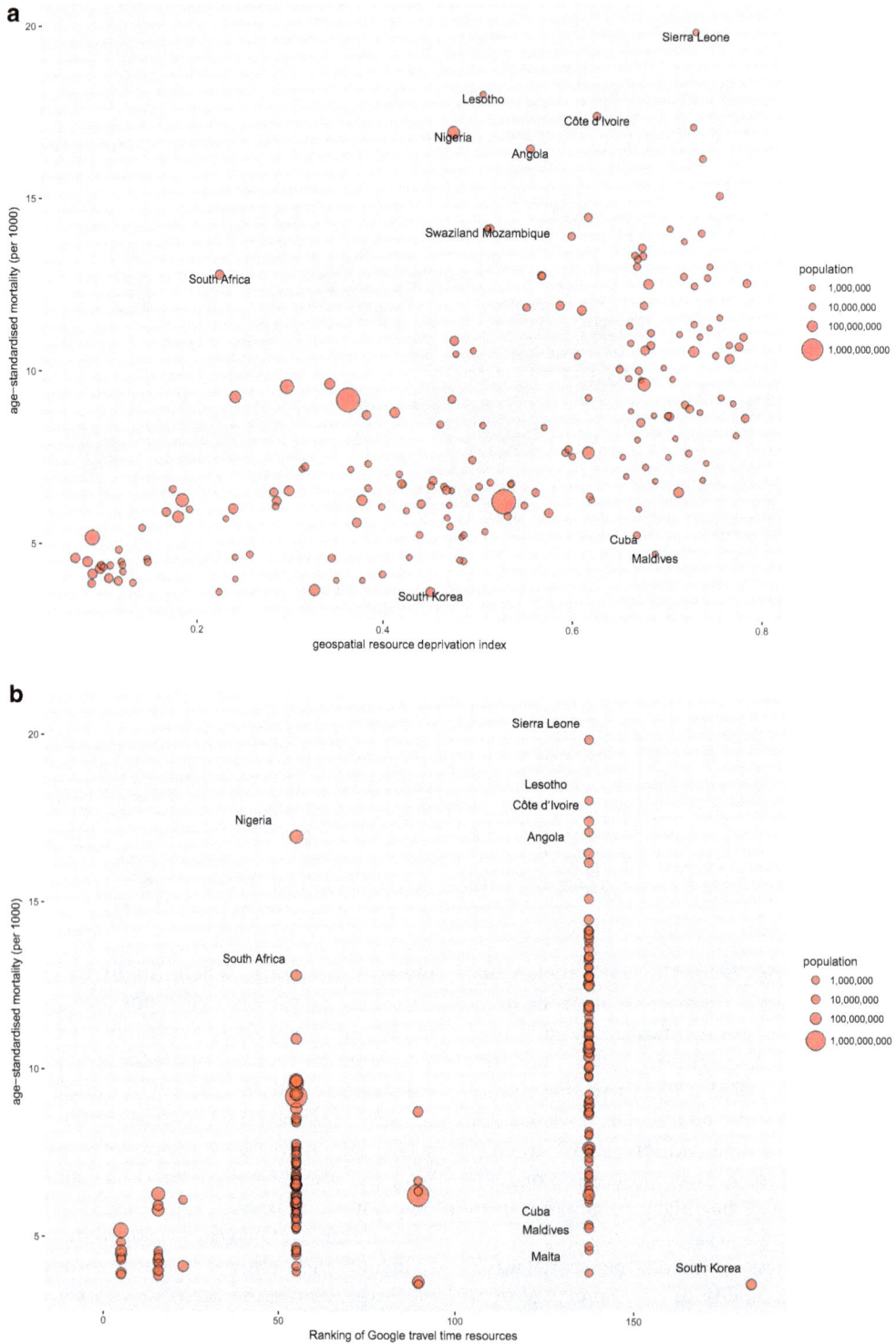

Fig. 2 Age-standardised all-cause mortality for 2015 versus **a** an index of commercial geospatial resource quality/availability; **b** ranked availability of Google Maps travel time resources (labelled countries were identified as outliers. Portions of this graphic are modifications based on work created and shared by Google and used according to terms described in the Creative Commons 3.0 Attribution License. Used with permission. Copyright © 2017 Esri, ArcGIS Online, HERE, Increment P, GlobeTech and the GIS User Community. All rights reserved. © 2017 Michael Bauer Research GmbH; © TomTom 2018)

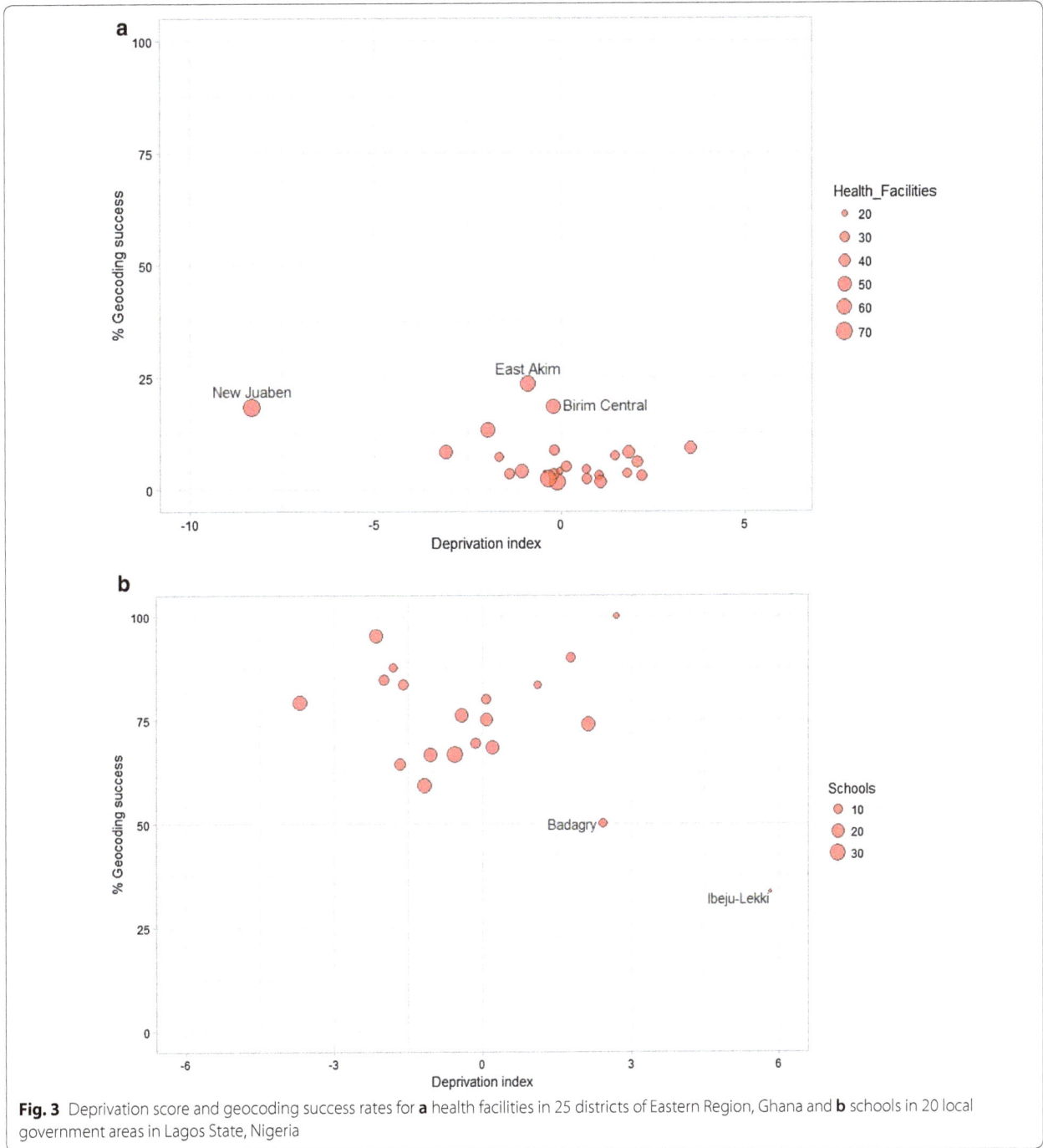

Fig. 3 Deprivation score and geocoding success rates for **a** health facilities in 25 districts of Eastern Region, Ghana and **b** schools in 20 local government areas in Lagos State, Nigeria

analysing LMIC patient data using inexact geocodes or areal statistics relating to large populations.

International organisations have invested heavily in geospatial infra-structure, capacity-building, and technology to address this paucity of commercial data and its affordability in low-resource settings. The WHO for example has developed AccessMod to estimate patient travel times to health facilities via a cost surface approach

[46]. Because of limited access to software and technical GIS skills, WHO also developed the HealthMapper software, which packages public domain spatial databases with a user-friendly interface to broaden uptake of GIS for healthcare planning. HealthMapper has been used in schistosomiasis control [47] and prioritising areas for filariasis elimination [48]. More recently, Measure Evaluation have supported health management information

Table 5 Inequalities in geocoding success rates, relative to area deprivation (for 984 health facilities in 25 districts in Eastern Region, Ghana and 298 schools in 20 LGAs in Lagos State, Nigeria)

Case study details	Relative concentration index	Slope index of inequality (95% confidence intervals)
Eastern Region, Ghana		
Geocoding success rate for health facilities		
Relative to UNICEF District League Table	0.14	6.87 (− 2.24 to 15.97)
Relative to bespoke district deprivation index	0.20	9.57 (0.93–18.21)
Lagos State, Nigeria		
Geocoding success rate for schools		
Relative to LGA deprivation index	0.00	− 1.99 (− 24.41 to 20.43)

systems by developing the Place Mapping plug-in for QGIS to ease handling and display of point data sets [49] and provided guidance on diagnosing positional errors [50].

We found less conclusive evidence that geocoding success rates were lower in deprived areas when considering the two sub-national case studies of Lagos State, Nigeria and Eastern Region, Ghana. There was no evidence of inequality in geocoding success in Lagos State, but mixed evidence of such inequality in Eastern Region. However, elsewhere an apparent inverse relationship between geocoding outcomes and area deprivation has been observed at local level in other LMICs. A study in the Brazilian city of Belo Horizonte, for example, found that geocoding precision via the Google geocoding API was lower in slum areas than in formal urban neighbourhoods [51]. In response to this issue, the What3Words georeferencing system, which uses an algorithm to assign three words as a unique, human-friendly georeference to each of 57 trillion grid squares globally, has been used to locate addresses in Brazilian favelas lacking conventional addressing systems [52].

Our findings are subject to several limitations. Our study assumes that the data provider's published country coverage information is an accurate reflection of geospatial data availability and precision across all countries. In reality, export of geospatial data from one country to another may be restricted by trade embargos, as has previously happened with satellite imagery exports to India for example [53], and where commercial geospatial data are available internationally, they may be unaffordable within the national health sector. In assessing the international availability of geodemographic classifications, we focussed on two major international data providers only, potentially omitting smaller data providers operating in individual countries. However, a recent study of the international availability of geodemographic classifications [54] showed very similar patterns to that found

here. Computed inequality indices are also likely to be lower for metrics of geospatial data availability and precision based on a small number of ordinal classes (e.g. for geodemographic data availability), than metrics on a ratio scale (e.g. mean population per areal unit). In our sub-national case studies, geocoding success rates for higher tier facilities (e.g. hospitals or large secondary schools) may be higher than for lower tier facilities (e.g. primary care facilities such as Community-Based Health Planning and Services compounds). Since such facilities are more often found in urban areas, such heterogeneity in facility type may lead to an over-estimate of inequality in geocoding resource access.

Given the rapid pace of change in the geospatial data sector, this analysis could be repeated in the future to monitor rapidly changing data availability in relation to health outcomes. We have only considered the relationship between commercial geospatial resources and mortality, but geospatial resource availability could also be examined in relation to underlying drivers of health outcomes, such as country income levels, internet access, and relevant government policies, or in relation to measures relevant for other sectors (such as infrastructure). There would also be scope to combine the country-level results presented here on commercial geospatial data with recent assessments of OSM completeness by country [15, 16]. These studies, based on stratified assessment of OSM road completeness [16] or saturation of user contributions [15], suggest that global commercial geospatial resources and OSM completeness patterns are somewhat different, with for example, China and Egypt having low OSM completeness [16]. The potential utility of commercial geospatial data resources for healthcare planning could also be explored through a case study country (e.g. South Africa), deliberately selected because of its high mortality and high geospatial data availability.

The comparatively richer commercial resources in west and southern African countries such as Nigeria and

South Africa merit further investigation for healthcare planning in these countries, subject to sufficient funds being available to support their use in a given project.

In contrast to analyses from elsewhere [51], our subnational analyses in Lagos State suggested only limited evidence that geocoding success was lower in deprived areas. Our inconclusive results may be because the large areal units we used to assess deprivation may mask localised pockets of deprivation, which have been identified via previous work in Accra [55]. In our analysis, we implicitly use geocoding success rates to assess spatial variation in the Google Maps API reference data set and geocoding algorithm performance. However, geocoding success also depends on the quality of the input address data [56] and this will have been affected by local variations in service provision tiers, language of place-names and place-name aliases in our Nigerian and Ghanaian case studies. Furthermore, in our two case studies, success rates in geocoding service locations in Eastern Region, Ghana, and Lagos State, Nigeria were very different, despite identical documented levels of geocoding service precision. Despite their growing potential, this suggests careful evaluation of such resources is needed prior to their application to healthcare management.

In many other countries with high mortality, commercial geospatial data availability was very low. By examining commercial geospatial resource availability alongside OSM completeness [16], such countries could be targeted via non-profit initiatives to increase the availability of open geospatial data availability, such as those undertaken through OSM-based volunteer mapping initiatives by humanitarian organisations [57, 58]. Whilst commercial geospatial resource availability may improve in these countries in the future, in the interim, there remains a need for innovative solutions to geocoding outpatient data, estimating patient travel times and characterising neighbourhoods in such countries as described above.

Conclusions

To our knowledge, our analysis is the first to examine global patterns of commercial geospatial data availability in relation to health outcomes. The relationship observed between commercial geospatial resource availability and health needs suggests LMICs still have inadequate geospatial resources for the type of granular analysis needed to drive the SDG agenda surrounding UHC. This inequality in data availability is more pronounced for mortality due to communicable diseases than for all-cause mortality. There were some outliers, however: several west and southern African countries such as Nigeria and South Africa had comparatively

high geospatial data availability and high mortality. In contrast, there were several countries with low mortality and comparatively geospatial data availability, often island states (e.g. the Maldives) or those with policy restrictions on geospatial data (e.g. South Korea). This analysis thus suggests some resources, particularly those for quantifying patient travel times, are penetrating countries with high all-cause mortality. In countries such as South Africa and Nigeria where there is high mortality but also comparatively rich commercial geospatial data, these data are a potential resource for examining healthcare utilisation that requires further evaluation. In countries such as Sierra Leone where there is high mortality but minimal commercial geospatial data, alternative approaches, for example based on open data such as OSM, are needed in quantifying patient travel times, geocoding patient addresses, and characterising patients' neighbourhoods.

In many instances, our examination of patterns of commercial geospatial availability confirms other studies of global digitalisation, with for example lower levels of digitalisation in the Gulf States for a given level of GDP per capita. However, even where this is comparatively high availability of relevant commercial geospatial data availability, this alleviates just one barrier among many that inhibit uptake of GIS in healthcare planning. Beyond increasing the availability of core data, further investments are needed in technical capacity-building, awareness-raising, guidelines, standards and protocols if the potential of such data is to be realised within the health sector.

Abbreviations
API: Application Programming Interface; DLT: District League Table; DHIMS: District Health Information Systems; ESRI: Environmental Systems Research Institute; GDP: gross domestic product; LGA: local government area; LMICs: low and middle-income countries; OSM: OpenStreetMap; SDGs: Sustainable Development Goals; SDI: spatial data infra-structure; UHC: universal health coverage; WHO: World Health Organisation.

Authors' contributions
WD, AA, NW, and JW designed the study. AA prepared and analysed the Nigerian case study data, WD prepared and analysed the Ghanaian case study data, and JW and MT prepared and analysed the international data sets. WD and JW drafted the manuscript, which was reviewed by all other authors. All authors read and approved the final manuscript.

Author details
Kibi Government Hospital, Ghana Health Service, Accra, Ghana. [2] Geography and Environment, University of Southampton, Highfield, Southampton SO17 1BJ, UK.

Competing interests
The authors declare that they have no competing interests.

Availability of data and materials

The mortality and Google-derived datasets analysed during the current study are available in the WHO Global Health Organisation repository at http://www.who.int/healthinfo/global_burden_disease/estimates/en/index1.html and the Google Maps Application Programming Interfaces documentation, https://developers.google.com/maps/coverage. Data concerning the percentage of internet users per country and GDP per country are available as open data from https://data.worldbank.org/ . The other web documentation that supports the findings of this study are available from ESRI, Pitney Bowes, MapBox, TomTom and Michael Bauer but restrictions apply to the availability of these web pages, which were used under license or with permission for the current study, and so are not publicly available. Data are however available from the authors upon reasonable request and with permission of the data providers. The deprivation datasets for Ghana are in the 2010 Population and housing census analytical reports available online for download, whilst names of healthcare facilities were provided with permission by Ghana Health Services. The District League Table data for Ghana are available for download from UNICEF Ghana and the Ghana Centre for Democratic Development: http://www.unicef.org/ghana/. 2006 census data for Nigeria were acquired under licence from the National Population Commission, whilst school names are available at https://9jaskulnews.blogspot.co.uk.

Funding

WD is a Commonwealth Scholar, and was funded by the UK government and University of Southampton. MT's contribution to the paper was supported by the Economic and Social Research Council (Grant No. ES/P000673/1). Neither funding body had a role in the design of the study.

References

1. United Nations. Sustainable development goal 3: ensure healthy lives and promote well-being for all at all ages. New York: Department of Economic and Social Affairs; 2018 [cited 2018 18 April 2018]. https://sustainabledevelopment.un.org/sdg3.

2. Roth S, Landry M, Ebener S, Marcelo A, Kijsanayotin B, Parry J. The geography of universal health coverage: why geographic information systems are needed to ensure equitable access to quality healthcare. Manila: Asian Development Bank; 2016.

3. Campbell O, Graham W. Strategies for reducing maternal mortality: getting on with what works. Lancet. 2006;368(9543):7–13.

4. Shaw N. Geographical information systems and health: current state and future directions. Healthc Inf Res. 2012;18(2):88–96.

5. Rosu A, Chen DM. An improved approach for geocoding Canadian postal code-based data in health-related studies. Can Geogr Geogr Can. 2016;60(2):270–81.

6. Edwards SE, Strauss B, Miranda ML. Geocoding large population-level administrative datasets at highly resolved spatial scales. Trans GIS. 2014;18(4):586–603.

7. Sharma DK, Vangaveti VN, Larkins S. Geographical access to radiation therapy in North Queensland: a retrospective analysis of patient travel to radiation therapy before and after the opening of an additional radiotherapy facility. Rural Remote Health. 2016;16(1):3640.

8. Chu S, Boxer R, Madison P, Kleinman L, Skolarus T, Altman L, et al. Veterans affairs telemedicine: bringing urologic care to remote clinics. Urology. 2015;86(2):255–60.

9. Nnoaham KE, Frater A, Roderick P, Moon G, Halloran S. Do geodemographic typologies explain variations in uptake in colorectal cancer screening? An assessment using routine screening data in the south of England. J Public Health. 2010;32(4):572–81.

10. Grubesic TH, Miller JA, Murray AT. Geospatial and geodemographic insights for diabetes in the United States. Appl Geogr. 2014;55:117–26.

11. Petersen J, Gibin M, Longley P, Mateos P, Atkinson P, Ashby D. Geodemographics as a tool for targeting neighbourhoods in public health campaigns. J Geogr Syst. 2011;13(2):173–92.

12. Hilbert M. The bad news is that the digital access divide is here to stay: domestically installed bandwidths among 172 countries for 1986–2014. Telecommun Policy. 2016;40(6):15.

13. Bishop ID, Escobar FJ, Karuppannan S, Williamson IP, Yates PM, Suwarnarat K, et al. Spatial data infrastructures for cities in developing countries—lessons from the Bangkok experience. Cities. 2000;17(2):85–96.

14. Williams S, Marcello E, Klopp JM. Toward open source Kenya: creating and sharing a GIS database of Nairobi. Ann Assoc Am Geogr. 2014;104(1):114–30.

15. Grochenig S, Brunauer R, Rehr K. Digging into the history of VGI data-sets: results from a worldwide study on OpenStreetMap mapping activity. J Locat Based Serv. 2014;8(3):198–210.

16. Barrington-Leigh C, Millard-Ball A. The world's user-generated road map is more than 80% complete. PLoS ONE. 2017;12(8):e0180698.

17. Hart JT. The inverse care law. Lancet. 1971;297(7696):8.

18. McLean G, Guthrie B, Mercer SW, Watt GCM. General practice funding underpins the persistence of the inverse care law: cross-sectional study in Scotland. Br J Gen Pract. 2015;65(641):E799–805.

19. Tansley G, Stewart BT, Gyedu A, Boakye G, Lewis D, Hoogerboord M, et al. The correlation between poverty and access to essential surgical care in Ghana: a geospatial analysis. World J Surg. 2017;41(3):639–43.

20. Chavehpour Y, Rashidian A, Raghfar H, Sefiddashti SE, Maroofi A. 'Seeking affluent neighbourhoods?' A time-trend analysis of geographical distribution of hospitals in the Megacity of Tehran. Health Policy Plan. 2017;32(5):669–75.

21. Wright J, Martin D, Cockings S, Polack C. Overall Quality of Outcomes Framework scores lower in practices in deprived areas. Br J Gen Pract. 2006;56(525):277–9.

22. World Health Organization. Global health estimates 2015: deaths by cause, age, sex, by country and by region, 2000–2015. In: World Health Organization, editor. Geneva: World Health Organization; 2016.

23. Regidor E. Methods for measuring health inequalities: part 2. J Epidemiol Community Health. 2004;58:4.

24. Public Health England. Excel tool for calculating various inequality measures, such as Slope Index of Inequality and Concentration Index. March 2014 ed. Redditch: Public Health England; 2014.

25. World Bank. World Bank Open Data Washington DC: World Bank; 2018 [17 April 2018]. https://data.worldbank.org/.

26. Anderson RT, Sorlie P, Backlund E, Johnson N, Kaplan GA. Mortality effects of community socio-economic status. Epidemiology. 1997;8(1):42–7.

27. Aanensen D. spatialepidemiology.net London: Imperial College; 2018 [29 March 2018]. http://www.spatialepidemiology.net/.

28. UNICEF, CDD Ghana. Ghana's District League Table. New York: UNICEF; 2017.

29. Wright G, Barnes H, Noble M, Dawes A. The South African index of multiple deprivation for children 2001 at datazone level. Pretoria: Department of Social Development; 2009.

30. Ghana Statistical Service. 2010 Population and housing census, Eastern region analytical report; 2013.

31. Anuoluwap B. List of registered schools in Lagos State Lagos: MySchoolNews; 2018 [29 March 2018]. https://9jaskulnews.blogspot.co.uk.

32. BatchGeo. BatchGeo Vancouver: BatchGeo; 2018 [29 March 2018]. https://batchgeo.com/.

33. Robison KK, Crenshaw EM. Reevaluating the global digital divide: sociodemographic and conflict barriers to the internet revolution. Sociol Inq. 2010;80(1):34–62.

34. International Telecommunications Union. Measuring the information society report 2015. Geneva: International Telecommunications Union; 2015.

35. Billon M, Lera-Lopez F, Marco R. Differences in digitalization levels: a multivariate analysis studying the global digital divide. Rev World Econ. 2010;146(1):39–73.

36. Associated Press. No driving directions: Google, South Korean Can't Reach Map Deal VOA News; 2016 [cited 2017 31 Oct 2017]. https://www.voanews.com/a/google-maps-data-south-korea/3602188.html.

37. Makanga PT, Schuurman N, Sacoor C, Boene H, Von Dadelszen P, Firoz T. Guidelines for creating framework data for GIS analysis in low- and middle-income countries. Can Geogr Geogr Can. 2016;60(3):320–32.

38. Ferguson WJ, Kemp K, Kost G. Using a geographic information system to enhance patient access to point-of-care diagnostics in a limited-resource setting. Int J Health Geogr. 2016;15:10.

39. Al-Taiar A, Clark A, Longenecker JC, Whitty CJM. Physical accessibility and utilization of health services in Yemen. Int J Health Geogr. 2010;9:38.

40. Stresman GH, Stevenson JC, Owaga C, Marube E, Anyango C, Drakeley C, et al. Validation of three geolocation strategies for health-facility attendees for research and public health surveillance in a rural setting in western Kenya. Epidemiol Infect. 2014;142(9):1978–89.

41. Beletsky L, Arredondo J, Werb D, Vera A, Abramovitz D, Amon JJ, et al. Utilization of Google enterprise tools to georeference survey data among hard-to-reach groups: strategic application in international settings. Int J Health Geogr. 2016;15:24.

42. Mao H, Shuai X, Ahn Y-Y, Bollen J. Quantifying socio-economic indicators in developing countries from mobile phone communication data: applications to Côte d'Ivoire. EPJ Data Sci. 2015;4:15.

43. Weeks JR, Hill A, Stow D, Getis A, Fugate D. Can we spot a neighborhood from the air? Defining neighborhood structure in Accra, Ghana. GeoJournal. 2007;69(1–2):9–22.

44. Ribeiro AI, Olhero A, Teixeira H, Magalhaes A, Pina MF. Tools for address georeferencing—limitations and opportunities every public health professional should be aware of. PLoS ONE. 2014;9(12):e114130.

45. Mazumdar S, Rushton G, Smith BJ, Zimmerman DL, Donham KJ. Geocoding accuracy and the recovery of relationships between environmental exposures and health. Int J Health Geogr. 2008;7:13.

46. Ray N, Ebener S. AccessMod 3.0: computing geographic coverage and accessibility to healthcare services using anisotropic movement of patients. Int J Health Geogr. 2008;7:63.

47. Chammartin F, Hurlimann E, Raso G, N'Goran E, Utzinger J, Vounatsou P. Statistical methodological issues in mapping historical schistosomiasis survey data. Acta Trop. 2013;128(2):345–52.

48. Ngwira B, Tambala P, Perez A, Bowie C, Molyneux D. The geographical distribution of lymphatic filariasis infection in Malawi. Filaria J. 2007;6:12.

49. Evaluation Measure. The place mapping tool: a plug-in for QGIS. Chapel Hill: University of North Carolina; 2017.

50. Measure Evaluation. Overview: spatial quality anomalies diagnosis (SQUAD) tool for QGIS. Chapel Hill, North Carolina: University of North Carolina, 2018 April 2018. Report No.

51. Davis CA, de Alencar RO. Evaluation of the quality of an online geocoding resource in the context of a large Brazilian city. Trans GIS. 2011;15(6):851–68.

52. Jones G. Human friendly coordinates. Geoinformatics. 2015;18(5):10–2.

53. Nagendra N. Industry participation in India's space program: current trends and perspectives for the future. Int J Space Politics Policy. 2016;14(2–3):237–55.

54. Ojo A. Geodemographic classification systems for the developing world: the case of Nigeria and the Philippines. Sheffield: University of Sheffield; 2010.

55. Aggrey-Korsah E, Oppong J. Researching urban slum health in Nima, a slum in Accra. In: Weeks JR, Hill A, Stoler J, editors. Spatial inequalities: health, poverty and place in Accra, Ghana. Dordrecht: Springer; 2013. p. 109–24.

56. Zanderbergen P. Geocoding quality and implications for spatial analysis. Geogr Compass. 2009;3(2):647–80.

57. de Albuquerque JP, Herfort B, Eckle M. The tasks of the crowd: a typology of tasks in geographic information crowdsourcing and a case study in Humanitarian mapping. Remote Sens. 2016;8(10):859.

58. Givoni M. Between micro mappers and missing maps: digital humanitarianism and the politics of material participation in disaster response. Environ Plan D Soc Space. 2016;34(6):1025–43.

3

Developing a data-driven spatial approach to assessment of neighbourhood influences on the spatial distribution of myocardial infarction

Wahida Kihal-Talantikite[1*], Christiane Weber[2], Gaelle Pedrono[3], Claire Segala[4], Dominique Arveiler[5], Clive E. Sabel[6], Séverine Deguen[7,8] and Denis Bard[9]

Abstract

Background: There is a growing understanding of the role played by 'neighbourhood' in influencing health status. Various neighbourhood characteristics—such as socioeconomic environment, availability of amenities, and social cohesion, may be combined—and this could contribute to rising health inequalities. This study aims to combine a data-driven approach with clustering analysis techniques, to investigate neighbourhood characteristics that may explain the geographical distribution of the onset of myocardial infarction (MI) risk.

Methods: All MI events in patients aged 35–74 years occurring in the Strasbourg metropolitan area (SMA), from January 1, 2000 to December 31, 2007 were obtained from the Bas-Rhin coronary heart disease register. All cases were geocoded to the census block for the residential address. Each areal unit, characterized by contextual neighbourhood profile, included socioeconomic environment, availability of amenities (including leisure centres, libraries and parks, and transport) and psychosocial environment as well as specific annual rates standardized (per 100,000 inhabitants). A spatial scan statistic implemented in SaTScan was then used to identify statistically significant spatial clusters of high and low risk of MI.

Result: MI incidence was non-randomly spatially distributed, with a cluster of high risk of MI in the northern part of the SMA [relative risk (RR) = 1.70, p = 0.001] and a cluster of low risk of MI located in the first and second periphery of SMA (RR 0.04, p value = 0.001). Our findings suggest that the location of low MI risk is characterized by a high socioeconomic level and a low level of access to various amenities; conversely, the location of high MI risk is characterized by a high level of socioeconomic deprivation—despite the fact that inhabitants have good access to the local recreational and leisure infrastructure.

Conclusion: Our data-driven approach highlights how the different contextual dimensions were inter-combined in the SMA. Our spatial approach allowed us to identify the neighbourhood characteristics of inhabitants living within a cluster of high versus low MI risk. Therefore, spatial data-driven analyses of routinely-collected data georeferenced by various sources may serve to guide policymakers in defining and promoting targeted actions at fine spatial level.

Keywords: Data-driven, Multidimensional, Spatial approach, Neighbourhood influences, Social health inequalities, Myocardial infarction

*Correspondence: wahida.kihal@live-cnrs.unistra.fr
[1] LIVE UMR 7362 CNRS (Laboratoire Image Ville Environnement),
University of Strasbourg, Strasbourg 6700, Strasbourg, France
Full list of author information is available at the end of the article

Background

Despite a succession of high-profile reports based on scientific studies demonstrating the links between social determinants and several health outcomes, health inequalities persist and still constitute a major public health issue [1–3]. Since the early 2000s, there has been a growing number of studies demonstrating the role played by 'place' where people live (also referred to as 'context') in influencing health status [4–7]. More precisely, the underlying idea is that the health effect of the environment exposure is complex, including both direct effect of specific environmental exposure (e.g. air pollution) and indirect consequences commonly addressed as the concept of "neighbourhood" [4, 6–8]. Many literature reviews support the significant effect of neighbourhood on a set of outcomes [9] such as mental health, birth [10], early childhood health [11], and obesity [12].

In order to explain the pathway via which neighbourhood may affect health, several papers have proposed conceptual models related to neighbourhood and to individuals' behaviours—such as physical activities [13], walkability [13], diet [14] and such bio-physiological events as stress [15]. For instance, the causal framework proposed by Pearce et al. [16] uses three distinct domains to describe the various components of neighbourhood: physical characteristics (quality of outdoor environment and housing, traffic and physical disorder, etc.), (2) social characteristics (social network, social cohesion, etc.), and (3) community resources access (leisure facilities, healthcare, etc.). More recently, Komeily et al. [17] have defined neighbourhood as a function of several variables selected from physical (street design, connectivity, building type and use, etc.), operational (transit stops, routes, etc.), socioeconomic (demographics, land use and density, etc.) environmental (climate, topography, etc.) and institutional points of view (policy, etc.). In the majority of studies, however, neighbourhood was characterized by a single variable such as, for instance, noise [18–20] or the presence of graffiti, [21] defining the physical domain in epidemiological studies investigating respiratory [18] or cardiovascular disease [18–20]. Characterization of neighbourhood in the domain of community resources access, food store accessibility [22], primary healthcare services, recreational facilities, and public open [23, 24] and green spaces [25, 26] has been investigated in the literature. The role of the social domain has so far been explored mainly through data on local violence [27, 28] and social cohesion (or social capital) [29].

Each of these domains has been recognized as being associated with health status beyond socioeconomic status. For instance, the association between a low social standing measurement for residential neighbourhood and blood pressure was found after adjusting for individual/neighbourhood socioeconomic status and individual risk factors for hypertension [30]. A recent systematic review revealed that the majority of studies show a reduced risk of cardiovascular disease mortality in areas having higher residential greenness [31]; a finding confirmed by another study investigating respiratory disease, which showed that children living in areas with more street trees have lower prevalence of asthma [32]. In addition, certain neighbourhood characteristics–such as proximity and/or access to green space or healthcare–are often not equitably distributed with regard to socioeconomic status [33]—and this could exacerbate health inequalities.

Fine neighbourhood characterization for the study of health effects now has major policy implications for the public health community, to promote development and application of policies and social action aimed at reducing health inequalities [34–36]. Moreover, the spatial identification of small geographical areas carrying a high health risk, and their contextual characteristics, could allow for action more closely targeted at those most at risk [37, 38].

In this context, the issue is the definition of relevant, evidence-based public health interventions, armed with precise knowledge of what truly influences health inequalities in a given setting and among specific, vulnerable population groups. It should be stressed that such knowledge may inform the "Health in all Policies" strategy advocated by WHO and the European Union [39, 40], through actions on urban planning, transport, educational services, social work, and amenities (including leisure centres, libraries and parks).

In this work, we sought to combine a data-driven approach with clustering analysis techniques, to investigate neighbourhood characteristics (including socioeconomic and public resources as well as the psychosocial dimension) that may explain the geographical distribution of onset of MI risk. This work is not intended to reveal any relationship or causal pathway between neighbourhood characteristics and MI risk; other, more appropriate studies were designed to answer this question [9].

Methods

Study setting

Our study setting was the Strasbourg metropolitan area (SMA), an urban area of $316 \, km^2$, located in the Bas-Rhin district of the Great-East region of north-eastern France, and having a population of 500,000. This area comprises 33 municipalities subdivided into 190 French census blocks named IRIS (Ilots Regroupés pour l'Information Statistique), each having an average of 2000 inhabitants.

This French census block/IRIS (a sub-municipal French census block) is defined by the National Institute of

Statistics and Economic Studies (INSEE). This is the smallest administrative unit in which socioeconomic and demographic data are available in France. In terms of population size, French census block is intermediate between US census tracts (about 4000 inhabitants) and US census block groups (about 1000 inhabitants).

Neighbourhood characteristics

To our knowledge, few groups have attempted to combine all the domains addressed above [41, 42]. For instance, the UK Department of the Environment, Transportation, and the Regions (DETR) [42] developed an Index of Multiple Deprivation (IMD) as an official measure of relative deprivation for small areas (or neighbourhoods) in England—based on a combination of six or seven domains.

As in the British contextual frameworks, we have undertaken a process of characterizing a neighbourhood in the SMA that includes the most common domains capable of supporting health studies of related to: socioeconomic, community resources (or public resource), and psychosocial (or social).

Data sources: Table 1

All socioeconomic data including employment, educational level, income, data about those receiving child benefit and also those receiving the French welfare allowance was obtained from the French National Census Bureau (INSEE-*Institut National de la Statistique et des Etudes Economiques*) and from the statistics department of the CAF (Caisse d'Allocations Familiales), family welfare system.

To characterize access to public resources, the regional health agency provided all the FINESS (French National Directory of Health and Social Establishments) files, which describe the healthcare system (physicians and facilities). The SMA made geocoded data available that allowed us to determine (1) transportation elements such as bus and tram stops and the number of lines served, as well as (2) geocoded data on location of public parks and green spaces. Lastly, the Great-East regional and district office DRDJS (Office of Youth and Sports) made available its database of all athletic equipment and facilities. However, no information concerning the usage of amenities was collected in this study.

To characterize the psychosocial environment, including the civic and community environments, local businesses and retail stores, and educational environment, we used SIRENE databases (INSEE), the educational facilities database available at the SMA authority and official education institutions, as well as data provided by the city's list of itinerant vendors (small markets). The CIGAL Spatial Data Infrastructure (Cooperation pour

l'Information Géographique en Alsace), provides a database describing land use and land cover coverage and categories (see Table 1).

Geographical information system analysis

Of the databases collected, some datasets were available at administrative spatial base level—such as census block. Such segmentation might, however, not be relevant for spatial analysis of other data produced for different purposes, at various scales. Instead of using the available French census block files, we therefore chose to design a specific spatial unit mesh, allowing us to manage the data's scale heterogeneity (that is, a square grid) for three reasons:

- Stability of the basic geographical unit; one advantage of cell-based over administrative borders (likely to change over time) is that it can be fixed: its borders do not change over time unless desired—in response for example to changing underlying population or land-use footprints.
- Administrative spatial units and their borders are not necessarily relevant for subsequent analysis other than that for which they were constructed.
- To homogenize contextual data; contextual data is extremely heterogeneous in terms of spatial scales, collection dates, and exhaustiveness. Use of the grid makes it possible to homogenize data to some extent, ahead of any statistical or spatial analysis.

To determine grid path size, we used the "nearest neighbour" method [43] to characterize the spatial distribution of the different patterns of geographical points (retail store, physicians, etc.). The mean distance separating points has been calculated as 270 m. Cell dimension was thus set at 250 m × 250 m to best approximate underlying data distribution, yielding 5127 cells for the SMA coverage. All contextual variables collected were assigned at this cell level.

Zonal data (such as the socioeconomic data obtained at IRIS scale for the 1999 census) was fitted to the 250 × 250 m grid using a clipping function. The "zone clipping" algorithm is then used to disaggregate the variable, according to a geometric overlap principle. The value of the information transferred to the cell is thus a function of the area common to the initial area (for example, the IRIS) and the grid cell.

In this desegregation approach, we assume equal density of the phenomenon across the area. The space considered, however, is not isotropic. This constraint was overcome using available geographic information (topographic database) to improve characterization of the disaggregation of the initial area.

Table 1 Data source to characterize the neighbourhood context

Domain	Category	Variables	Provider (Year)	Exhaustivity of location data
Domain 1: socioeconomic environment	Population	Total population % of born abroad	French National Census Bureau (INSEE-Institut National de la Statistique et des Etudes Economiques) (1999)	Data available from census block level
	Employment	Unemployment rate % of Blue collars among the active population with permanent jobs Non-permanent job rate		
	Education	% Persons aged 15+ without qualification People aged 15 years or older with at least a lower tertiary education People aged 15 years or older who did not go beyond an elementary education		—
	Family	% of single-parent families		
	Household	% of households with no car % of households with 2 cars		
	Income	% of population entitled to family allowance % of population entitled to safety net income	Statistics department of CAF (Caisse d'Allocations Familiales) (2007)	
Domain 2: public resources	Healthcare system	Location of doctors' surgeries—Location of health-care centres	Regional health agency/French National Directory of Health and Social Establishments (2007)	Systematic census of all doctor and health-care centre addresses located in the SMA
	Public transportation supply	Location of bus and tram stop and the number of lines served at each	SMA authority (2008)	Exact location ground-truthing
	Public parks and gardens	Location and area of public parks and gardens	SMA authority et CIGAL Spatial Data Infrastructure (Coopération pour l'Information Géographique en Alsace) (2008)	Systematic census conducted by the SMA authority (using ground-truthing) of all public parks (where inhabitants may practice sport)
	Sport facilities	Location of sport facilities	Great-East regional and district office DRDJS (Office of Youth and Sports) (2008)	Systematic census of all sports facilities by the Office of Youth and Sports, using ground-truthing
Domain 3: psychosocial environment	Local businesses	Location of retail outlets Location of food markets	SMA authority (2008)	Systematic census of retail outlets and food markets conducted by the SMA authority using ground-truthing of itinerant vendors only (small markets)
	Characterization of educational facilities	Number and type of Violence in schools	Official education institutions (Ministère de l'éducation). (2007)	Exact location and characteristics of education facilities provided by the official educational institutions that manage these schools
		Schools' social scores	Inspection d'académie (Ministère de l'éducation) (2007)	

Table 1 continued

Domain	Category	Variables	Provider (Year)	Exhaustivity of location data
		Primary/middle and secondary (high) schools ZEP (priority) and successful (AR) middle schools	SMA authority and official education institutions (2007)	
		Map showing primary and middle schools Secondary (High) schools	General Council of the Bas-Rhin and official education institutions (2007) SMA authority and official education institutions (2007)	
	Voting rates	Voting rates	The City Halls of Strasbourg (2000–2008)	–
	Civic associations	Location of civic associations	SMA authority and SIRENE databases (2000–2008)	
		Type of civic associations: Religious, political, volunteer		Exact location of association without use of ground-truthing

SMA Strasbourg metropolitan area

In our study, we postulate that the equidistribution of data was a function of the buildings' volume: in this case, we estimated the population of the cells proportionally to the habitable area of the buildings included in the cells, according to the following formula:

$$\text{Population} = \sum_{N}^{i-1} P_{\text{IRIS}_i} \times \frac{\sum_{n}^{i-1} \text{Area of housing}_i}{\text{Total area of housing in IRS}_i}$$

where Area of housing = Building footprint area of housing × Number of habitable floors. Number of habitable floors = housing height/3.

Once all socioeconomic variables had been desegregated at cell level, we calculated the socioeconomic indicator for each cell (e.g. unemployment rate, % of blue-collars among the active population with permanent jobs, non-permanent job rate).

For all spatial analyses described below, each cell was represented by the centroid of the inhabited built area.

A data-driven approach to neighbourhood characterization

First, the 25 variables described in Table 1 were geolocated and analysed in line with the approaches proposed by various studies (Table 2).

Second, we aimed to create a multidimensional profile with which to characterize each neighbourhood based on the underlying data structure using a data-driven approach, and without any a priori models.

Consider a data set composed of each domain within the same unit as group of variables. As we had several groups of both quantitative and qualitative contextual variables (socioeconomic, public resource, psychosocial) and because we wanted to give each equal weight regardless of the number of variables in it, we used Multiple Factor Analysis (MFA) [44]—a technique well-suited to this situation.

The MFA entailed performing either a Principal Component Analysis (PCA) for each subset, if the group is composed of quantitative variables (sets of both socioeconomic and public resources domain variables), or a Multiple Correspondence Analysis (MCA) if the group is composed of qualitative variables (sets psychosocial domain of variables). This first step allowed us to compute distance between units by giving a specific weight to each variable, based on use of the highest eigenvalue of the PCA or the MCA for each group, thus obtaining a particular metric. In the second step of the MFA, we used the previously obtained metric to perform a PCA on the whole data set. This allowed us to compare groups of different types of variables.

Following the MFA, we applied Hierarchical Ascendant Clustering (HAC) [45] to create meaningful contextual profile (cf. Appendix for Fig. 4). HAC is an unsupervised clustering method that creates a hierarchy of classes (clusters), and is frequently used after MFA. Given a set of variables created by the MFA, the HC algorithm creates a hierarchy of categories, step by step—at each step merging the two categories that are closest, according to a given distance between categories. When it is a particular distance (Ward distance), this algorithm aims to obtain categories that are homogeneous within and heterogeneous between one another, with respect to an inertia-based criterion.

These approaches therefore allow us to build a partition of our unit into homogeneous clusters (low within-variability) that are different from one another (high between-variability), ultimately producing a categorical indicator, referred to in our previous work as the Neighbourhood Deprivation Index (NDI) [46] (for more detail, see Sabel et al. [46]). These analyses were performed using SPAD 7.0 statistical software.

Synthetic neighbourhood design

To evaluate spatial implication of neighbourhood planning, we have chosen to define specific boundaries of the neighbourhood, so as to use (1) a more homogeneous area (with high intra-zone homogeneity and inter-zone heterogeneity), and (2) an area with population size set to 2000 inhabitants, similar to the French census blocks, ensuring health data confidentiality.

To produce these synthetic neighbourhoods, we used the AZTool zone design program provided by David Martin (University of Southampton, UK) to aggregate contiguous and homogeneous spatial units (cells) for generating optimal geographies [47, 48]. To produce a synthetic homogeneous neighbourhood, three criteria were considered: (1) output zone homogeneity (and inter-zone heterogeneity), using our NDindex as the homogeneity criterion; (2) population target size equal to 2000 inhabitants (similar to French census blocks) to ensure health data confidentiality; (3) shape compactness, avoiding linear or quasi-linear output zones. To design the new zones, we used different combinations of relative weighting of parameters (criteria) in the AZTool (population target, shape and homogeneity) to create candidate sets of pseudo-blocks (in total six experimental conditions were tested). To improve AZT performance, we used simulated annealing (SA). Next, we evaluated the zonal system (each criterion defined below) to identify the optimal solution using a measure of within-area homogeneity (IAC) and measure shape compactness (P2A score) for each experimental condition. International experience and AZTool parameter setting advice accepts an IAC of greater than 0.5 as representing a very reasonable degree of homogeneity. Then, to improve AZT's solution and

Table 2 Spatial characterization of different field of neighbourhood

Domain	Category	Variables	Spatial shape	Geographic Information System (GIS) analysis
Domain 1: socio-economic environment	Population	Total population; All socio-economic variables	Zonal data available at census block level (2000 inhabitants on average)	Using the ArcGIS software zone-clipping algorithm, we disaggregated the variables according to real weighting interpolation methods. Because the value of the information transferred to the cell was thus a function of the area common to both the initial area (here, the census block) and the grid cell, these variables were able to be integrated into the final analysis
Domain 2 : public resources	Healthcare system	Location of doctors' surgeries; Location of healthcare centres	Point data: address	We assigned to each cell centroid the road distance (non-Euclidian) to the nearest healthcare centre or doctor's surgery
	Public parks and gardens	Location and area of public parks and gardens	Polygon data: Location and size	We built an attractiveness index for public parks and gardens, derived from French studies showing that attractiveness is a function of size. Using GIS tools, we drew concentric zones of attractiveness by area: 100 m (area less than 1 ha), 500 m (area 1–10 ha), and 1000 m for larger areas. We subsequently computed this index for each cell
	Sports facilities	Location of sport facilities	Point data: address and coordinate X, Y	The road network distance to the nearest sports facility was attributed to each cell centroid
	Public transportation supply	Location of bus and tram stop and the number of lines served at each	Point data: coordinate X, Y	Using GIS tools, and on the basis of modal differential attractiveness between these two types of public transportation, we constructed a public transportation availability indicator, with a catchment area attributed to each stop (300 m for a bus stop, 400 m for a tram station), weighted by the number of lines at each stop or station. This indicator was then assigned to each cell
Domain 3: psychosocial environment	Local businesses	Location of retail outlets	Point data: address and coordinate X,Y	Using GIS tools, we attributed to each unit the quantity of retail stores relative to all available retail space within a radius of 200 m around the spatial unit centroids. The resulting values associated with the retail store scoring (quantity of retail stores relative to all available retail space) by category (itinerant vendors; retail food stores; retail non-food stores and other services) were attributed to each unit[a]
		Location of food markets	Point data: address and coordinate X, Y	
	Characterization of educational facilities	Violence in schools; Schools' social scores; Primary/middle and secondary (high) schools; ZEP (priority) and successful (AR) middle schools; Map showing primary and middle schools; Secondary (High) schools	Point data: address and coordinate X, Y	The French school environment is graded as: (1) Priority education zones (ZEP-Zone d'éducation prioritaire), where establishments receive additional resources and have greater autonomy for dealing with educational and social difficulties, (2) "successful ambition" zones (AR), having fewer (but definite) needs and thus fewer resources), and (3) others. All non-private schools in the city and their catchment area were geocoded, using information provided by local authorities. We computed an indicator taking into account school density and classification (primary/middle or secondary/high schools)
	Voting rates	Voting rates	Zonal data available for each center of vote	
	Civic associations	Civic associations	Point data: address and coordinate X, Y	The fairly exhaustive and georeferenced SIRENE database allowed calculation of the ratio of the number of (official) civic associations per 100 inhabitants in each unit, taking into consideration their type (religious, political, other)
		Type of civic associations: religious, political, volunteer	Point data: address and coordinate X, Y	

a 200 m is the distance for which 50% of the cells have at least one market the found optimum solution, we sought to optimise two conditions for which IC >0.5 and which also presented a shape that was more compact than linear, by increasing the number of iterations. For more details, see Sabel et al. [46].

Health data: MI

All MI events [International Classification of Diseases, 9th Revision (ICD-9): 410] occurring in the SMA, among the population aged 35–74 years, collected by the Bas-Rhin coronary heart disease register [49] between January 1, 2000 and December 31, 2007 were geocoded at their residential address areal unit (see below). Specific annual rates, standardized by age and gender (per 100,000 inhabitants), were calculated for each neighbourhood by contextual profile. Khi^2 tests were performed to compare the annual rate between the five contextual profiles.

Spatial method

In order to explore the geographic pattern of the MI risk, we used the spatial scan statistics (implemented in the SaTScan software [50]) to statistically and significantly detect the presence of potential clusters for both high and low risk. This approach, used in an increasing number of applications in the field of spatial epidemiology [51–55], allowed us to (1) identify the specific spatial location of the clusters and (2) evaluate and understand the implications of neighbourhood characteristics in the spatial distribution of MI risk [56, 57].

The procedure works as follows: a circle (or windows) of variable radius (from zero up to 50% of population size [56]) is placed at every centroid of the synthetic neighbourhood and moves across the whole study area to compare the MI rate in the windows with what would be expected under a random distribution.

In our study, the Poisson probability model implemented in the SaTScan software [50] was chosen as *cluster analysis method*. The number of cases in each census block is assumed to follow a Poisson distribution. Our cluster detection approach identified clusters of both high and low rates with maximum circle window size, to include up to 50% of the population at risk. Identification of the most-likely clusters is based on a likelihood ratio test [56] with an associated p value obtained using Monte Carlo replications [58]. The number of Monte Carlo replications was set to 999 to ensure adequate power for defining clusters and considered a 0.05 level of significance (p value derived from 999 replications).

If we detect a significant most-likely cluster (with p < 0.05) using this method, a logical next step is to take account of the individual characteristics acknowledged in the literature and available in our studies, to see whether the significant cluster can be explained by suspected risk factors. Spatial analyses were thus performed in two stages (step by step):

1. Unadjusted analysis, to identify and localize the most-likely cluster of high/low risk of MI.
2. Analysis adjusted for age and sex included this information directly in the SaTScan model [50].

Results

The MFA was applied on the 27 selected variables covering the three contextual groups described above. The first four components explain only 17, 8, 5 and 5% of total variance respectively (Table 3). These components can be interpreted using the contributions made by both groups and variables to the components or their graphical representations. To explain 60% of total variance, we needed to use ten components, because all ten were used as a basis for the HC in order to preserve all the variability of the initial information.

In line with the MFA, we performed an HAC—and according to both the dendrogram and the Ward distance (Fig. 1), we chose a 5-category partition. From the HAC analysis, then, five clusters (or contextual profiles Table 4), were determined using the coordinates of the cells for the first ten factorial axes of the MFA. Using the characteristics of each category by variable (Table 4), five contextual profiles can be identified in the SMA.

In total, we have identified: Two profiles (A and B) characterized by favourable socioeconomic conditions, low psychosocial cohesion, and poor access to public resources; two profiles (D and E) characterized by low socioeconomic conditions, very strong psychosocial cohesion and very good access to public resources, and profile (C) characterized by medium socioeconomic conditions, high psychosocial cohesion and average access to public resources.

Table 4 shows neighbourhood characteristics for the five contextual profiles, determined through multidimensional analysis (MFA and HAC).

Figure 2 shows the spatial distribution of these five contextual profiles from 'A' (least deprived) to 'E' (most deprived). Mapping these profiles shows that neighbourhood planning is spread unevenly across our study area. We have highlighted a centre-periphery gradient with two groups (C and D) characterizing the city centre and the old urban cores. A first periphery of SMA (profile E) concentrated on inner city neighbourhoods, which tend to be more distant from the historic city centre. A second periphery of SMA (profiles A and B) correspond to the urban extensions of the last decade and the urban spread in the SMA.

Table 3 Eigenvalue and variance explained by the ten first components of the MFA

Axe	Eigen-value	% Variance	% Cumul	
1	1.9973	17.39	17.39	**
2	0.9973	8.69	26.08	***
3	0.6796	5.92	32.00	*****************************
4	0.6029	5.25	37.25	*************************
5	0.5052	4.43	41.68	*********************
6	0.4693	4.09	45.77	******************
7	0.4439	3.87	49.64	*****************
8	0.4256	3.74	53.38	*****************
9	0.4184	3.64	57.02	****************
10	0.4065	3.54	60.56	****************

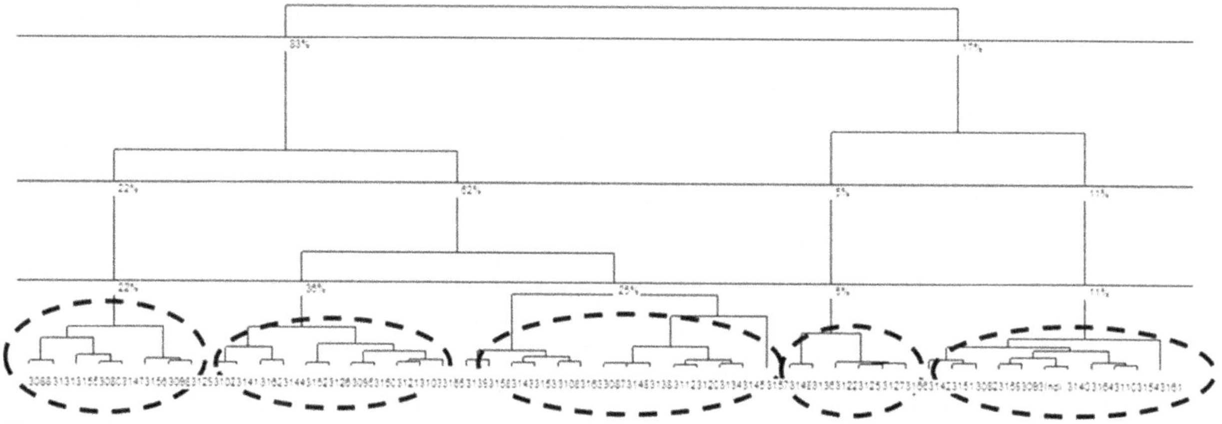

Fig. 1 Dendrogram showing the classification of 5 contextual profiles

Table 5 presents the age-standardized mean annual rates (per 100,000 inhabitants) by gender and by neighbourhood contextual profile. Regardless of contextual profile, MI rates in women are always lower than those in men, at all ages, and MI rates are always much higher among the elderly. Secondly, profile A and B neighbourhoods are characterized by lower rates than the other profiles. Finally, MI rates differ significantly between contextual profiles among women.

Identification of MI risk cluster

Spatial distribution of MI risk is not random, either across all SMA or between the five contextual profiles.

We identified three spatial clusters of high risk of MI (Fig. 3; Table 6) located mainly in the Strasbourg centre and first periphery of Strasbourg. These clusters are presented in order of most-likely cluster to least likely cluster in Fig. 3. Risk in the most-likely cluster (in the northern SMA) is 1.70 times greater than in the rest of the study area (p value = 0.001). The second cluster, also identified within the northern part

of the metropolitan area (RR = 1.28) was not statistically significant, while the third cluster was located in the southern part of the metropolitan area (RR 2.02). After adjustment for gender and age group, we found the same most-likely cluster [relative risk (RR) 1.64; p value = 0.001] with a slightly lower likelihood value (down from 22.56 to 19.73), indicating that age and sex can explain some of the excess risk of MI observed in the unadjusted analysis (Fig. 3).

On the other hand, we identified two spatial clusters of low MI risk (Fig. 3; Table 6) located mainly in the Strasbourg first and second peripheries. These clusters are presented from most-likely cluster to least likely cluster in Fig. 3. The most-likely cluster, in the western SMA, has lower risk that than in the rest of the study area (RR 0.04; p value = 0.001). The second cluster was also in the northern part of the metropolitan area, and was also statistically significant (RR 0.68; p value = 0.001). After adjustment for gender and age group, we found the same most-likely cluster, with a slightly lower likelihood value decreasing from 46.94 to 46.19 (Fig. 3).

Table 4 Description of neighbourhood characteristics of five contextual profiles

	Class A	Class B	Class C	Class D	Class E
Socio economic feature					
Proportion of population covered by CAF	42.2%	44.7%	50.24%	51.40%	62.16%
Proportion of population covered by RMI	1.9%	1.5%	5.19%	4.64%	10.88%
Population density	71.13	180.24	556.10	706.04	470.48
Proportion of precarious jobs	8.62%	9.33%	13.32%	14.46%	16.58%
Proportion of stable jobs	76%	75%	68%	65%	59%
Unemployment rate	5.95%	6.61%	10.04%	11%	19.83%
Proportion of blue-collar workers	18.77%	18%	17%	16%	32%
Proportion of high school graduates	10.38%	10%	6.68%	9.70%	5.29%
Proportion of single-parent families	8.19%	9.11%	13.01%	13.5%	19.79%
Proportion of foreigners	4.03%	4.5%	8.79%	9.45%	17.60%
Proportion of people without cars	9.02%	10.5%	23.38%	30.6%	29.04%
Proportion of people with 2 cars	43.54%	38.41%	20.69%	17.05%	17.64%
Access to resources					
Availability of green space	5.48	2.06	4.75	8.89	6.91
Distance to healthcare facilities (m)	−1385.55	478.25	263.71	214.88	399.00
Public transportation coverage	2.28	7.75	20.88	23.19	15.12
Distance to sports facilities (m)	996.96	522.37	353.44	339.95	349.59
Psychosocial environment					
Quantity of civic associations	Very low	Low	high	Very high	Medium
Local school socio-educational classification	Very high	High	Low	Medium	Very low
Local retail store score	Very low	Low	High	Very high	Medium
Urban fabric (housing types)	Single-family homes	Mixed buildings	Mixed buildings	Center-city homes and Mixed	Multiple-dwelling unit buildings

Very high: very good social support, high: good social support; low: low social support; very low: very low social support

The first two axes of the MFA explained 29.14% of the variance. From the HAC analysis, 5 clusters or contextual profiles were determined from the coordinates of the cells for the first ten factorial axes of the MFA, so as to preserve all the variability of the initial information

CAF fund for family allocations, RMI minimum insertion income

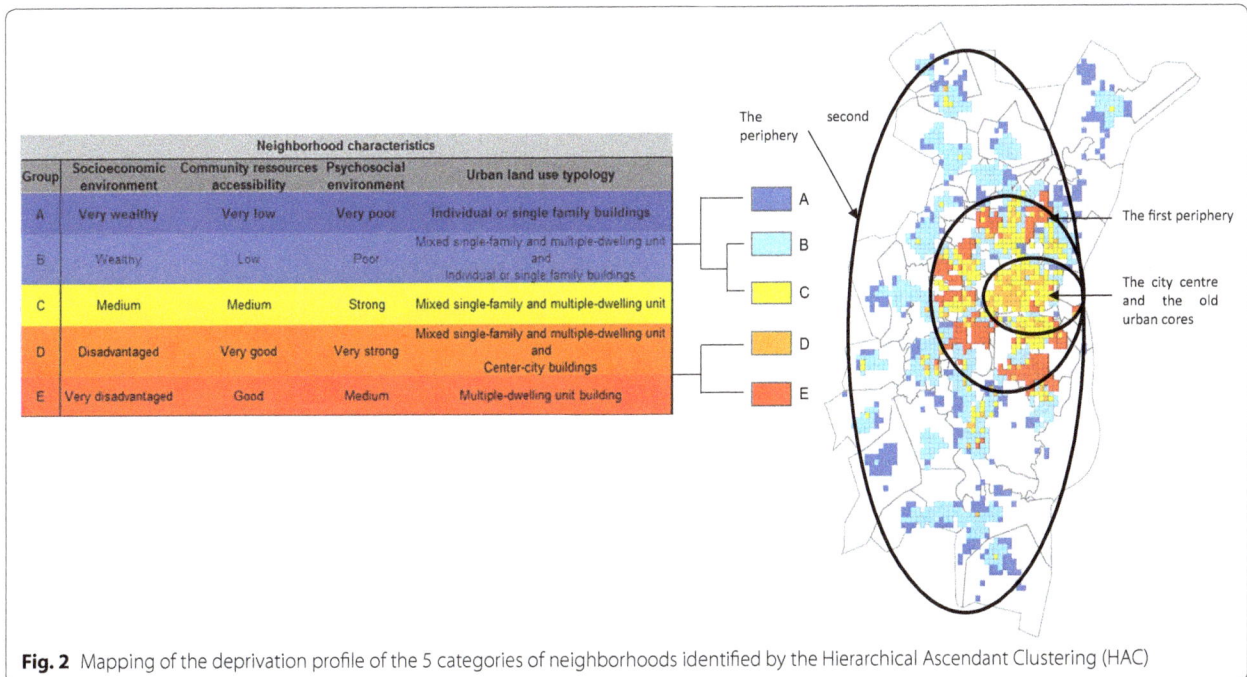

Fig. 2 Mapping of the deprivation profile of the 5 categories of neighborhoods identified by the Hierarchical Ascendant Clustering (HAC)

Table 5 Distribution of myocardial infarction event rates according to contextual profiles

Mean annual event rates, per 100,000 (CI 95%)	A	B	C	D	E	p values*
Neighbourhood contextual profiles (years)						
Females 35–74	382 (240–523)	383 (333–466)	459 (381–537)	548 (402–694)	720 (600–840)	0.0008**
35–54	88 (2–174)	143 (98–201)	204 (137–271)	175 (72–278)	430 (314–546)	0.0121**
55–74	859 (515–1202)	777 (654–961)	855 (685–1025)	1202 (843–1562)	1241 (977–1505)	0.0320**
Males 35–74	1424 (1147–1702)	1612 (1540–1822)	1773 (1610–1936)	1678 (1411–1944)	2171 (1955–2387)	0.0794
35–54	737 (486–989)	834 (743–997)	1230 (1062–1398)	1112 (849–1374)	1283 (1079–1488)	0.2081
55–74	2601 (1983–3219)	2980 (2787–3423)	2785 (2440–331)	2909 (2283–3535)	3880 (3386–4374)	0.2104

* Khi² test

** Significant p value <5%

Spatial implication of neighbourhood characteristics of the clusters

In the clusters for high MI risk, the population profile is mainly 'D & E' which is socioeconomically very disadvantaged, with weak psychosocial cohesion and good access to public resources (see Tables 2, 7). Thus, compared to inhabitants in the rest of the study area, people living in those clusters identified as high MI risk, which had the highest proportion of population covered by welfare benefits (family allowances/child benefits, and the French "safety net" welfare allowance for people with resources below the poverty line), high rates of insecure employment, and the highest proportion of foreigners. These spatial units are characterized by good access to sports

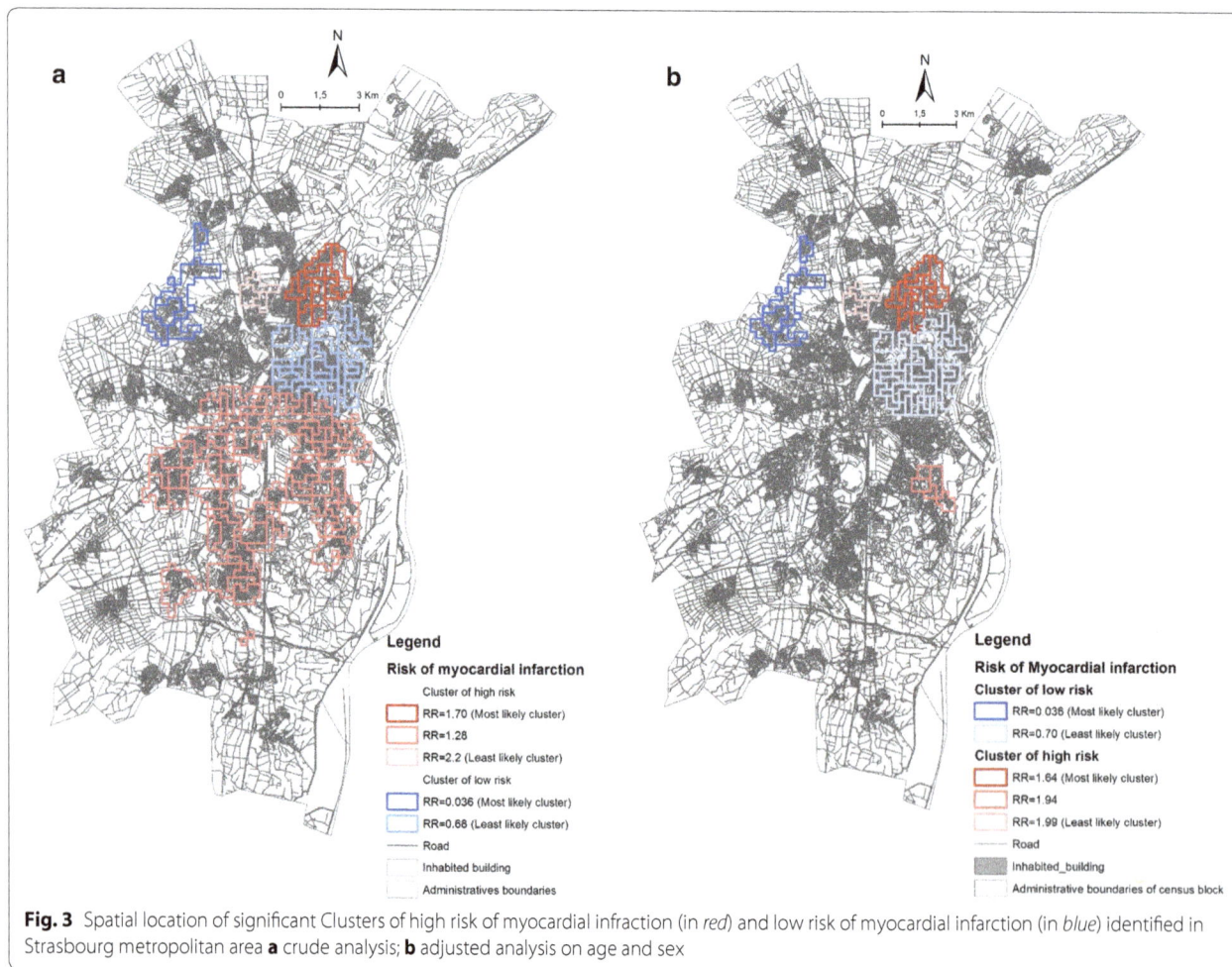

Fig. 3 Spatial location of significant Clusters of high risk of myocardial infraction (in *red*) and low risk of myocardial infarction (in *blue*) identified in Strasbourg metropolitan area **a** crude analysis; **b** adjusted analysis on age and sex

Table 6 The most likely clusters of high and low risk

	Radius (m)	Area included/population	Expected cases	Observed cases	RR[a]	LLr[b]	p value
Most likely cluster of high risk	1207.74	10/11,486	125.68	205	1.70	22.56	0.001
Most likely cluster of low risk	1978.61	5/5018	54.91	2	0.036	46.95	0.001

[a] *rr* Relative risk

[b] *LLr* Log likelihood ratio

Table 7 Comparison between neighbourhood characteristics of inhabitant of cluster of high risk and inhabitant of cluster of high risk

Main characteristics	Most likely cluster		p value*
	Cluster of high risk[a]	Cluster of low risk[b]	
No civic associations	1.2%	99%	<0.0001
No school graded ZEP[c]	22.11	96%	<0.0001
Proportion of population covered by CAF higher that 60%	67%	13.62	<0.0001
Multiple–dwelling unit buildings	58.79	2.90	<0.0001
Single–family homes	24.6	90.43	<0.0001
Distance to healthcare facilities (<500)	76.8	4.93	<0.0001
No public transportation	10	60	<0.0001
Availability of green space	26	14	<0.05

[a] Neighbourhood characteristics of profile "E" and "C" which composed cluster of high risk

[b] Neighbourhood characteristic of profile "A" which composed cluster of low risk

[c] *ZEP* Priority education zones: where establishments receive additional resources, and have greater autonomy for dealing with educational and social difficulties

* Khi test

facilities and high retail store scores. This group is distinguished by the highest availability of green spaces, high public transportation coverage and weak community/civic fabric.

However, in the low MI risk cluster, the population profile is mainly 'A'—which describes the most socioeconomically advantaged areas having low psychosocial cohesion and very poor access to public resources (see Tables 2, 7). This most-likely cluster identified for low MI risk (n = 5018 inhabitants in the significant spatial clusters) had a significantly lower proportion of inhabitant rates of unemployment and of insecure (or temporary) jobs: on the contrary, the employment rate is stable and the proportion of high school graduates is highest. This group is characterized by the longest distances to healthcare facilities, and very poor access to public transport. It has an extremely favourable socioeconomic profile with low psychosocial cohesion and very poor access to public resources.

Discussion

Our study confirms work we previously conducted on the SMA [59], which demonstrated that, whatever the level of deprivation, the rates of events in men were always clearly higher than those in women, at all ages. The literature reported that the relationship between neighbourhood characteristics may vary by gender, as our findings suggest. For instance, several studies have found stronger associations of neighbourhood characteristics with CHD outcomes in women than in men [60–62]. These gender differences could result from gender differences in health-related behavioural responses to neighbourhood perceptions. In addition, we observed a clear increase to the event rate with age, even after stratification by gender and deprivation.

Our study's data-driven approach has allowed us to provide a fine description of the neighbourhood, using a set of contextual data. It highlights several neighbourhood profiles and provides us with evidence on the different combinations of dimensions within the SMA. In comparison with the literature, our profiles reveal differences—especially with regard to how the socioeconomic, social cohesion and access to amenities dimensions are combined.

Several studies show that individuals living in deprived socioeconomic environments have less access to businesses, sports leisure and other infrastructure. For instance, some have revealed that people living in deprived neighbourhoods are less likely to make use of green spaces because they do not perceive the need to do so [63, 64]. We revealed an inverse relation in the SMA: neighbourhoods with a deprived socioeconomic environment are characterized by a substantial presence of sports leisure infrastructure, unlike neighbourhoods with an advantaged socioeconomic environment.

Another aspect highlighted by the literature concerns the relationship between social capital and socioeconomic deprivation. Research projects have demonstrated that socioeconomic deprivation is associated with reduced levels of social capital [65]. Our study, however, shows the opposite result. In the SMA, neighbourhoods with an advantaged socioeconomic environment are characterized by a low level of social cohesion in comparison with neighbourhoods with a deprived socioeconomic environment, which are characterized by a high level of social cohesion.

Regarding the geospatial analysis performed (based on the Kulldorff approach), our study characterized the neighbourhoods of inhabitants living within a cluster of high MI risk, in comparison with those living within a cluster of low MI risk. Although our study allows us to precisely characterize the neighbourhoods included in the cluster with higher MI risk, it was not designed to reveal the MI risk factor among neighbourhood characteristics. Our spatial analysis is more suited to the formulation of certain hypotheses aimed at improving our understanding of the unequal spatial distribution of MI risk using the contextual data panel.

- First, the neighbourhood characteristics of inhabitants living within a cluster of high or low MI risk seem to have more disadvantaged and advantaged conditions respectively, confirming the results of previous studies [66]. Indeed, MI risk was significantly higher among: those whose education ceased after primary or secondary school, compared with those with a higher level of education (university) [66]; the unemployed [67], and men in the lowest socioeconomic group [68].
- Secondly, using only the accessibility and attractiveness of amenities indicator, our study revealed that within high MI risk clusters, inhabitants have excellent access to various amenities (including transport, green space and park and sports facilities)—in contrast to the low MI risk clusters. In the literature, results are contrasted depending on the measure used to describe availability/proximity of the infrastructure. For instance, some studies reported protective associations of green space against high blood pressure [69], coronary heart disease *and* cardiovascular disease mortality [70]. In New Zealand, however, Richardson et al. found no evidence that cardiovascular disease mortality was related to availability of either total or usable green space. In Tamosiunas et al. [71] found that the prevalence of cardiovascular

risk factors was not related to the distance from people's homes to green spaces—but was significantly lower among park users than among non-park-users.

- Lastly, the characterization of neighbourhoods of inhabitants living within a cluster of high MI risk show that they have high psychosocial cohesion in comparison with inhabitants within a cluster of low MI risk. This finding is incoherent with other studies which found that lower neighbourhood cohesion predicted higher coronary artery calcification prevalence [72].

What this research adds in public health?

Beyond the geospatial approach applied on the local territory in France, this study answers to a major problem identified today by WHO to which classical epidemiological approaches do not respond. The European Union, supported by the World Health Organization (WHO), recognizes that it is time to move from the research about risk factors of health disparities to actions which aim to reduce them. Research conducted in public health policy issues supply little evidence for effective interventions aiming to improve population health and to reduce health inequalities.

This paper is attempts to fill the gap regarding a need for powerful tool to support priority setting and guide policy makers in their choice of health interventions, and that maximizes social welfare.

Today, more and more international and European institutions suggest certain actions on place that could improve health and thus tend to reduce health inequalities, such as improving access to, and quality of, green space, particularly in deprived areas—providing places for play, physical activity and favouring social interaction. For instance, the World Health Organization has also announced that access to green spaces can reduce health inequalities, improve well-being [73]. More recently, NHS Health Scotland stated, in the "Place and Communities Report" that policy and practice should continue to integrate health, housing, environment, transport, and community and spatial planning to improve health outcomes and promote sustainability [74].

In the majority of epidemiological research projects investigating health inequalities, sophisticated analyses are implemented to measure the strength of the association between risk factors and outcomes. These research findings may be pivotal to public health policy, but an attempt to distinguish between correlational and causal associations does not form the basis of effective interventions aimed at improving population health and reducing health inequalities. These classic epidemiological approaches offer limited guidance to policymakers in their choice of intervention, and suggest the need for spatial approaches to the investigation of social health inequalities.

Our study describes an approach that may guide policymakers in selecting which priority setting to use, and in choosing and developing the most appropriate local intervention if, for instance, they decide to apply the 'proportionate universalism' strategy described by Marmot in 2010. Policymakers are thus enabled to plan targeted interventions, choosing one of two appropriate broad approaches to action that are commonly accepted today as reducing health inequalities [36].

The present paper permits to novel way to investigate the social health inequalities:

1. Our work highlights that the investigation of the spatial distribution of multiple risk factors, including social, economic and contextual factors, can help policy makers to choose appropriately between two or more broad approaches which will be performed for the whole population, but with a scale and intensity proportionate to need.

2. The local diagnosis can assist policy makers to focus the scope of prevention/intervention programs and changes to the health care system, thus providing more effective interventions in order to response to individual needs, and public resources can be distributed more efficiently. Thereby, this spatial tool may assist the policy maker to tackle the social gradient in health if they choose to apply the strategy named 'proportionate universalism' and described by Marmot in 2010 [75].

3. In addition, our study show that the use of a routinely-collected data set within a data-driven approach to characterize neighbourhood, alongside a geospatial tool combined with GIS will be particularly relevant and of interest to policymakers involved in the identification, definition and promotion of targeted health inequality actions at varying spatial levels.

4. This study illustrates the usefulness of the geospatial approach using routinely-collected data to support policy makers in planning more focused community interventions in appropriate areas and to choose if public health interventions should be declined either at a national level, at a local level, or both.

Strengths

The areal unit we constructed at a very small scale allowed us to consistently accommodate data produced at different scales. Our use of a single grid allowed us to minimize the effect of scale associated with the modifiable areal unit problem (MAUP), [76] because all the basic spatial units (cells) were constructed to have the same

area. These new spatial units offer three benefits: (1) they make it possible to homogenize the best of the data collected, prior to any statistical or spatial analysis; (2) they allow us to spread the value of a piece of geographic information initially noted or represented according to a specific unit, in values calculated according to regular spatial units, while preserving the integrity of the initial information; and finally (3) the point of using these cells as statistical units is to allow an extremely detailed analysis while preserving total health data anonymity in the subsequent analysis.

Weaknesses

Our approach did have certain limitations in terms of the contextual data used. Data availability necessarily constrains the variables integrated to this analysis, so that the number of contextual dimensions used to characterize neighbourhood context is also constrained.

We acknowledge that some data could not be included in our analysis. This is the case, for example, for violence in neighbourhoods, the presence of exterior annoyances and substandard housing. Traffic noise data, for instance, is considered politically sensitive when displayed at a fine scale, and we were unable to obtain access to this. The collection of data regarding quality of housing and exterior annoyances is available only for the City of Strasbourg, and is not available across the SMA scale. In addition the health data was collected between 2000 and 2008, while the contextual data was mainly available between 2007 and 2008, with the exception of the socioeconomic data, obtained from the 1999 census. The collection of data according to availability may result in a temporal gap between contextual data and its outcome data, which could influence the result observed. In our study, we are however unable to measure this misclassification.

Conclusion

We proposed a data-driven approach developed at fine spatial scale level, aimed at the investigation of neighbourhood characteristics capable of explaining geographical distribution of the onset of MI risk. In our study, we characterized the neighbourhood free of any a priori hypothesis, and without weighting certain contextual neighbourhood components, privileging the use of diverse contextual neighbourhood profiles and the ad hoc synthetic neighbourhood areal unit. Our spatial approach allowed us to identify the neighbourhood characteristics of inhabitants living within a high MI risk cluster in comparison with those living within a low MI risk cluster.

Therefore, spatial data-driven analyses of routinely-collected data georeferenced by various sources may serve to guide policymakers in defining and promoting targeted actions at fine spatial level. Armed with local characterization of the combination between the socio-economic dimension, social cohesion and access to amenities relating to social inequalities in health, policy-makers may be able to promote more accurately-targeted actions aimed at reducing health inequalities, and promote a better understanding of social, healthy behaviour among deprived populations. An open question worthy of further research would be to determine the minimal set of data (according to the principle of parsimony and for the sake of efficiency) needed to appropriately characterize neighbourhood influences, given that what holds true in a given area may differ across geographical settings having different historical and sociological contexts.

Authors' contributions

WKT collected all contextual and health data, geocoded the cases to the IRIS level, undertook the statistical and spatial analysis, produced the map, carried out the literature review and drafted the paper. CW, head of the unit TETIS UMR 9000 monitored the general work, helped with the analysis and interpretation of the results and contributed to draft and finalize the paper. GP implemented the data-driven approach to neighbourhood characterization and helped to finalize the paper. CS helped with the interpretation of the results and contributed finalize the paper. DA head of the Bas-Rhin coronary heart disease register, were responsible of the collected health data, contribute to design of the work and draft and finalize the paper. CES contributed to Synthetic neighbourhood design, the interpretation of the results and helped to draft and finalize the paper. SD contributed to spatial analysis and helped with the interpretation of the results and finalize the paper. DB principal investigator of the PAISARC + Project, was responsible for quality assurance and rigor in the data analysis, contributed to interpret the results and reviewed the drafts of the article and contributed to finalize it. All authors read and approved the final manuscript.

Author details

[1] LIVE UMR 7362 CNRS (Laboratoire Image Ville Environnement), University of Strasbourg, Strasbourg 6700, Strasbourg, France. [2] UMR Tetis (Territoires, environnement, télédétection et information spatiale), Montpelier, France. [3] The French National Public Health agency, Saint-Maurice, France. [4] SEPIA-Santé, Baud, France. [5] Department of Epidemiology and Public Health, EA 3430, FMTS, Strasbourg University, Strasbourg, France. [6] School of Geographical Sciences, University of Bristol, Bristol BS8 1SS, UK. [7] Department of Environmental and Occupational Health, School of Public Health (EHESP), Sorbonne Paris Cité, Rennes, France. [8] Department of Social Epidemiology, Sorbonne Universités, UPMC Univ Paris 06, INSERM, Institut Pierre Louis d'Epidémiologie et de Santé Publique (UMRS 1136), Paris, France. [9] Department of Quantitative Methods in Public Health, School of Public Health (EHESP), Sorbonne Paris Cité, Rennes, Paris, France.

Acknowledgements

The authors gratefully acknowledge the use of the AZTool software, which is copyright David Martin, Samantha Cockings and University of Southampton.

Competing interests

The authors declare that they have no competing interests.

Funding

This work was supported by French Agency for Food, Environmental and Occupational Health & Safety (ANSES); Institute for Public Health Research (IRESP); French Environment and Energy Management Agency (ADEME); and SITA Corporation. The funders had no role in study design, data collection and analysis, decision to publish, or preparation of the manuscript.

Appendix

See Fig. 4

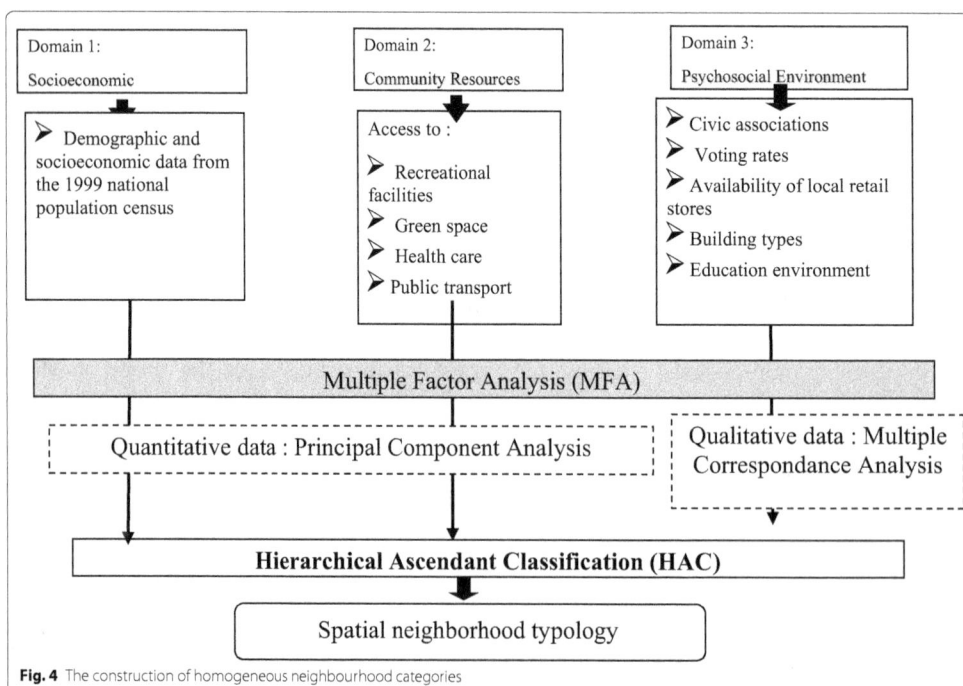

Fig. 4 The construction of homogeneous neighbourhood categories

References

1. Judge K, Platt S, Costongs C, Jurczak K. Health inequalities: a challenge for Europe. Discussion Paper. London: UK Presidency of the EU. 2006. http://ec.europa.eu/health/ph_determinants/socio_economics/documents/ev_060302_rd05_en.pdf.
2. Sheiham A. Closing the gap in a generation: health equity through action on the social determinants of health. A report of the WHO Commission on Social Determinants of Health (CSDH) 2008. Community Dent Health. 2009;26:2–3.
3. Marmot M, Allen J, Bell R, Bloomer E, Goldblatt P. Consortium for the European review of social determinants of health and the health divide. WHO European review of social determinants of health and the health divide. Lancet. 2012;380:1011–29.
4. Macintyre S, Ellaway A, Cummins S. Place effects on health: How can we conceptualise, operationalise and measure them? Soc Sci Med. 2002;55:125–39.
5. Diez Roux AV. Neighborhoods and health: Where are we and were do we go from here? Rev Epidemiol Sante Publique. 2007;55:13–21.
6. Diez Roux AV. Residential environments and cardiovascular risk. J Urban Health. 2003;80:569–89.
7. Kawachi IB. Neighborhoods and health. New York: Oxford University Press; 2003.
8. Pickett KE, Pearl M. Multilevel analyses of neighbourhood socioeconomic context and health outcomes: a critical review. J Epidemiol Community Health. 2001;55:111–22.
9. Arcaya MC, Tucker-Seeley RD, Kim R, Schnake-Mahl A, So M, Subramanian SV. Research on neighborhood effects on health in the United States: a systematic review of study characteristics. Soc Sci Med. 2016;168:16–29.
10. Vos AA, Posthumus AG, Bonsel GJ, Steegers EAP, Denktaş S. Deprived neighborhoods and adverse perinatal outcome: a systematic review and meta-analysis. Acta Obstet Gynecol Scand. 2014;93:727–40.
11. Truong KD, Ma S. A systematic review of relations between neighborhoods and mental health. J Ment Health Policy Econ. 2006;9:137–54.
12. Corral I, Landrine H, Hall MB, Bess JJ, Mills KR, Efird JT. Residential segregation and overweight/obesity among African–American adults: a critical review. Front Public Health. 2015;3:169.
13. Owen N, Humpel N, Leslie E, Bauman A, Sallis JF. Understanding environmental influences on walking: review and research agenda. Am J Prev Med. 2004;27:67–76.
14. Rose D, Richards R. Food store access and household fruit and vegetable use among participants in the US food stamp program. Public Health Nutr. 2004;7:1081–8.
15. Matthews SA, Yang T-C. Exploring the role of the built and social neighborhood environment in moderating stress and health. Ann Behav Med. 2010;39:170–83.
16. Pearce J, Witten K, Hiscock R, Blakely T. Are socially disadvantaged neighbourhoods deprived of health-related community resources? Int J Epidemiol. 2007;36:348–55.
17. Komeily A, Srinivasan RS. What is neighborhood context and why does it matter in sustainability assessment? Proc Eng. 2016;145:876–83.
18. Niemann H, Bonnefoy X, Braubach M, Hecht K, Maschke C, Rodrigues C, et al. Noise-induced annoyance and morbidity results from the pan-European LARES study. Noise Health. 2006;8:63–79.
19. Van kempen E, van Kamp I, Fischer P, Davies H, Houthuijs D, Stellato R, et al. Noise exposure and children's blood pressure and heart rate: the RANCH project. Occup Environ Med. 2006;63:632–9.
20. Willich SN, Wegscheider K, Stallmann M, Keil T. Noise burden and the risk of myocardial infarction. Eur Heart J. 2006;27:276–82.
21. Aneshensel CS, Sucoff CA. The neighborhood context of adolescent mental health. J Health Soc Behav. 1996;37:293–310.
22. Pearce J, Hiscock R, Blakely T, Witten K. The contextual effects of neighbourhood access to supermarkets and convenience stores on individual fruit and vegetable consumption. J Epidemiol Community Health. 2008;62:198–201.
23. Giles-Corti B, Broomhall MH, Knuiman M, Collins C, Douglas K, Ng K, et al. Increasing walking: How important is distance to, attractiveness, and size of public open space? Am J Prev Med. 2005;28:169–76.
24. Witten K, Hiscock R, Pearce J, Blakely T. Neighbourhood access to open spaces and the physical activity of residents: a national study. Prev Med. 2008;47:299–303.
25. Maas J, Verheij RA, Groenewegen PP, de Vries S, Spreeuwenberg P. Green space, urbanity, and health: How strong is the relation? J Epidemiol Community Health. 2006;60:587–92.
26. van den Berg AE, Maas J, Verheij RA, Groenewegen PP. Green space as a buffer between stressful life events and health. Social Sci Med. 2010;70:1203–10.
27. Augustin T, Glass TA, James BD, Schwartz BS. Neighborhood psychosocial hazards and cardiovascular disease: the Baltimore Memory Study. Am J Public Health. 2008;98:1664–70.
28. Sundquist K, Theobald H, Yang M, Li X, Johansson SE, Sundquist J. Neighborhood violent crime and unemployment increase the risk of coronary heart disease: a multilevel study in an urban setting. Soc Sci Med. 2006;62:2061–71.
29. Sundquist J, Johansson SE, Yang M, Sundquist K. Low linking social capital as a predictor of coronary heart disease in Sweden: a cohort study of 2.8 million people. Soc Sci Med. 2006;62:954–63.
30. Van Hulst A, Thomas F, Barnett TA, Kestens Y, Gauvin L, Pannier B, et al. A typology of neighborhoods and blood pressure in the RECORD Cohort Study. J Hypertens. 2012;30:1336–46.
31. Gascon M, Triguero-Mas M, Martínez D, Dadvand P, Rojas-Rueda D, Plasència A, et al. Residential green spaces and mortality: a systematic review. Environ Int. 2016;86:60–7.
32. Lovasi GS, Quinn JW, Neckerman KM, Perzanowski MS, Rundle A. Children living in areas with more street trees have lower prevalence of asthma. J Epidemiol Community Health. 2008;62:647–9.
33. Wolch JR, Byrne J, Newell JP. Urban green space, public health, and environmental justice: the challenge of making cities "just green enough". Landsc Urban Plan. 2014;125:234–44.
34. Frieden TR. A framework for public health action: the health impact pyramid. Am J Public Health. 2010;100:590–5.
35. Arcaya MC, Arcaya AL, Subramanian SV. Inequalities in health: definitions, concepts, and theories. Glob Health Action [Internet]; 2015 [cited 2017 Mar 29]; 8. http://www.ncbi.nlm.nih.gov/pmc/articles/PMC4481045/.
36. Marmot M, Friel S, Bell R, Houweling TA, Taylor S. Closing the gap in a generation: health equity through action on the social determinants of health. Lancet. 2008;372:1661–9.
37. Kihal W, Padilla C, Deguen S. Spatial planning of green space as a local intervention aimed at tackling social health inequalities: adverse pregnancy issues. Geoinform Geostat Overv. 1011;2016:2.
38. Kihal W, Padilla C, Deguen S. The need for, and value of, a spatial scan statistical tool for tackling social health inequalities. Glob Health Promot. 2016. doi:10.1177/1757975916656358.
39. Ollila E, Ståhl T, Wismar M, Lahtinen E, Melkas T, Leppo K. Health in all policies in the European union and its member states. 2006. http://ec.europa.eu/health/ph_projects/2005/action1/docs/2005_1_18_frep_a4_en.pdf.
40. WHO. Health in all policies |Publications| UNRISD [Internet]. 2013. http://www.unrisd.org/80256B3C005BCCF9/search/5416E4680AD46606C1257B730038FAC1?OpenDocument.
41. Eibner C, Sturm R. US-based indices of area-level deprivation: results from healthcare for communities. Soc Sci Med. 2006;62:348–59.
42. Departement of Environment T. Indices of deprivation. Departement of Environment, Transport, and the Region, London. 2000 http://www.odpm.gov.uk/stellent/groups/odpm_urbanpolicy/documents/downloadable/odpm_urbpol_021680.pdf.
43. Clark PJ, Evans FC. Distance to nearest neighbor as a measure of spatial relationships in populations. Ecology. 1954;35:445–53.
44. Escofier B, Pagès J. Multiple factor analysis (AFMULT package). Comput Stat Data Anal. 1994;1:121–40.
45. Hastie T, Tibshirani R, Friedman J. The elements of statistical learning. Berlin: Springer; 2001.
46. Sabel CE, Kihal W, Bard D, Weber C. Creation of synthetic homogeneous neighbourhoods using zone design algorithms to explore relationships between asthma and deprivation in Strasbourg, France. Soc Sci Med. 2013;91:110–21.
47. Martin D. Automatic neighbourhood identification from population surfaces. Comput Environ Urban Syst. 1998;22:107–20.
48. Martin D. Optimizing census geography: the separation of collection and output geographies. Int J Geogr Inf Sci. 1998;12:673–85.
49. Tunstall-Pedoe H, Kuulasmaa K, Mahonen M, Tolonen H, Ruokokoski E, Amouyel P. Contribution of trends in survival and coronary-event rates to changes in coronary heart disease mortality: 10-year results from 37 WHO

MONICA project populations. Monitoring trends and determinants in cardiovascular disease. Lancet. 1999;353:1547–57.

50. Kulldorff M. Information management services, Inc. SaTScan: software for the spatial, temporal, and space-time scan statistics, version 6.0. 2005. 2009. http://www.satscan.org/.

51. Kihal-Talantikite W, Deguen S, Padilla C, Siebert M, Couchoud C, Vigneau C, et al. Spatial distribution of end-stage renal disease (ESRD) and social inequalities in mixed urban and rural areas: a study in the Bretagne administrative region of France. Clin Kidney J. 2015;8:7–13.

52. Kihal-Talantikite W, Padilla CM, Lalloué B, Gelormini M, Zmirou-Navier D, Deguen S. Green space, social inequalities and neonatal mortality in France. BMC Pregnancy Childbirth. 2013;13:191.

53. Kihal-Talantikite W, Padilla CM, Lalloue B, Rougier C, Defrance J, Zmirou-Navier D, et al. An exploratory spatial analysis to assess the relationship between deprivation, noise and infant mortality: an ecological study. Environ Health. 2013;12:109.

54. Kulldorff M, Feuer EJ, Miller BA, Freedman LS. Breast cancer clusters in the northeast United States: a geographic analysis. Am J Epidemiol. 1997;146:161–70.

55. Sabel CE, Wilson JG, Kingham S, Tisch C, Epton M. Spatial implications of covariate adjustment on patterns of risk: respiratory hospital admissions in Christchurch, New Zealand. Social Sci Med. 2007;65:43–59.

56. Kulldorff M, Nagarwalla N. Spatial disease clusters: detection and inference. Stat Med. 1995;14:799–810.

57. Kulldorff M. Spatial scan statistics: models, calculations, and application. In: Glaz J, Balakrishnan N, editors. Scan statistics and applications. Boston: Birkhäuser; 1999. p. 303–22.

58. Dwass M. Modified randomization tests for nonparametric hypotheses. Ann Math Stat. 1957;28:181–7.

59. Havard S, Deguen S, Bodin J, Louis K, Laurent O, Bard D. A small-area index of socioeconomic deprivation to capture health inequalities in France. Soc Sci Med. 2008;67:2007–16.

60. Diez Roux AV, Merkin SS, Arnett D, Chambless L, Massing M, Nieto FJ, et al. Neighborhood of residence and incidence of coronary heart disease. N Engl J Med. 2001;345:99–106.

61. Winkleby M, Sundquist K, Cubbin C. Inequities in CHD incidence and case fatality by neighborhood deprivation. Am J Prev Med. 2007;32:97–106.

62. Sundquist K, Malmström M, Johansson S-E. Neighbourhood deprivation and incidence of coronary heart disease: a multilevel study of 2.6 million women and men in Sweden. J Epidemiol Community Health. 2004;58:71–7.

63. Takano T, Nakamura K, Watanabe M. Urban residential environments and senior citizens' longevity in megacity areas: the importance of walkable green spaces. J Epidemiol Community Health. 2002;56:913–8.

64. Jones A, Hillsdon M, Coombes E. Greenspace access, use, and physical activity: understanding the effects of area deprivation. Prev Med. 2009;49:500–5.

65. van der Linden J, Drukker M, Gunther N, Feron F, van Os J. Children's mental health service use, neighbourhood socioeconomic deprivation, and social capital. Soc Psychiatry Psychiatr Epidemiol. 2003;38:507–14.

66. González-Zobl G, Grau M, Muñoz MA, Martí R, Sanz H, Sala J, et al. Socioeconomic status and risk of acute myocardial infarction. Population-based case-control study. Rev Esp Cardiol. 2010;63:1045–53.

67. Dupre ME, George LK, Liu G, Peterson ED. The cumulative effect of unemployment on risks for acute myocardial infarction. Arch Intern Med. 2012;172:1731–7.

68. Machón M, Aldasoro E, Martínez-Camblor P, Calvo M, Basterretxea M, Audicana C, et al. Socioeconomic differences in incidence and relative survival after a first acute myocardial infarction in the Basque Country, Spain. Gac Sanit. 2012;26:16–23.

69. Hartig T, Evans GW, Jamner LD, Davis DS, Gärling T. Tracking restoration in natural and urban field settings. J Environ Psychol. 2003;23:109–23.

70. Mitchell R, Popham F. Effect of exposure to natural environment on health inequalities: an observational population study. Lancet. 2008;372:1655–60.

71. Tamosiunas A, Grazuleviciene R, Luksiene D, Dedele A, Reklaitiene R, Baceviciene M, et al. Accessibility and use of urban green spaces, and cardiovascular health: findings from a Kaunas cohort study. Environ Health. 2014;13:20.

72. Kim D, Diez Roux AV, Kiefe CI, Kawachi I, Liu K. Do neighborhood socioeconomic deprivation and low social cohesion predict coronary calcification? Am J Epidemiol. 2010;172:288–98.

73. WHO. Urban green spaces. http://www.who.int/sustainable-development/cities/health-risks/urban-green-space/en/.

74. NHS Health Scotland. Place and communities report. 2016. http://www.healthscotland.scot/media/1088/27414-place-and-communties-06-16.pdf.

75. Marmot M. Fair society, healthy lives: strategic review of health inequalities in England post-2010. London: Marmot Review. https://www.google.fr/search?q=Marmot+M+(2010).+Fair+Society,+Healthy+Lives:+Strategic+review+of+health+inequalities+in+England+post-2010.+London:+Marmot+Review.&ie=utf-8&oe=utf-8&gws_rd=cr&ei=EGvxVefKBsO3a5bmo8AE.

76. Openshaw S. A geographical solution to scale and aggregation problems in region-building, partitioning and spatial modelling. Inst Br Geogr Trans New Ser. 1977;2(4):459–72.

4

Does exposure to the food environment differ by socioeconomic position? Comparing area-based and person-centred metrics in the Fenland Study, UK

Eva R. Maguire[1], Thomas Burgoine[1], Tarra L. Penney[1], Nita G. Forouhi[2] and Pablo Monsivais[1,3*] ⓘ

Abstract

Background: Retail food environments (foodscapes) are a recognised determinant of eating behaviours and may contribute to inequalities in diet. However, findings from studies measuring socioeconomic inequality in the foodscape have been mixed, which may be due to methodological differences. The aim of this cross-sectional study was to compare exposure to the foodscape by socioeconomic position using different measures, to test whether the presence, direction or amplitude of differences was sensitive to the choice of foodscape metric or socioeconomic indicator.

Methods: A sample of 10,429 adults aged 30–64 years with valid home address data were obtained from the Fenland Study, UK. Of this sample, 7270 participants also had valid work location data. The sample was linked to data on food outlets obtained from local government records. Foodscape metrics included count, density and proximity of takeaway outlets and supermarkets, and the percentage of takeaway outlets relative to all food outlets. Exposure metrics were area-based (lower super output areas), and person-centred (proximity to nearest; Euclidean and Network buffers at 800 m, 1 km, and 1 mile). Person-centred buffers were constructed using home and work locations. Socioeconomic status was measured at the area-level (2010 Index of Multiple Deprivation) and the individual-level (highest educational attainment; equivalised household income). Participants were classified into socioeconomic groups and average exposures estimated. Results were analysed using the statistical and percent differences between the highest and lowest socioeconomic groups.

Results: In area-based measures, the most deprived areas contained higher takeaway outlet densities ($p < 0.001$). However, in person-centred metrics lower socioeconomic status was associated with lower exposure to takeaway outlets and supermarkets (all home-based exposures $p < 0.001$) and socioeconomic differences were greatest at the smallest buffer sizes. Socioeconomic differences in exposure was similar for home and combined home and work measures. Measuring takeaway exposure as a percentage of all outlets reversed the socioeconomic differences; the lowest socioeconomic groups had a higher percentage of takeaway outlets compared to the middle and highest groups ($p < 0.001$).

Conclusions: We compared approaches to measuring socioeconomic variation in the foodscape and found that the association was sensitive to the metric used. In particular, the direction of association varied between area- and person-centred measures and between absolute and relative outlet measures. Studies need to consider the most

*Correspondence: p.monsivais@wsu.edu
[1] UKCRC Centre for Diet and Activity Research (CEDAR), MRC
Epidemiology Unit, University of Cambridge School of Clinical Medicine,
Institute of Metabolic Science, Cambridge Biomedical Campus,
Cambridge CB2 0QQ, UK
Full list of author information is available at the end of the article

appropriate measure for the research question, and may need to consider multiple measures as a single measure may be context dependent.

Keywords: Diet inequalities, Food environment, Fast food, Supermarkets, Socioeconomic status, Area deprivation, Geographic information systems, Density, Proximity, Food access

Background

Socioeconomic disparities in diet quality have been identified [1–3] and likely contribute to inequalities in health outcomes including obesity, type 2 diabetes and cardiovascular disease [4–7]. Pervasive inequalities in diet have led researchers to seek modifiable determinants as potential targets of public health policies and interventions. The built environment, including the local retail food environment, or 'foodscape', may influence dietary behaviours and as a consequence contribute to rising levels of obesity, through shaping the context in which people make their food decisions [8–11]. The foodscape may be important for explaining socioeconomic disparities in diet, with some evidence of foodscapes varying by socioeconomic status (SES) [11, 12].

Much of the evidence on disparities in food retail access has centred on supermarkets and takeaway food ('fast-food') outlets. Specifically, supermarkets are seen to offer a range of affordable fresh produce for preparation at home [13, 14]. The ready-prepared hot foods typically served in takeaway outlets have been positively associated with energy and fat intakes [15], with frequent consumption associated with weight gain over time [16, 17]. In the United States (US) systematic reviews have identified consistent evidence of limited supermarket access and high takeaway food outlet access in low-income and racially-segregated neighbourhoods [18–20]. However, outside of the US, the picture has been more mixed. In the United Kingdom (UK), Canada and Australia, a limited number of studies have found more takeaway outlets in deprived areas [21–25], with one exception from Glasgow, Scotland [26]. No UK studies have identified socioeconomic disparities in the geographic accessibility of supermarkets [23, 27, 28]. In New Zealand, findings have shown that all food outlets are more prevalent in deprived areas [29]. These studies tend to use area-based measures of SES, limiting further association of these exposures to individual-level dietary behaviours and health outcomes. Socioeconomic differences in foodscape exposure based on individual level measures are therefore important to understand.

Furthermore, a number of studies have recognised the importance of considering a wider range of food outlets when assessing potential neighbourhood impacts on diet [30–34]. It may be that outlets offering both 'healthy' and 'unhealthy' options are commonly co-located, given

food outlets tend to cluster in commercial areas [30]. Few previous studies have examined the socioeconomic differences in foodscape exposure using a relative measure of the retail food landscape [35, 36]. A recent Canadian study reported how more deprived neighbourhoods in Waterloo were more likely to have a less healthy food retail mix [36], however these findings were in contrast to previous Canadian research [35], may not reflect the wider international context, and were not based on person-centred estimates of either food access or indicators of SES.

The majority of foodscape studies use Geographic Information Systems (GIS), which is now a common tool in public health research [8]. However, a number of review articles have noted that methodological differences limit comparisons between food environment studies [8, 9, 12]. As a result, such reviews have called for greater consistency across methods used, as well as consideration of specific aspects of the methods, when assessing associations between measures of the foodscape and both SES and other outcomes including diet and obesity.

The purpose of this study was to compare socioeconomic differences in foodscape exposure using a number of commonly-used GIS-based metrics to better understand the implications of selecting different metrics. Using a cohort sample of UK adults, we compared area-based ('ecological') and person-centred ('egocentric') methods. Moreover, as much of the person-centred methods published in the literature is based on exposures around the residence only, we analysed person-centred metrics derived from both residential exposures and combined home- and work-based exposures. We also examined both absolute measures of takeaway outlet and supermarket exposure and relative measures of takeaway outlet exposure across three socioeconomic indicators.

Methods
Study sample

The Fenland Study is a population-based, observational cross-sectional cohort study, which aims to understand the genetic, behavioural and environmental factors relating to obesity and diabetes in adults. Eligible participants were men and women born between the years 1950 and 1975, aged 30–62 years at recruitment, who were registered at participating general practices across Fenland

and East Cambridgeshire. Exclusion criteria were diagnosed diabetes, psychotic or terminal illness, pregnancy and being unable to walk unaided. Recruitment ran from 2005 to 2014 [37].

At the time of requesting data for this study, data were available for 11,857 Fenland Study participants. Participant home and work postcodes were geocoded using GeoConvert [38], and mapped using a GIS software package (ArcMAP 10, ESRI). UK postcodes contain 15 addresses on average, and therefore represent addresses with relative precision [39]. Participants whose home postcodes were missing (n = 1276), incomplete or invalid (n = 121), or outside the study area (n = 31) were removed, leaving an analytic sample of 10,429 with complete home address data. For work-based exposure assessments, we further excluded those not in work (n = 963) or where work status data was missing (n = 94), as well as those missing work postcodes, who provided incomplete work postcodes, or whose work address was outside the study area (n = 2102), resulting in a sub-sample of 7270.

Food outlet data

Food outlet data collection and classification for use alongside Fenland Study data has been previously reported [40]. Briefly, food outlet data were collected in November and December 2011 from ten local councils covering the study area. All food outlet owners in the UK are required to register their premises with local Environmental Health departments, and to notify the department if they are closing. Local councils therefore hold records of food outlets that are regularly updated [41]. These are considered the most accurate source of food outlet data in the UK [42]. For this study we focussed on the locations of takeaways, supermarkets, convenience stores, restaurants, and cafés, which together account for the majority of household food shopping and out-of-home eating [40].

Foodscape exposure metrics

Two broad and commonly employed approaches to assessing the foodscape were compared [43–45]: area-based metrics and person-centred (individual-level) metrics. Area-based metrics define neighbourhoods using administrative boundaries, which in this study were lower super output areas (LSOAs) designed to contain an average of 1500 residents and 650 households [46]. There were 801 LSOAs within the Fenland Study area. When using area-based metrics, outlet counts are generally standardised by resident population to give a density measure of exposure. In this study, takeaway and supermarket outlet counts were standardised against mid-2011 LSOA population estimates [47].

Person-centred metrics capture a neighbourhood specific to the individual, typically centred on a study participants' home location. In addition to home, we considered the workplace an important daily anchor point and therefore also assessed the inclusion of workplace exposure to capture wider exposure to the foodscape [48]. We counted numbers of food outlets within Euclidean (straight-line) buffers and street network buffers, which measure distance along the road network and thus account for land use, for the reported home and work postcodes of Fenland Study participants. Buffers were constructed at three distances: 800, 1000, and 1609 m (1 mile), based on common precedent for their use in the published literature, wherein they have been theorised as 'walkable' for an average adult in 10–15 min [49–52]. In addition, person-centred exposure was also measured as proximity to the nearest takeaway outlet and supermarket, calculated as the shortest street network distance using ArcGIS Network Analyst.

Socioeconomic indicators

Area-level SES was defined using the 2010 Index of Multiple Deprivation (IMD) [53]. IMD is a composite measure of deprivation calculated from indicators in seven domains: income; employment; health and disability; education skills and training; barriers to housing and other services; crime; living environment. IMD assigns relative scores to LSOAs, with higher scores reflecting greater deprivation. Fenland Study LSOAs ranged in score from 1.01 (least deprived) to 61.39 (most deprived), spanning the first and ninety-eighth centiles of all scores across England. LSOAs were divided into tertiles of deprivation based on their IMD score.

Two common indicators of individual-level SES were used: highest educational attainment and equivalised income. These data were provided by Fenland Study participants in a self-completed general questionnaire. Participants' highest educational attainment was collapsed into three categories ('Low', includes compulsory school education and equivalent qualifications, typically completed at 16 years of age; 'Medium', includes academic or vocational qualifications gained during further education, such as those that allow university entry; 'High', degree-level or equivalent qualifications). To adjust for household size, annual household income was equivalised using the OECD's modified equivalence scale [54]. Equivalised income was calculated for each participant from the midpoint of the available household income categories and collapsed into three bands (<£23,000; £23,000–£42,999; ≥£43,000).

As this was a complete case analysis, missing socioeconomic data reduced sample sizes in person-centred models that included educational attainment and equivalised income to 10,276 and 9617 respectively for home-based assessments, and to 7169 and 6774 respectively for combined home and work assessments.

Data analysis

Average counts of, and distances to the nearest of each supermarket and takeaway were calculated across socioeconomic groups (highest educational attainment and household income groups for person-centred exposure metrics; tertiles of IMD scores for area-based metrics). Average proximity to the nearest supermarket and takeaway outlet from home was calculated for each socioeconomic group. Relative differences in exposures between the highest and lowest socioeconomic groups were also calculated. Takeaway density as a percentage of the sum of all food outlet types (takeaways, supermarkets, convenience stores, restaurants, cafés) was calculated. This calculation resulted in missing values where there were both no takeaway outlets and no other outlets, that is, both the numerator and denominator were zero. This was a complete case analysis, such that missing values resulted in list wise exclusion from respective analyses. For example, where person-based residential neighbourhood food environment exposures were derived in relation to participant educational attainment, we included all participants with data for education, home address, and associated covariates. Participants included in these analyses could have been lacking income data and work addresses. The number of missing values also varied according to the size of spatial buffer used, as detailed in Appendix Table 6. Linear tests for trends were used to test differences in means across socioeconomic groups, with $p < 0.05$ considered statistically significant. All analyses were conducted in Stata 13 (StataCorp., 2013).

Sensitivity analyses

As every LSOA for the total Fenland Study geographic area was included in main area-based analyses (n = 801 LSOAs)—including both LSOAs where Fenland participants lived and those where they did not—there was a potential for bias. Thus, we conducted a sensitivity analysis of only the subsample of LSOAs where Fenland Study participants lived (n = 285 LSOAs).

Results

Sample characteristics

Characteristics of the analytic sample are provided in Table 1. Of the home-based sample, 89.9% reported being in work. The home and the combined home and work samples were similar across key age, sex, education and income profiles (Table 1).

Area-based exposures

The population-adjusted density of takeaway outlets was greatest in the most deprived LSOAs (Table 2), with 76%

Table 1 Descriptive statistics for the Fenland Study analytic sample (n = 10,429)

Variable	n	%	Missing n (%)
Female	5392	51.7	0
Age (years)	10,429	100	0
29–39	1652	15.8	
40–49	4338	41.6	
50–64	4439	42.6	
Educational attainment[a]	10,276	98.5	153 (1.5)
Low	2091	20.1	
Medium	4698	45.1	
High	3487	33.4	
Equivalised income[b]	9617	92.2	812 (7.8)
<£23,000	2372	22.7	
£23,000–£42,999	3991	38.3	
≥£43,000	3254	31.2	
Work address reported	7927	76.0	2502 (24.0)
Work status	10,335	99.1	94 (0.9)
In work[c]	9372	89.9	
Not in work[d]	963	9.2	

[a] Educational attainment: 'Low' indicates compulsory school education and corresponding qualifications; 'Medium' indicates further education academic or vocational qualifications; 'High' represents degree or higher qualifications

[b] Total household income equivalised using a version of the OECD's modified equivalence scale

[c] Listed as working 'full time', 'part time', 'obtained new job'

[d] Listed as 'retired', 'keeping house', 'unemployed', 'sick leave'

fewer outlets in the least deprived tertile of areas compared to the most, and with a significant gradient across the deprivation tertiles ($p < 0.001$). There was no significant difference in area-based supermarket density by deprivation ($p = 0.126$). When measured as a percentage of all outlets, takeaway outlets made up 21.5% in the most deprived tertile compared to 12.4% in the least deprived tertile.

Person-centred exposures
Comparing geographic boundaries for home-based exposures

Around the home, mean takeaway exposure was significantly and positively associated with both equivalised income and level of education at each scale of Euclidean and Network buffers (Table 3). Of the two socioeconomic indicators, educational attainment revealed larger differences in takeaway exposure than equivalised income. For example, within 1 mile Euclidean buffers, the percentage increase in takeaway outlets between the lowest and highest socioeconomic group was 56% for level of education and 17% for equivalised income. While absolute counts of outlets were greater in the larger buffers, relative socioeconomic differentials were greater at the

Table 2 Area-based takeaway outlet and supermarket densities (mean, 95% CI) per 10,000 population

LSOAs[a]	Takeaway outlets (n)	Supermarkets (n)	Takeaway outlets (% all outlets)[d]
Most deprived	9.4 (7.4, 11.5)	1.4 (1.0, 1.8)	21.5 (18.6, 24.4)
Medium	4.9 (3.6, 6.1)	1.0 (0.7, 1.3)	15.0 (12.1, 17.9)
Least deprived	2.3 (1.7, 2.8)	1.0 (0.7, 1.3)	12.4 (9.7, 15.2)
p-Trend[b]	<0.001	0.126	<0.001
% Difference[c]	-76	-29	-42

[a] Lower super output areas (n = 801) in tertiles of deprivation, defined using 2010 Index of Multiple Deprivation

[b] Test for trend based on linear regression with tertiles of deprivation treated as a continuous variable

[c] Percent difference computed as 100*((least deprived-most deprived)/most deprived)

[d] All food outlets = takeaways, supermarkets, convenience stores, restaurants, cafes

Table 3 Home-based takeaway exposure by groups of educational attainment and equivalised income

	Euclidean buffers (no. of outlets)			Network buffers (no. of outlets)			Proximity to nearest (km)
	800 m	1 km	1 mile	800 m	1 km	1 mile	Mean
Educational attainment[a]*(n = 10,276)*							
Low	2.6 (2.4, 2.8)	3.8 (3.6, 4.1)	7.8 (7.4, 8.2)	1.3 (1.2, 1.4)	1.9 (1.8, 2.13)	4.7 (4.5, 5.0)	1.55 (1.50, 1.60)
Medium	2.5 (2.4, 2.6)	3.6 (3.4, 3.7)	7.0 (6.7, 7.3)	1.24 (1.2, 1.3)	1.9 (1.8, 2.0)	4.3 (4.1, 4.5)	1.64 (1.59, 1.69)
High	4.3 (4.1, 4.5)	6.1 (5.9, 6.4)	12.2 (11.7, 12.6)	2.2 (2.0, 2.3)	3.2 (3.1, 3.4)	7.0 (6.7, 7.3)	1.45 (1.39, 1.51)
p (Highest to lowest)	<0.001	<0.001	<0.001	<0.001	<0.001	<0.001	0.012
% Difference[c]	65	61	56	69	68	49	-7
Equivalised income[b]*(n = 9617)*							
<£23,000	2.9 (2.7, 3.1)	4.2 (4.0, 4.5)	8.6 (8.2, 9.0)	1.5 (1.4, 1.6)	2.3 (2.1, 2.4)	5.1 (4.8, 5.4)	1.55 (1.48, 1.62)
£23,000–£42,999	3.0 (2.8, 3.1)	4.3 (4.1, 4.5)	8.3 (7.9, 8.6)	1.5 (1.4, 1.6)	2.3 (2.1, 2.4)	5.1 (4.8, 5.3)	1.58 (1.52, 1.63)
≥£43,000	3.6 (3.4, 3.8)	5.1 (4.8, 5.3)	10.1 (9.7, 10.6)	1.8 (1.6, 1.9)	2.6 (2.5, 2.8)	5.9 (5.6, 6.1)	1.52 (1.46, 1.58)
p (Highest to lowest)	<0.001	<0.001	<0.001	<0.001	<0.001	<0.001	0.915
% Difference[c]	24	21	17	20	13	16	-2

Mean values (95% confidence intervals), and statistical and percent difference between the lowest and highest socioeconomic groups

[a] Educational attainment: 'Low' indicates compulsory school education and corresponding qualifications; 'Medium' indicates further education academic or vocational qualifications; 'High' represents degree or higher qualifications

[b] Total household income equivalised using a version of the OECD's modified equivalence scale

[c] Percent difference computed as 100*((Higher SES-Lower SES)/lower SES)

smallest buffer sizes. Within Network buffers across level of education, for example, the difference in takeaway outlets at 800 m was 69% and at 1 mile was 49%. Outlet counts were greater in Euclidean than Network buffers. Proximity to the nearest takeaway was 7% shorter for the most educated participants than the least educated, which was significantly different ($p = 0.012$). There was no significant difference between equivalised income groups in proximity to the nearest takeaway outlet.

Results for supermarkets were similar (Table 4). Supermarket exposures were significantly and positively associated with both socioeconomic indicators, with educational attainment showing larger differentials than equivalised income. Within 1 mile Euclidean buffers, for example, between the lowest and highest socioeconomic group, the difference was 136% for level of education and 37% for equivalised income. The absolute outlet counts

were greater in larger Euclidean and Network buffer sizes, and the relative differences were greater for smaller buffer sizes. Distances to the nearest supermarket were significantly shorter for highly-educated participants (23% shorter) compared to those least educated, and for higher income participants (9% shorter) compared to those in the lowest income group.

Geographic boundaries and combined home and work exposures

With combined home and work exposures, there was a consistent association between level of education and takeaway exposure, which was positive and significant for all Euclidean buffers and for 1 mile Network buffers (Table 5). For example, within the 1 mile Network buffer highest educated participants had 16% greater takeaway exposure than lowest educated participants ($p < 0.001$).

Table 4 Home-based supermarket exposure by groups of educational attainment and equivalised income

	Euclidean buffer counts (no. of outlets)			Network buffer counts (no. of outlets)			Proximity to nearest (km)
	800 m	1 km	1 mile	800 m	1 km	1 mile	Mean
Educational attainment[a]*(n = 10,276)*							
Low	0.4 (0.4, 0.5)	0.7 (0.6, 0.7)	1.4 (1.4, 1.5)	0.2 (0.2, 0.2)	0.3 (0.2, 0.4)	1.7 (1.6, 1.8)	3.73 (3.59, 3.88)
Medium	0.5 (0.5, 0.5)	0.7 (0.7, 0.7)	1.5 (1.4, 1.5)	0.2 (0.2, 0.2)	0.3 (0.3, 0.4)	1.7 (1.6, 1.8)	3.90 (3.80, 3.99)
High	1.1 (1.0, 1.1)	1.6 (1.5, 1.6)	3.3 (3.2, 3.4)	0.5 (0.4, 0.5)	0.7 (0.7, 0.8)	3.8 (3.7, 4.0)	2.87 (2.76, 2.98)
p (Highest to lowest)	<0.001	<0.001	<0.001	<0.001	<0.001	<0.001	<0.001
% Difference[c]	1175	129	136	150	133	124	-23
Equivalised income[b]*(n = 9617)*							
<£23,000	0.6 (0.5, 0.6)	0.8 (0.8, 0.9)	1.9 (1.8, 2.0)	0.3 (0.2, 0.3)	0.4 (0.4, 0.4)	2.2 (2.0, 2.3)	3.67 (3.54, 3.81)
£23,000–£42,999	0.6 (0.6, 0.7)	0.9 (0.9, 1.0)	2.0 (1.9, 2.1)	0.3 (0.3, 0.3)	0.5 (0.5, 0.5)	2.3 (2.2, 2.4)	3.60 (3.49, 3.71)
≥£43,000	0.8 (0.8, 0.9)	1.2 (1.1, 1.3)	2.6 (2.4, 2.7)	0.4 (0.3, 0.4)	0.6 (0.5, 0.6)	2.9 (2.8, 3.1)	3.34 (3.22, 3.46)
p (Highest to lowest)	<0.001	<0.001	<0.001	<0.001	<0.001	<0.001	<0.001
% Difference[c]	33	50	37	33	50	32	-9

Mean values (95% confidence intervals), and statistical and percent difference between the lowest and highest socioeconomic groups

[a] Educational attainment: 'Low' indicates compulsory school education and corresponding qualifications; 'Medium' indicates further education academic or vocational qualifications; 'High' represents degree or higher qualifications

[b] Total household income equivalised using a version of the OECD's modified equivalence scale

[c] Percent difference computed as 100*((Higher SES-Lower SES)/lower SES)

The association between equivalised income and takeaway exposure was positive and significant within 1 mile Euclidean and Network buffers, with a 11% and 7% difference between the highest and lowest income groups, respectively.

Absolute takeaway outlet counts for the combined home and work exposures were greater than home-only exposures. For example, within the 800 m Euclidean buffer, combined home and work exposures were two to three times greater than home-based exposures alone. However, the relative differences between socioeconomic groups were smaller than for home-based exposures. In addition, the relative differences were greater in larger than smaller buffer sizes. Highest educated participants had an additional 8% of takeaway outlets within 800 m buffers and 24% within 1 mile Euclidean buffers. In common with home-based exposures, outlet counts were greater in Euclidean than Network buffers.

Results for combined home and work exposures were similar for supermarkets, although unlike takeaway outlets, there were significant and positive associations with both socioeconomic indicators at every Euclidean and Network buffer scale. Educational attainment showed larger differentials than equivalised income, with a relative difference at the 1 mile Euclidean buffer of 78% between lowest and highest level of education and 32% between lowest and highest equivalised income. Similar to takeaway outlets, absolute counts were two to three times greater compared to home-based exposures only. Further, the relative differences in supermarket exposures were greater at larger buffer sizes. For example, compared

to lowest educated participants, highest educated participants had 59% greater numbers of supermarkets within 800 m Euclidean buffers and 78% more supermarkets within 1 mile.

Takeaway outlets as a percentage of all food outlets

Takeaway exposure as a percentage of all outlets was negatively and significantly associated with both indicators of individual SES. This association was found for both home and combined home and work exposures. For example, in the 1 mile home-based Euclidean buffer (Fig. 1), takeaway outlets constituted 21.4% of all outlets for the least educated and 16.5% of all outlets for the most educated. There was a smaller but significant difference between low income (20.3%) and high income (18.0%) groups. Results were similar for combined home and work exposure showing that takeaway outlets comprised 21.7% of all outlets for the least educated participants compared to 16.9% for the most educated, and 20.9% for the lowest compared to 18.4% for the highest income participants.

Similar results were found for all other Euclidean and Network buffers (Appendix Table 6). Average home-based and combined home and work-based exposures by SES to convenience stores, restaurants, cafés and all outlets are also shown in Appendix Table 7.

Sensitivity analysis

In sensitivity analyses, we compared these results, which were derived from analyses of all LSOAs (n = 801) within the extent of the Fenland Study area, to those obtained

Table 5 Combined home and work exposure to takeaway outlets and supermarkets, by groups of educational attainment and equivalised income

	Euclidean buffer counts (no. of outlets)			Network buffer counts (no. of outlets)		
	800 m	1 km	1 mile	800 m	1 km	1 mile
Takeaway outlets						
Educational attainment[a] (n = 7169)						
Low	7.86 (7.39, 8.32)	10.73 (10.16, 11.29)	20.22 (19.29, 21.14)	4.55 (4.23, 4.87)	6.29 (5.89, 6.69)	12.74 (12.09, 13.38)
Medium	7.01 (6.72, 7.29)	9.53 (9.18, 9.89)	18.05 (17.46, 18.64)	4.00 (3.80, 4.20)	5.54 (5.29, 5.79)	11.34 (10.93, 11.76)
High	8.49 (8.15, 8.83)	12.35 (11.90, 12.81)	25.14 (24.32, 25.95)	4.48 (4.27, 4.70)	6.62 (6.32, 6.91)	14.82 (14.27, 15.37)
p (Highest to lowest)	0.026	<0.001	<0.001	0.725	0.191	<0.001
% Difference[c]	8	15	24	-2	5	16
Equivalised income[b] (n = 6774)						
<£23,000	7.73 (7.28, 8.17)	10.59 (10.04, 11.14)	20.31 (19.38, 21.24)	4.47 (4.17, 4.77)	6.23 (5.84, 6.61)	12.62 (11.98, 13.26)
£23,000–£42,999	7.51 (7.20, 7.82)	10.47 (10.06, 10.88)	20.18 (19.48, 20.87)	4.16 (3.95, 4.37)	5.89 (5.62, 6.16)	12.50 (12.02, 12.99)
≥£43,000	7.91 (7.57, 8.25)	11.28 (10.83, 11.72)	22.49 (21.71, 23.27)	4.25 (4.03, 4.47)	6.13 (5.84, 6.42)	13.46 (12.93, 13.98)
p (Highest to lowest)	0.510	0.057	<0.001	0.236	0.686	0.048
% Difference[c]	2	7	11	-5	-2	7
Supermarkets						
Educational attainment[a] (n = 7169)						
Low	1.38 (1.30, 1.46)	1.94 (1.84, 2.05)	3.74 (3.54, 3.94)	0.75 (0.70, 0.81)	1.05 (0.98, 1.12)	3.22 (3.04, 3.39)
Medium	1.32 (1.27, 1.37)	1.86 (1.79, 1.94)	3.65 (3.51, 3.79)	0.71 (0.68, 0.75)	1.00 (0.96, 1.05)	3.10 (2.98, 3.23)
High	2.20 (2.11, 2.28)	3.23 (3.12, 3.35)	6.66 (6.42, 6.90)	1.07 (1.02, 1.12)	1.60 (1.53, 1.66)	5.90 (5.67, 6.12)
p (Highest to lowest)	<0.001	<0.001	<0.001	<0.001	<0.001	<0.001
% Difference[c]	59	67	78	45	52	83
Equivalised income[b] (n = 6774)						
<£23,000	1.43 (1.35, 1.51)	2.08 (1.96, 2.19)	4.15 (3.92, 4.38)	0.77 (0.71, 0.82)	1.08 (1.01, 1.14)	3.63 (3.43, 3.83)
£23,000–£42,999	1.61 (1.55, 1.68)	2.32 (2.23, 2.42)	4.56 (4.37, 4.74)	0.84 (0.80, 0.89)	1.21 (1.15, 1.26)	3.96 (3.79, 4.13)
≥£43,000	1.87 (1.79, 1.94)	2.68 (2.57, 2.79)	5.47 (5.25, 5.69)	0.93 (0.88, 0.98)	1.37 (1.30, 1.43)	4.75 (4.55, 4.95)
p (Highest to lowest)	<0.001	<0.001	<0.001	<0.001	<0.001	<0.001
% Difference[c]	31	29	32	21	27	31

Mean values (95% confidence intervals), trend statistics and percent difference between the lowest and highest socioeconomic groups

[a] Educational attainment: 'Low' indicates compulsory school education and corresponding qualifications; 'Medium' indicates further education academic or vocational qualifications; 'High' represents degree or higher qualifications

[b] Total household income equivalised using a version of the OECD's modified equivalence scale

[c] Percent difference computed as 100*((Higher SES-Lower SES)/lower SES)

from analyses which only included LSOAs (n = 285) containing Fenland Study participants. These alternate results (not shown) were not materially different from those presented here.

Discussion

Summary of findings

We compared the socioeconomic differences in foodscape exposure across a number of GIS-based metrics, and found that the direction and magnitude of socioeconomic differences was metric dependent. Using an area-based metric, takeaway outlets were more concentrated in more deprived areas. This is consistent with the majority of existing area-based work across international contexts [21, 22, 24, 25, 55, 56]. Area-based analysis of

supermarkets showed no association between density and area deprivation, consistent with findings from previous UK-based research [23, 27, 28].

The most notable finding in this study is the contrast between the area-based and person-centred measures, when person-centred exposure was characterised as counts of outlets. The area-based results provided evidence that deprived areas have more takeaway outlets, and numbers of supermarkets equivalent to those found in less deprived areas, whereas using person-centred measures, takeaway and supermarket counts were greater for those with higher levels of education and income. There are multiple potential explanations for this discordance. Firstly, an individual's own SES (based on income or educational attainment) may not be aligned

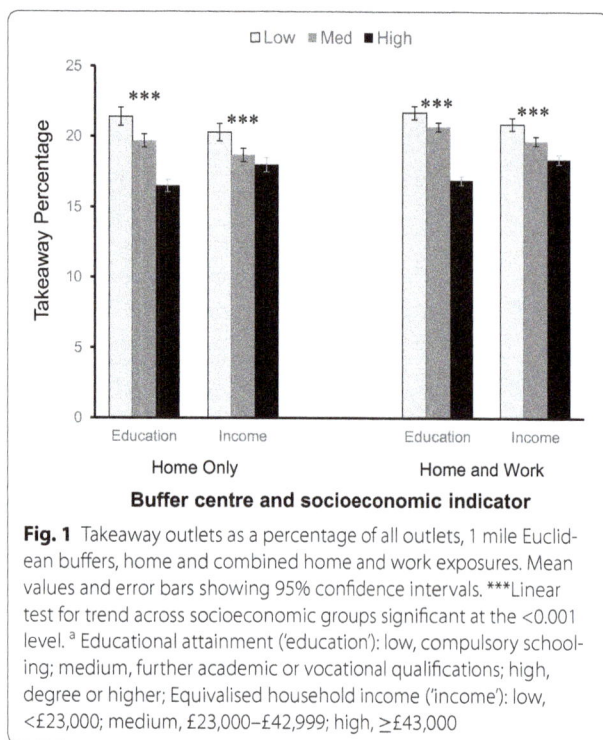

Fig. 1 Takeaway outlets as a percentage of all outlets, 1 mile Euclidean buffers, home and combined home and work exposures. Mean values and error bars showing 95% confidence intervals. ***Linear test for trend across socioeconomic groups significant at the <0.001 level. [a] Educational attainment ('education'): low, compulsory schooling; medium, further academic or vocational qualifications; high, degree or higher; Equivalised household income ('income'): low, <£23,000; medium, £23,000–£42,999; high, ≥£43,000

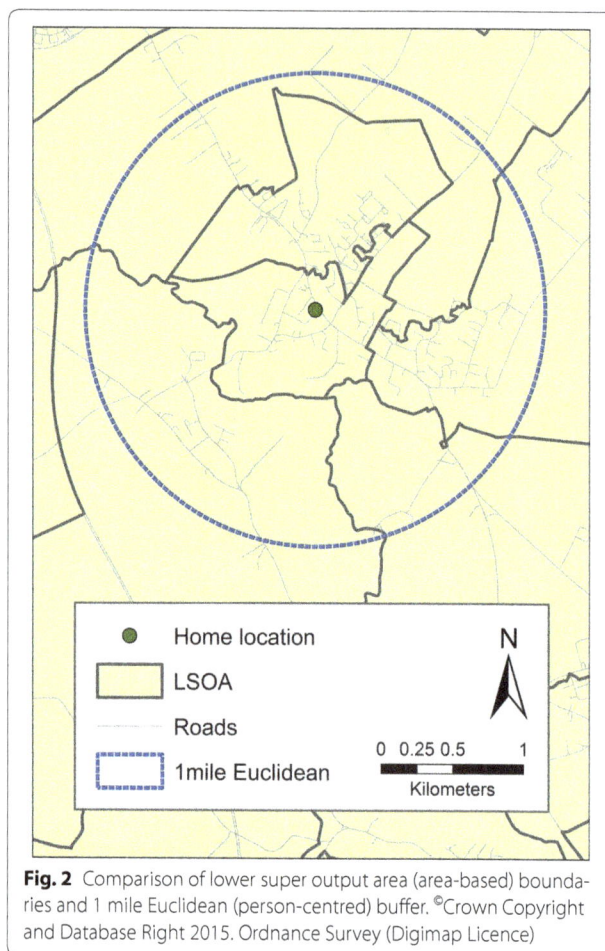

Fig. 2 Comparison of lower super output area (area-based) boundaries and 1 mile Euclidean (person-centred) buffer. ©Crown Copyright and Database Right 2015. Ordnance Survey (Digimap Licence)

with the SES of their assigned 'neighbourhood' (i.e. the deprivation level of their LSOA of residence) [57], or even their specific location *within* their assigned neighbourhood. There will inevitably exist unmeasured variation in levels of deprivation especially within and across larger administrative areas, such that these estimates cannot be attributed confidently to all residents [58]. Secondly, administrative boundaries such as LSOAs were not designed to capture the extent of their resident's movements [44, 59], in the way that our person-based metrics of exposure are a better (although imperfect) approximation [60]. For smaller administrative boundaries in particular, individuals' 'activity spaces' (defined as "the sub-set of all locations within which an individual has direct contact as a result of his or her day-to-day activities" [61]) are likely to extend beyond their limits [62], potentially resulting in foodscape exposure that is not reflected in estimates based solely on their assigned residential LSOA (Fig 2). These activity spaces would also likely be heterogeneous in socioeconomic conditions, with the individual exposed to neighborhoods socioeconomically disimilar to their own. This uncertain geographic context problem [63] may partly explain why socioeconomic differentials in absolute person-based food exposure are attenuated when accounting for food outlets around the work place.

By contrast, relative takeaway outlet exposure (takeaways as a percentage of all outlets), which better accounts

for wider food environment context, showed the same (negative) socioeconomic gradient in both person- and area-level analyses, and this relationship was not attenuated by the addition of work-based exposure estimates. This relative approach has precedent [31, 33–36, 64–68], and has the potential to minimise residual confounding in analyses relating food outlet exposure to health [55]. In addition, relative access may be a more important conceptualisation of the impact of food outlet exposure on dietary behaviours than absolute numbers [12]. For example, while a high concentration of takeaway outlets offering a range of takeaway options might encourage more frequent consumption, the salience of this exposure may be reduced in the presence of retailers who are offering healthier food options [33]. Prior studies have associated higher relative takeaway outlet densities with low neighbourhood SES [36, 65], higher weight status [33, 34, 64, 67], and lower diet quality [68]. Our findings support the hypothesis that absolute counts of individual outlet types do not provide a complete picture of foodscape exposures.

Our neighbourhood foodscape exposure estimates also showed sensitivity to buffer scale and type specifications, emerging from what has been described in the geographical literature the modifiable areal unit problem's (MAUP's) 'scale' and 'zonation' effects [69]. As illustrated in Fig. 3, irrespective of buffer type larger buffers tend to contain greater numbers of food outlets, resulting in greater estimates of exposure to the foodscape. Similarly, at any given scale, network buffers (that account for land use and may be considered more realistic delineators of neighbourhood than Euclidean buffers [70] generally have a smaller footprint than Euclidean equivalents (Fig. 3), and are therefore likely to contain fewer outlets, resulting in reduced estimates of foodscape exposure. The MAUP is a common consideration in the statistical analysis of geographical data, but has received limited attention in the food environments literature, wherein exposure estimates driven by methodological choices may reveal differential associations with individual-level outcomes of interest. Importantly however, the relative differences between socioeconomic groups in outlet counts remained present across all combinations of buffer scale and type, and were particularly similar across buffers of equal size irrespective of type (i.e., little evidence of MAUP zonation effect was observed when determining differences in outlet densities across socioeconomic groups).

There was also some sensitivity in our findings across the two indicators of individual SES tested, with larger differences between the groups highest and lowest educated, than between those on highest and lowest incomes. This suggests that the foodscape is structured according to local residents' education more so than their income, and may reflect a greater spatial segregation among participants on the basis of their educational background. Alternatively or in addition, it may also reflect the targeting of stores according to neighbourhood sociodemographics.

Finally, the food outlet proximity measures tested also showed evidence of socioeconomic difference. The observed consistency with density measures is consistent with the findings of previous work, which has shown a strong correlation in this regard [71]. However, while proximity measures are useful for assessing geographic access to the closest outlet, they do not address the wider issues of the concentration or mix of outlets in the neighbourhood, which may be important to consider.

Implications for further research

Given that the choice of GIS metric and specifications thereof can influence results, it is important that studies using GIS-based measures of the foodscape are aware of whether and to what extent methodological choices matter, and to conduct sensitivity analyses accordingly. For example, the null associations observed among smaller Network buffers for combined home and work exposure

to takeaway outlets suggests that at smaller scales, Type-II errors may be introduced, where an association that exists is not identified, an issue previously identified by Thornton et al. [52]. The choice of metric should be informed by theories of the expected mechanisms by which the foodscape influences diet, and which features of the foodscape are seen as important. For example, takeaway outlets are increasingly seen as particularly relevant within the context of the work 'neighbourhood', with behavioural evidence from a US study showing that trips to fast-food outlets occur frequently on workdays [72]. However, given the time constraints of breaks at work, it may be that smaller buffer sizes are more appropriate in this context, in order to capture where workers are able to travel for food purchases, when examining the potential influence of takeaway outlets around the workplace [40]. On the other hand, the appropriate scale for assessing supermarket access may be larger given evidence that shoppers travel longer distances for grocery shopping trips [72], and that they are less likely to use their local supermarket if it is not also economically accessible to them [73]. Proximity measures could inform the size of spatial buffers to capture specific outlet types. Here, the median distance from residents to takeaway outlets was less than 1 km and to supermarkets was up to 2 km. Studies may use such distances to specify exposures by outlet type, as seen in a recent paper examining restaurant and supermarket exposures in relation to dietary behaviours and body mass index [32].

Methodological considerations and limitations

This study is not without limitations. Some degree of temporal mismatch is possible, as the Fenland Study data collection ran from 2005 to 2014 and the food outlet data were collected in 2011. As relative SES is understood as a fairly stable construct [74], the level of error from changes in SES should be minimal. However inaccuracies may still result from any moves in participants' home or work location. Further, addressing food environment exposure around the workplace does not provide a full assessment of exposure within broader activity spaces. While GIS techniques allow proxy measures, recording the extent of people's actual activity spaces is possible with global positioning systems (GPS) technologies, an approach that is gradually becoming more common [62, 75, 76]. In addition, participants who did not report being in work were excluded from this wider assessment, and their exposure restricted to the residential neighbourhood. This has potential implications for understanding socioeconomic differences in exposure, as those not in work for certain reasons (e.g. unemployed or on sick leave) may be more likely to be disadvantaged more generally, thus skewing the sample towards higher SES

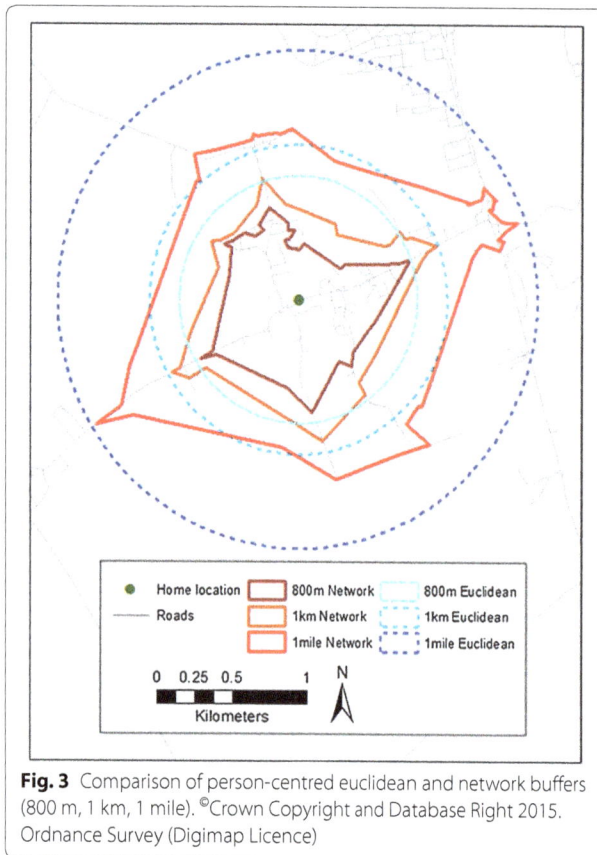

Fig. 3 Comparison of person-centred euclidean and network buffers (800 m, 1 km, 1 mile). ©Crown Copyright and Database Right 2015. Ordnance Survey (Digimap Licence)

participants. However, there is some evidence that being out-of-work is predictive of having a smaller daily activity space [75], potentially resulting in more accurate approximations of activity space exposure to food outlets when only addressing residential neighbourhood exposure for this group. While 24% of our sample did not have valid work addresses, we found that this percentage did not vary by area deprivation (data not shown), suggesting the lack of this information did not bias the socioeconomic profile of the sample.

The Fenland Study area includes urban and rural areas, and as such is fairly typical of many regions of the United Kingdom. The spread of LSOAs in this sample across the first and ninety-eighth percentile of IMD scores for England, further suggests that our findings are generalisable. With regard to the individual SES measures, the proportions of study participants in the highest education and income groups were also similar to the national average. For example, in 2012/13, 40% of non-retired households in England had an equivalised income upwards of £39,000 [77], while in 2011, 30% of the population held a degree qualification [78]. However, our sample contained a smaller representation of individuals with lower income and less education. For example, in 2011, 13% of residents

in the same region had no qualifications [78]. However, the underrepresentation of lower socioeconomic groups among study cohorts is a general concern not unique to our study [79]. Moreover, underrepresentation of low SES groups may only have served to underestimate the scale of inequalities in foodscape exposures between the highest and lowest income groups.

The study also has a number of strengths. Most importantly, we systematically assessed multiple commonly-used foodscape exposure metrics using a large study cohort with detailed sociodemographic information, allowing two indicators of individual-level SES to be used. In addition, the inclusion of workplace location in the cohort allows an important additional anchor point in people's regular activity space to be included in the measured exposure. In measuring the foodscape, food outlet data were collected from a validated source [41], the accuracy of which is comparable to other secondary food outlet location datasets commonly utilised in food environments research [80].

Conclusions

This study showed associations between socioeconomic status and absolute exposure to takeaway outlets and supermarkets, and relative exposure to takeaway outlets, around home and work locations in a large UK sample of working age adults. The study provides a reference to health researchers interested in measuring the socioeconomic differences in exposure to the food environment and the impact that the choice of metric can have on results. As such, the results presented here can inform further investigations of associations between SES and foodscape exposure , to explore the role that the neighbourhood retail food environment plays in dietary inequalities.

Abbreviations
IMD: Index of Multiple Deprivation; GIS: geographical information systems; GPS: global positioning systems; LSOA: lower super output area; MAUP: modifiable areal unit problem; OECD: Organisation for Economic Co-operation and Development; SES: socioeconomic status; UK: United Kingdom; US: United States.

Authors' contributions
ERM, TB and PM conceived of the study. ERM conducted the spatial and statistical analyses and drafted the manuscript. TLP contributed to the statistical analysis. TB collected and categorised the food outlet data, and contributed to the spatial and statistical analysis. PM provided input on the statistical analysis and interpretation of results. NGF is a principal investigator of the Fenland Study. All authors contributed considerably to critical revisions and have read and approved the final manuscript.

Author details
[1] UKCRC Centre for Diet and Activity Research (CEDAR), MRC Epidemiology Unit, University of Cambridge School of Clinical Medicine, Institute of Metabolic Science, Cambridge Biomedical Campus, Cambridge CB2 0QQ, UK. [2] MRC Epidemiology Unit, University of Cambridge School of Clinical Medicine, Institute of Metabolic Science, Cambridge Biomedical Campus,

Does exposure to the food environment differ by socioeconomic position? Comparing area-based...

57

Cambridge CB2 0QQ, UK. [3] Present Address: Department of Nutrition and Exercise Physiology, Washington State University Elson S Floyd College of Medicine, Spokane WA 99210, USA.

Acknowledgements
We thank all the volunteers who have participated in the Fenland Study, the Fenland PIs and the MRC Epidemiology Unit Study Coordination, Field Epidemiology, and Data Management teams. The Fenland study is funded by the MRC (MC_UU-12,015/1).

Competing interests
The authors declare that they have no competing interests and no financial disclosures to make.

Funding
This work was undertaken by the Centre for Diet and Activity Research (CEDAR), a UKCRC Public Health Research Centre of Excellence. Funding from Cancer Research UK, the British Heart Foundation, the Economic and Social Research Council, the Medical Research Council, the National Institute for Health Research [ES/G007462/1], and the Wellcome Trust [087636/Z/08/Z], under the auspices of the UK Clinical Research Collaboration, is gratefully acknowledged. TLP's Ph.D. studentship is generously supported by the Cambridge International Scholarship, a scheme funded by the Cambridge Commonwealth, European & International Trust. Core Medical Research Council Epidemiology Unit for NGF (MC_UU_12015/5) is also acknowledged. The Fenland Study is funded by the Wellcome Trust and the Medical Research Council.

Appendix

See Tables 6 and 7.

Table 6 Home and combined home and work exposures (mean, 95% CI) to takeaway outlets as a percentage of all food outlets

	Home			Home and Work		
	800 m	1 km	1 mile	800 m	1 km	1 mile
Educational attainment[a]						
Euclidean	N = 9276[d]	N = 9568[d]	N = 9929[d]	N = 6890[d]	N = 6961[d]	N = 7067[d]
Low	22.2 (21.2, 23.2)	23 (22.1, 23.9)	21.4 (20.8, 22.1)	21.1 (20.4, 21.8)	21.7 (21.1, 22.3)	21.7 (21.2, 22.2)
Medium	20.0 (19.4, 20.7)	19.9 (19.4, 20.5)	19.7 (19.2, 20.1)	20.2 (19.8, 20.7)	20.5 (20.1, 20.9)	20.7 (20.4, 21)
High	18.1 (17.5, 18.7)	17.9 (17.4, 18.4)	16.5 (16, 16.9)	17.1 (16.6, 17.5)	17.0 (16.6, 17.3)	16.9 (16.6, 17.2)
p-trend[c]	<0.001	<0.001	<0.001	<0.001	<0.001	<0.001
Network	N = 7850[d]	N = 8717[d]	N = 9592[d]	N = 6479[d]	N = 6769[d]	N = 7002[d]
Low	20.4 (19.1, 21.8)	22.2 (21.3, 23)	21.9 (21.4, 22.5)	20.5 (19.6, 21.4)	20.8 (20.1, 21.6)	21.3 (20.8, 21.8)
Medium	18.4 (17.5, 19.2)	20.3 (19.7, 20.8)	20.5 (20.1, 20.9)	19.1 (18.5, 19.7)	19.7 (19.2, 20.2)	20.2 (19.9, 20.6)
High	16.8 (16.1, 17.5)	17 (16.5, 17.5)	16.6 (16.2, 16.9)	15.9 (15.4, 16.5)	16.5 (16, 17)	16.4 (16.1, 16.7)
p-trend[c]	<0.001	<0.001	<0.001	<0.001	<0.001	<0.001
Equivalised income[b]						
Euclidean	N = 8,609[d]	N = 8,856[d]	N = 9,189[d]	N = 6,524[d]	N = 6,588[d]	N = 6,686[d]
<£23,000	21.3 (20.4, 22.2)	21.7 (20.9, 22.5)	20.3 (19.7, 21)	20.3 (19.6, 20.9)	20.8 (20.3, 21.4)	20.9 (20.4, 21.3)
£23,000–£42,999	19.5 (18.9, 20.2)	19.6 (19, 20.2)	18.7 (18.3, 19.2)	19.5 (19, 20)	19.6 (19.2, 20)	19.7 (19.3, 20)
≥£43,000	19.1 (18.4, 19.8)	18.9 (18.3, 19.5)	18.0 (17.5, 18.5)	18.4 (17.9, 18.9)	18.3 (17.9, 18.8)	18.4 (18, 18.7)
p-trend[c]	<0.001	<0.001	<0.001	<0.001	<0.001	<0.001
Network	N = 7498[d]	N = 8281[d]	N = 9014[d]	N = 6153[d]	N = 6424[d]	N = 6627[d]
<£23,000	18.7 (17.5, 19.9)	21.0 (20.2, 21.7)	21 (20.5, 21.5)	19.3 (18.4, 20.1)	19.8 (19.1, 20.6)	20.4 (19.9, 20.9)
£23,000–£42,999	18.2 (17.4, 19.1)	19.6 (19, 20.1)	19.4 (19, 19.8)	18.5 (17.9, 19.1)	19 (18.4, 19.5)	19.2 (18.8, 19.5)
≥£43,000	17.8 (16.9, 18.7)	18.1 (17.6, 18.7)	18.2 (17.8, 18.6)	17.2 (16.5, 17.8)	17.7 (17.1, 18.2)	17.9 (17.5, 18.3)
p-trend[c]	0.071	<0.001	<0.001	<0.001	<0.001	<0.001

All food outlets = takeaways, supermarkets, convenience stores, restaurants, cafes

[a] Educational attainment: 'Low' indicates compulsory school education and corresponding qualifications; 'Medium' indicates further education academic or vocational qualifications; 'High' represents degree or higher qualifications

[b] Total household income equivalised using a version of the OECD's modified equivalence scale

[c] Test for trend based on linear regression with groups of education/income treated as a continuous variable

[d] Analytic sample size restricted to person-centred neighbourhoods containing a minimum of one none takeaway food outlet

Table 7 Home-based exposures (mean, 95% CI) to convenience stores, restaurants, cafés and all outlets, Euclidean and Network 1 mile buffers

Home	Convenience stores		Restaurants		Cafés		All outlets	
	1 mile euclidean	1 mile network	1 mile euclidean	1 mile network	1 mile euclidean	1 mile network	1 mile euclidean	1 mile network
Educational attainment[a] (n = 10,276)								
Low	9.0 (8.5, 9.5)	5.3 (5.0, 5.6)	10.2 (9.5, 11.0)	5.6 (5.2, 6.0)	5.8 (5.3, 6.3)	3.0 (2.6, 3.3)	34.3 (32.3, 36.3)	20.2 (19.0, 21.5)
Medium	8.0 (7.7, 8.2)	4.8 (4.6, 4.9)	10.7 (10.1, 11.3)	5.9 (5.6, 6.3)	6.4 (6.0, 6.8)	3.3 (3.0, 3.5)	33.5 (32.0, 35.0)	19.9 (19.0, 20.8)
High	13.3 (12.8, 13.7)	7.5 (7.2, 7.8)	30.1 (28.7, 31.5)	15.7 (14.9, 16.6)	20.0 (19.0, 20.9)	9.8 (9.2, 10.4)	78.8 (75.4, 82.2)	43.8 (41.7, 45.9)
p-trend[c]	<0.001	<0.001	<0.001	<0.001	<0.001	<0.001	<0.001	<0.001
% Difference[d]	48	42	195	180	245	227	129	117
Equivalised income[b] (n = 9617)								
<£23,000	9.9 (9.5, 10.4)	5.8 (5.5, 6.1)	14.2 (13.1, 15.2)	7.6 (7.0, 8.2)	8.5 (7.8, 9.2)	4.2 (3.8, 4.7)	43.0 (40.4, 45.7)	24.9 (23.2, 26.5)
£23,000–£42,999	9.4 (9.0, 9.7)	5.6 (5.3, 5.8)	15.7 (14.8, 16.6)	8.5 (8.0, 9.1)	9.6 (9.0, 10.3)	4.8 (4.5, 5.2)	44.9 (42.6, 47.2)	26.3 (24.9, 27.7)
≥£43,000	11.2 (10.7, 11.6)	6.3 (6.1, 6.6)	22.0 (20.8, 23.3)	11.4 (10.7, 12.2)	14.3 (13.4, 15.1)	6.9 (6.4, 7.5)	60.2 (57.2, 63.2)	33.5 (31.7, 35.3)
p-trend[c]	<0.001	<0.001	<0.001	<0.001	<0.001	<0.001	<0.001	<0.001
% Difference[d]	13	9	55	50	68	64	50	35
Home and work[e]								
Educational attainment[a] (n = 7169)								
Low	23.0 (21.9, 24.1)	14.2 (13.5, 15.0)	32.6 (30.4, 34.8)	21.0 (19.4, 22.6)	19.3 (17.8, 20.8)	12.7 (11.5, 13.8)	98.8 (93.4, 104.2)	63.8 (59.9, 67.7)
Medium	20.3 (19.6, 21.0)	12.6 (12.1, 13.1)	33.2 (31.6, 34.8)	21.4 (20.3, 22.5)	20.4 (19.3, 21.4)	13.2 (12.4, 14.0)	95.5 (91.7, 99.3)	61.7 (59.0, 64.4)
High	27.7 (26.8, 28.6)	16.2 (15.6, 16.7)	69.1 (66.2, 72.0)	42.7 (40.6, 44.7)	45.3 (43.3, 47.2)	27.9 (26.5, 29.3)	173.9 (167.3, 180.5)	107.4 (102.8, 112.1)
p-trend[c]	<0.001	<0.001	<0.001	<0.001	<0.001	<0.001	<0.001	<0.001
% Difference[d]	20	14	112	103	135	120	76	68
Equivalised income[b] (n = 6774)								
<£23,000	23.0 (21.9, 24.1)	14.2 (13.5, 14.9)	36.6 (34.1, 39.2)	22.9 (21.1, 24.6)	22.3 (20.6, 24.0)	14.0 (12.8, 15.2)	106.4 (100.3, 112.5)	67.3 (63.1, 71.4)
£23,000–£42,999	22.7 (21.9, 23.5)	13.9 (13.3, 14.4)	43.2 (41.1, 45.4)	27.5 (26.0, 29.1)	26.9 (25.4, 28.3)	17.2 (16.1, 18.3)	117.5 (112.6, 122.5)	75.1 (71.5, 78.6)
≥£43,000	25.1 (24.2, 26.0)	14.9 (14.3, 15.5)	55.2 (52.6, 57.9)	34.4 (32.6, 36.2)	35.5 (33.8, 37.3)	22.1 (20.9, 23.4)	143.8 (137.8, 149.9)	89.6 (85.4, 93.8)
p-trend[c]	0.001	0.084	<0.001	<0.001	<0.001	<0.001	<0.001	<0.001
% Difference[d]	9	5	51	50	59	58	35	33

[a] Educational attainment: 'Low' indicates compulsory school education and corresponding qualifications; 'Medium' indicates further education academic or vocational qualifications; 'High' represents degree or higher qualifications

[b] Total household income equivalised using a version of the OECD's modified equivalence scale

[c] Test for trend based on linear regression with groups of education/income treated as a continuous variable

[d] Percent difference is of the additional exposure in the highest socioeconomic group compared to the lowest

[e] Participants included if they had a valid work postcode and were in work

All food outlets = takeaways, supermarkets, convenience stores, restaurants, cafes

References

1. James WP, Nelson M, Ralph A, Leather S. Socioeconomic determinants of health. The contribution of nutrition to inequalities in health. BMJ. 1997;314:1545–9.
2. Dowler E. Inequalities in diet and physical activity in Europe. Public Health Nutr. 2001;4:701–9.
3. Ball K, Mishra GD, Thane CW, Hodge A. How well do Australian women comply with dietary guidelines? Public Health Nutr. 2004;7:443–52.
4. Giskes K, Avendano M, Brug J, Kunst AE. A systematic review of studies on socioeconomic inequalities in dietary intakes associated with weight gain and overweight/obesity conducted among European adults. Obes Rev. 2010;11:413–29.
5. Drewnowski A. Obesity, diets, and social inequalities. Nutr Rev. 2009;67(Suppl 1):S36–9.
6. Mejean C, Droomers M, van der Schouw YT, Sluijs I, Czernichow S, Grobbee DE, Bueno-de-Mesquita HB, Beulens JW. The contribution of diet and lifestyle to socioeconomic inequalities in cardiovascular morbidity and mortality. Int J Cardiol. 2013;168:5190–5.
7. Stringhini S, Tabak AG, Akbaraly TN, Sabia S, Shipley MJ, Marmot MG, Brunner EJ, Batty GD, Bovet P, Kivimaki M. Contribution of modifiable risk factors to social inequalities in type 2 diabetes: prospective Whitehall II cohort study. BMJ. 2012;345:e5452.
8. Caspi CE, Sorensen G, Subramanian SV, Kawachi I. The local food environment and diet: a systematic review. Health Place. 2012;18:1172–87.
9. Feng J, Glass TA, Curriero FC, Stewart WF, Schwartz BS. The built environment and obesity: a systematic review of the epidemiologic evidence. Health Place. 2010;16:175–90.
10. Swinburn B, Vandevijvere S, Kraak V, Sacks G, Snowdon W, Hawkes C, Barquera S, Friel S, Kelly B, Kumanyika S, et al. Monitoring and benchmarking government policies and actions to improve the healthiness of food environments: a proposed Government Healthy Food Environment Policy Index. Obes Rev. 2013;14:24–37.
11. Popkin BM, Duffey K, Gordon-Larsen P. Environmental influences on food choice, physical activity and energy balance. Physiol Behav. 2005;86:603–13.
12. Black C, Moon G, Baird J. Dietary inequalities: what is the evidence for the effect of the neighbourhood food environment? Health Place. 2014;27:229–42.
13. Burns CM, Inglis AD. Measuring food access in Melbourne: access to healthy and fast foods by car, bus and foot in an urban municipality in Melbourne. Health Place. 2007;13:877–85.
14. Morland K, Diez Roux AV, Wing S. Supermarkets, other food stores, and obesity: the atherosclerosis risk in communities study. Am J Prev Med. 2006;30:333–9.
15. Lachat C, Nago E, Verstraeten R, Roberfroid D, Van Camp J, Kolsteren P. Eating out of home and its association with dietary intake: a systematic review of the evidence. Obes Rev. 2012;13:329–46.
16. Prentice AM, Jebb SA. Fast foods, energy density and obesity: a possible mechanistic link. Obes Rev. 2003;4:187–94.
17. Rosenheck R. Fast food consumption and increased caloric intake: a systematic review of a trajectory towards weight gain and obesity risk. Obes Rev. 2008;9:535–47.
18. Fleischhacker SE, Evenson KR, Rodriguez DA, Ammerman AS. A systematic review of fast food access studies. Obes Rev. 2011;12:e460–71.
19. Morland K, Wing S, Diez Roux A, Poole C. Neighborhood characteristics associated with the location of food stores and food service places. Am J Prev Med. 2002;22:23–9.
20. Filomena S, Scanlin K, Morland KB. Brooklyn, New York foodscape 2007–2011: a five-year analysis of stability in food retail environments. Int J Behav Nutr Phys Act. 2013;10:46.
21. Cummins SC, McKay L, MacIntyre S. McDonald's restaurants and neighborhood deprivation in Scotland and England. Am J Prev Med. 2005;29:308–10.
22. Macdonald L, Cummins S, Macintyre S. Neighbourhood fast food environment and area deprivation-substitution or concentration? Appetite. 2007;49:251–4.
23. Maguire ER, Burgoine T, Monsivais P. Area deprivation and the food environment over time: a repeated cross-sectional study on takeaway outlet density and supermarket presence in Norfolk, UK, 1990–2008. Health Place. 2015;33:142–7.
24. Smoyer-Tomic KE, Spence JC, Raine KD, Amrhein C, Cameron N, Yasenovskiy V, Cutumisu N, Hemphill E, Healy J. The association between neighborhood socioeconomic status and exposure to supermarkets and fast food outlets. Health Place. 2008;14:740–54.
25. Reidpath DD, Burns C, Garrard J, Mahoney M, Townsend M. An ecological study of the relationship between social and environmental determinants of obesity. Health Place. 2002;8:141–5.
26. Macintyre S, McKay L, Cummins S, Burns C. Out-of-home food outlets and area deprivation: case study in Glasgow, UK. Int J Behav Nutr Phys Act. 2005;2:16.
27. White M, Bunting J, Mathers J, Williams L, Adamson A. Do 'food deserts' exist A multi-level, geographical analysis of the relationship between retail food access, socio-economic position and dietary intake. Newcastle: University of Newcastle; 2004.
28. Cummins S, Macintyre S. A systematic study of an urban foodscape: the price and availability of food in Greater Glasgow. Urban Stud. 2002;39:2115–30.
29. Pearce J, Day P, Witten K. Neighbourhood Provision of food and alcohol retailing and social deprivation in Urban New Zealand. Urban Policy Res. 2008;26:213–27.
30. Kestens Y, Daniel M. Social inequalities in food exposure around schools in an urban area. Am J Prev Med. 2010;39:33–40.
31. Clary CM, Ramos Y, Shareck M, Kestens Y. Should we use absolute or relative measures when assessing foodscape exposure in relation to fruit and vegetable intake? Evidence from a wide-scale Canadian study. Prev Med. 2015;71:83–7.
32. Richardson AS, Meyer KA, Howard AG, Boone-Heinonen J, Popkin BM, Evenson KR, Shikany JM, Lewis CE, Gordon-Larsen P. Multiple pathways from the neighborhood food environment to increased body mass index through dietary behaviors: a structural equation-based analysis in the CARDIA study. Health Place. 2015;36:74–87.
33. Polsky J, Moineddin R, Dunn JR, Glazier RH, Booth GL. Absolute and relative densities of fast-food versus other restaurants in relation to weight status: Does restaurant mix matter? Prev Med (Baltim) 2015;82:28–34
34. Stark JH, Neckerman K, Lovasi GS, Konty K, Quinn J, Arno P, Viola D, Harris TG, Weiss CC, Bader MD, Rundle A. Neighbourhood food environments and body mass index among New York City adults. J Epidemiol Commun Health. 2013;67:736–42.
35. Mercille G, Richard L, Gauvin L, Kestens Y, Payette H, Daniel M. Comparison of two indices of availability of fruits/vegetable and fast food outlets. J Urban Health. 2012;90:240–5.
36. Luan H, Minaker LM, Law J. Do marginalized neigbourhoods have less healthy retail food environments? An analysis using Bayesian spatial latent factor and hurdle models. Int J Health Geographys. 2016;15:1–16.
37. Fenland Study. http://www.mrc-epid.cam.ac.uk/research/studies/fenland.
38. UK Data Service Census Support. GeoConvert. In Book GeoConvert (Editor ed.^eds.); 2015.
39. Smith D, Cummins S, Clark C, Stansfeld S. Does the local food environment around schools affect diet? Longitudinal associations in adolescents attending secondary schools in East London. BMC Public Health. 2013;13:70.
40. Burgoine T, Monsivais P. Characterising food environment exposure at home, at work, and along commuting journeys using data on adults in the UK. Int J Behav Nut Phys Act. 2013;10:85.
41. Lake AA, Burgoine T, Greenhalgh F, Stamp E, Tyrrell R. The foodscape: classification and field validation of secondary data sources. Health Place. 2010;16:666–73.
42. Lake AA, Burgoine T, Stamp E, Grieve R. The foodscape: classification and field validation of secondary data sources across urban/rural and socioeconomic classifications in England. Int J Behav Nut Phys Act. 2012;9:37.
43. Charreire H, Casey R, Salze P, Simon C, Chaix B, Banos A, Badariotti D, Weber C, Oppert J-M. Measuring the food environment using geographical information systems: a methodological review. Public Health Nutr. 2010;13:1773–85.
44. Thornton LE, Pearce JR, Kavanagh AM. Using geographic information systems (GIS) to assess the role of the built environment in influencing obesity: a glossary. Int J Behav Nutr Phys Activ. 2011;8:71.
45. Burgoine T, Alvanides S, Lake AA. Creating 'obesogenic realities'; Do our methodological choices make a difference when measuring the food environment? Int J Health Geograph. 2013;12:1–9.
46. Super Output Area. http://www.ons.gov.uk/ons/guide-method/geography/beginner-s-guide/census/super-output-areas--soas-/index.html

47. Office for National Statistics. Super output Area mid-year population estimates for England and Wales, Mid-2011 (Census based); 2013. https://www.ons.gov.uk/peoplepopulationandcommunity/populationandmigration/populationestimates/datasets/lowersuperoutputareamidyearpopulationestimates. Accessed 28 Apr 2017.

48. Chaix B, Merlo J, Evans D, Leal C, Havard S. Neighbourhoods in eco-epidemiologic research: delimiting personal exposure areas. A response to Riva, Gauvin, Apparicio and Brodeur. Soc Sci Med. 2009;69:1306–10.

49. Jeffery RW, Baxter J, McGuire M, Linde J. Are fast food restaurants an environmental risk factor for obesity? Int J Behav Nutr Phys Act. 2006;3:2.

50. An R, Sturm R. School and residential neighborhood food environment and diet among California youth. Am J Prev Med. 2012;42:129–35.

51. Bodor JN, Rose D, Farley TA, Swalm C, Scott SK. Neighbourhood fruit and vegetable availability and consumption: the role of small food stores in an urban environment. Public Health Nutr. 2008;11:413–20.

52. Thornton LE, Pearce JR, Macdonald L, Lamb KE, Ellaway A. Does the choice of neighbourhood supermarket access measure influence associations with individual-level fruit and vegetable consumption? A case study from Glasgow. Int J Health Geogr. 2012;11:29.

53. English Indices of Deprivation 2010. http://data.gov.uk/dataset/index-of-multiple-deprivation.

54. Anyaegbu G. Using the OECD equivalence scale in taxes and benefits analysis. Econ Labour Mark Rev. 2010;4:49–54.

55. Pearce J, Blakely T, Witten K, Bartie P. Neighborhood deprivation and access to fast-food retailing: a national study. Am J Prev Med. 2007;32:375–82.

56. Richardson AS, Boone-Heinonen J, Popkin BM, Gordon-Larsen P. Are neighbourhood food resources distributed inequitably by income and race in the USA? Epidemiological findings across the urban spectrum. BMJ Open. 2012;2:e000698.

57. Blakely T, Woodward AJ. Ecological effects in multi-level studies. J Epidemiol Commun Health. 2000;54:367–74.

58. Riva M, Gauvin L, Apparicio P, Brodeur J-M. Disentangling the relative influence of built and socioeconomic environments on walking: the contribution of areas homogenous along exposures of interest. Soc Sci Med. 2009;69:1296–305.

59. Boyle MH, Willms JD. Place effects for areas defined by administrative boundaries. Am J Epidemiol. 1999;149:577–85.

60. Smith G, Gidlow C, Davey R, Foster C. What is my walking neighbourhood? A pilot study of English adults' definitions of their local walking neighbourhoods. Int J Behav Nutr Phys Act. 2010;. doi:10.1186/1479-5868-1187-1134.

61. Golledge RG, Stimson RJ. Spatial behavior: a geographic perspective. New York: The Guilford Press; 1997.

62. Kestens Y, Lebel A, Daniel M, Thériault M, Pampalon R. Using experienced activity spaces to measure foodscape exposure. Health Place. 2010;16:1094–103.

63. Kwan M-P. The uncertain geographic context problem. Ann Assoc Am Geogr. 2012;102:37–41.

64. Mehta NK, Chang VW. Weight status and restaurant availability a multilevel analysis. Am J Prev Med. 2008;34:127–33.

65. Powell LM, Chaloupka FJ, Bao Y. The availability of fast-food and full-service restaurants in the United States: associations with neighborhood characteristics. Am J Prev Med. 2007;33:S240–5.

66. Mason KE, Bentley RJ, Kavanagh AM. Fruit and vegetable purchasing and the relative density of healthy and unhealthy food stores: evidence from an Australian multilevel study. J Epidemiol Commun Health. 2013;67:231–6.

67. Kestens Y, Lebel A, Chaix B, Clary C, Daniel M, Pampalon R, Theriault M. SVPS: association between activity space exposure to food establishments and individual risk of overweight. PLoS One. 2012;7:e41418.

68. Mercille G, Richard L, Gauvin L, Kestens Y, Shatenstein B, Daniel M, Payette H. Associations between residential food environment and dietary patterns in urban-dwelling older adults: results from the VoisiNuAge study. Public Health Nutr. 2012;15:2026–39.

69. Flowerdew R, Manley DJ, Sabel CE. Neighbourhood effects on health: does it matter where you draw the boundaries? Soc Sci Med. 2008;66:1241–55.

70. Oliver LN, Schuurman N, Hall AW. Comparing circular and network buffers to examine the influence of land use on walking for leisure anderrands. Int J Health Geogr 2007;6:1–11.

71. Burgoine T, Alvanides S, Lake AA. Creating 'obesogenic realities'; Do our methodological choices make a difference when measuring the food environment? Int J Health Geogr. 2013;12:33.

72. Kerr J, Frank L, Sallis JF, Saelens B, Glanz K, Chapman J. Predictors of trips to food destinations. Int J Behav Nutr Phys Act. 2012;9:58.

73. Drewnowski A, Aggarwal A, Hurvitz PM, Monsivais P, Moudon AV. Obesity and supermarket access: proximity or price? Am J Public Health. 2012;102:e74–80.

74. Sampson R, Morenoff J. Durable inequality: spatial dynamics, social processes and the persistence of poverty in Chicago neighborhoods. In: Bowles S, Durlauf S, Hoff K, editors. Poverty traps. Princeton: Princeton University Press; 2006. p. 176–203.

75. Zenk SN, Schulz AJ, Matthews SA, Odoms-Young A, Wilbur J, Wegrzyn L, Gibbs K, Braunschweig C, Stokes C. Activity space environment and dietary and physical activity behaviors: a pilot study. Health Place. 2011;17:1150–61.

76. Christian WJ. Using geospatial technologies to explore activity-based retail food environments. Spat Spatiotemporal Epidemiol. 2012;3:287–95.

77. The effects of taxes and benefits on household income. https://www.ons.gov.uk/peoplepopulationandcommunity/personalandhouseholdfinances/incomeandwealth/datasets/theeffectsoftaxesandbenefitsonhouseholdincomefinancialyearending2014.

78. Local Area Analysis of Qualifications Across England and Wales. http://webarchive.nationalarchives.gov.uk/20160105160709/http://www.ons.gov.uk/ons/dcp171776_355401.pdf.

79. Choudhury Y, Hussain I, Parsons S, Rahman A, Eldridge S, Underwood M. Methodological challenges and approaches to improving response rates in population surveys in areas of extreme deprivation. Prim Health Care Res Dev. 2012;13:211–8.

80. Lebel A, Daepp MIG, Block JP, Walker R, Lalonde B, Kestens Y, Subramanian SV. Quantifying the foodscape: a systematic review and meta-analysis of the validity of commercially available business data. PLoS ONE. 2017;12:1–17.

5

Modelling and mapping tick dynamics using volunteered observations

Irene Garcia-Martí[1*] ⓘ, Raúl Zurita-Milla[1], Arnold J. H. van Vliet[2] and Willem Takken[3]

Abstract

Background: Tick populations and tick-borne infections have steadily increased since the mid-1990s posing an ever-increasing risk to public health. Yet, modelling tick dynamics remains challenging because of the lack of data and knowledge on this complex phenomenon. Here we present an approach to model and map tick dynamics using volunteered data. This approach is illustrated with 9 years of data collected by a group of trained volunteers who sampled active questing ticks (AQT) on a monthly basis and for 15 locations in the Netherlands. We aimed at finding the main environmental drivers of AQT at multiple time-scales, and to devise daily AQT maps at the national level for 2014.

Method: Tick dynamics is a complex ecological problem driven by biotic (e.g. pathogens, wildlife, humans) and abiotic (e.g. weather, landscape) factors. We enriched the volunteered AQT collection with six types of weather variables (aggregated at 11 temporal scales), three types of satellite-derived vegetation indices, land cover, and mast years. Then, we applied a feature engineering process to derive a set of 101 features to characterize the conditions that yielded a particular count of AQT on a date and location. To devise models predicting the AQT, we use a time-aware Random Forest regression method, which is suitable to find non-linear relationships in complex ecological problems, and provides an estimation of the most important features to predict the AQT.

Results: We trained a model capable of fitting AQT with reduced statistical metrics. The multi-temporal study on the feature importance indicates that variables linked to water levels in the atmosphere (i.e. evapotranspiration, relative humidity) consistently showed a higher explanatory power than previous works using temperature. As a product of this study, we are able of mapping daily tick dynamics at the national level.

Conclusions: This study paves the way towards the design of new applications in the fields of environmental research, nature management, and public health. It also illustrates how Citizen Science initiatives produce geospatial data collections that can support scientific analysis, thus enabling the monitoring of complex environmental phenomena.

Keywords: Tick dynamics, Random forest, Volunteered geographic information (VGI), Data analysis, Environmental modelling

Background

Tick populations and tick-borne infections like Lyme borreliosis have steadily increased since the mid-1990s. This concurrent increase has been observed in various European countries [19, 23], in the US [48] and in Canada

*Correspondence: i.garciamarti@utwente.nl
[1] Department of Geo-Information Processing (GIP), Faculty of Geo-Information and Earth Observation (ITC), University of Twente, Enschede, The Netherlands
Full list of author information is available at the end of the article

[31]. In the Netherlands, periodic national studies among general practitioners (GPs), revealed a consistent two-decade rising trend in the number of tick bites consultations and Lyme borreliosis diagnoses [22], that only showed a first sign of stabilization recently. Still, more than 20,000 people per year develop Lyme borreliosis in the Netherlands and its disease burden is substantial, especially in patients who develop chronical symptoms [21].

Scientists of different fields have investigated this global increase of tick populations and tick-borne infections, converging upon two main causes: global environmental changes are altering the spatio-temporal dynamics of ticks [29, 47] and socio-economic changes are changing the spatial patterns of human populations around urbanized areas, increasing the human exposure to ticks [38, 40, 53]. Tick dynamics are complex ecological processes driven by numerous factors (i.e. wildlife, weather, vegetation, landscape). Understanding the interactions between these factors and tick dynamics is crucial to develop models capable of forecasting the incidence and distribution of ticks and tick-borne diseases [12, 33].

Models predicting the spatio-temporal distribution of ticks are needed to implement control measures which mitigate future disease infections [9, 18] or help managing public health risks [29]. However, the development of such models is not straightforward due to several issues. First, it is unclear what the best set of environmental predictors are. Past studies have found correlations between different combinations of biotic and abiotic factors and tick dynamics, but the spatio-temporal scale of these experiments is diverse enough to pose difficulties in drawing general conclusions. For instance, Berger et al. [2, 3] found a link between relative humidity and the seasonal abundance of ticks at the regional level. Dantas-Torres and Otranto [10] found weak correlations at local scale between monthly temperature, evapotranspiration and saturation deficit with tick abundances, whereas [42] found links (in laboratory conditions) between the saturation deficit and the number of questing ticks. Second, it is often unclear at what time scales the different predictors operate. Previous studies have found linear correlations between tick abundances and environmental predictors at multiple temporal scales [2, 3, 50]. However, the temporal sparsity of the tick sampling or the use of short-term time series question if these correlations are scalable to long-term time series at the country level. Third, tick dynamics are complex phenomena that traditionally have been modelled with linear methods. Two of the well-known disadvantages of classical linear methods is that they are not capable of finding non-linear interactions between variables (except when explicitly included a priori), and do not properly handle large numbers of predictors (e.g. due to collinearity). However, such data are a reality when modelling complex natural phenomena.

In this work, we address the above-mentioned issues by modelling nine years of monthly data on Active Questing Ticks (AQT) collected by volunteers on 15 different locations in the Netherlands. This modelling exercise includes a wide array of (a) biotic predictors and, by applying an ensemble regression method (i.e. random

forest), we aim at identifying the most important variables to model AQT at multiple time-scales. Building such AQT dynamic model allows us to explore and map tick's seasonality across the Netherlands. We envision applications of this model in the fields of environmental and ecological research, nature management and public health, which hopefully will reduce the incidence of Lyme disease.

Ticks and environment
Tick sampling

Ticks are blood sucking arthropods capable of transmitting a wide variety of pathogens (e.g. bacteria, viruses) which cause disease in humans [19]. Deciduous or mixed forests in temperate and humid regions, which are inhabited by different mammalian species (e.g. deer, rodents), create optimal habitats sustaining ticks life cycle [33]. Ticks quest at the top of vegetation or litter layer, waiting for a human or animal host to attach and feed. This behavior is used to determine tick populations in a particular location. To do so, two manual monitoring techniques are used: flagging and dragging. Flagging consists on sweeping a squared cloth attached to a pole on one side upon the litter or vegetation layers, whereas dragging consists in attaching the previous material to a rope, which the investigator can pull along the study area [45]. In both cases, ticks that are touched by the cloth attach to it, allowing researchers to count the number of ticks in its different life stages (i.e. larvae, nymph, or adult). Both techniques have been widely used in small scale biological studies to acquire raw data on tick counts that can be later incorporated in a scientific workflow [10, 11, 13, 15, 41].

Environmental factors

Ticks are particularly susceptible to environmental conditions because of their high surface-to-volume ratio, which makes them experience water losses through their exoskeleton, and their lack of thermal inertia, which makes them vulnerable to extreme weather conditions [33]. The following sub sections list the environmental variables used in our work and sketch their impact on tick dynamics.

Weather data

Temperature determines the start of the questing season, tick population development rate and the chances of survival through the winter season [32, 40, 52]. Precipitation and relative humidity are crucial to sustain tick populations in nature. Precipitation is necessary during the summer season [25], but extreme precipitation events (i.e. drought and heavy rain) may prevent the development of new tick populations [33]. Long-lasting and adverse humidity conditions have been linked to an increased mortality among nymphal ticks and this, in turn, may decrease the total number of cases of Lyme disease [2, 3]. Some studies suggest that nymphal ticks can desiccate within 48 h if the humidity conditions at ground level are suboptimal [2, 3]. Additionally, relative humidity and temperature can be used to calculate the saturation deficit and vapor pressure. Saturation deficit has been used in a previous and thorough study to understand the role of humidity in tick survival [42] and vapor pressure has been identified as a major indicator of tick habitat suitability [8]. In some studies, evapotranspiration has been used as a proxy for vapor pressure deficit [44].

Weather datasets are publicly available at the online data center of the Royal Netherlands Meteorological Institute (KNMI).[1] We downloaded daily gridded layers of temperature, precipitation, evapotranspiration and relative humidity for the period 2005–2014. From temperature and relative humidity, we obtained saturation deficit and vapour pressure [30, 42]. The temporal resolution of the weather datasets and the tick sampling is different, since the former are available at daily temporal resolution, whereas the latter is carried out on a unique day each month. To match both resolutions, it is necessary to aggregate the weather variables to a coarser temporal scale in a way that reflect the impact later caused on the tick count.

Vegetation data from satellites

Ticks are sensitive to local environmental conditions, such as the thickness of forest canopy or soil moisture at the ground level [29]. Earth observation satellites allow the monitoring of these environmental conditions over large areas. In this work, we used three vegetation indices to characterize local environmental conditions: the Normalized Difference Vegetation Index (NDVI), the Enhanced Vegetation Index (EVI) and the Normalized Difference Water Index (NDWI). Previous studies have demonstrated that fluctuations in NDVI, which has traditionally been used to measure the greenness and the density of vegetation, correlate well with fluctuations in the number of nymphs and adult ticks and that NDVI can be used as a proxy to find suitable tick habitats [11, 39]. More recent studies show that novel vegetation indices like EVI or NDWI are better estimators of tick populations [1] and Lyme disease incidence [37].

Vegetation indices are publicly available in the Google Earth Engine (GEE) platform.[2],[3] GEE is a free image pro-

cessing cloud platform for environmental analysis, which aggregates and integrates products coming from different Earth observation sensors, such as the Moderate-Resolution Imaging Spectroradiometer (MODIS). MODIS provides daily global imagery at 250, 500 and 1000 m of spatial resolution. However, due to the persistent cloud coverage over the Netherlands we used MODIS composite products. In particular, we used the MCD43A4 product, which provides the NDVI, EVI and NDWI indices derived from the daily surface reflectance at a pixel size of 500 m, using data of the previous 16 days. It is important to note that this product is released every 8 days, so there is a 50% of temporal overlap between each composite, meaning that the vegetation signal will contain smooth changes.

Land cover, tick habitat and mast years

Land cover is another important factor in the field of tick ecology because it influences tick survival and determines the chances of human-tick contact. Ticks prefer habitats where the vegetation prevents reaching desiccation conditions and where hosts (e.g. deer, rodents, mice) species are present. Complex landscapes, in which multiple land covers are intertwined in a small area unit, increase the probability of contact between ticks and their human or animal hosts [17, 26, 27, 51]. For land cover we use the 7th release of the national land cover database or LGN (Landelijk Grondgebruik Nederland[4]). This database was produced in 2012 and contains information for 39 classes at 25 m.

The sampling sites are located in forested areas with specific types of vegetation (i.e. deciduous and coniferous forest, grasses, and bushlands). The plant associations in these sites contribute determining the presence of wildlife species in each location, by providing forage or shelter, and subsequently, tick populations move with them. Previous studies have demonstrated that deciduous forests present higher abundances of AQT than coniferous forest, and also that a dense shrub layer has a positive effect on tick populations [49]. Gassner et al. [15] gives a thorough description of the plant associations and habitat characteristics found in the surroundings of each transect of the flagging sites.

Mast seeding is a natural phenomenon in which certain plant species synchronously produce an abnormal amount of acorns and nuts [46]. This overproduction feeds a wide range of animal species and contributes to a steep increase of their populations for the next season. When the populations of rodents, deer and other tick host species increase, the same occurs with tick populations [34, 36]. Dutch volunteers from the Mammal

---

[1] https://data.knmi.nl/datasets.

[2] https://code.earthengine.google.com/.

[3] https://earthengine.google.com/.

[4] http://tinyurl.com/j47m2ol.

Association (http://www.zoogdiervereniging.nl) quantify each year the amount of acorns produced for beech, oak and American oak. The amount of acorns is classified in a categorical scale that goes from 0 to 5 depending on how strong the mast year.

Data

This work relies on a unique dataset of tick dynamics collected by volunteers in the context of a project of participatory modelling. This dataset was enriched with a set of environmental variables extracted for each sampling location. For this, we collected and preprocessed weather and satellite data, and included biological data regarding habitat and mast years. The remaining of this section first contains a description of the volunteered tick counts data ("Volunteered tick counts reports" section), and then we explain the process of feature engineering carried out to create a series of predictors that characterize tick dynamics as monitored by volunteers.

Volunteered tick counts reports

In the context of the Dutch phenological network Nature's Calendar (www.natuurkalender.nl) every month

since July 2006, a group of volunteers sampled AQT on 24 forest sites. This joint effort aimed to quantify and understand the spatial and temporal dynamics of ticks and the Borrelia bacteria that can cause Lyme disease [15]. Out of the 24 sites participating in the research project, we were able to include data from 15 sites, which represent a total of 3073 observations collected by volunteers. We excluded the sites in which the sampling stopped in an early stage of the project, or the site was sparsely sampled in time. At each site, volunteers sampled two transects, separated from each other several hundred meters. Ticks were collected using a technique called "dragging", in which the volunteer drags a 1 m² cloth over the low vegetation of each transect for 100 m, turning the cloth every 25 m to count the number of larvae, nymphs and adult ticks. This study focuses on the nymphs because they pose the highest risk for humans to get a tick bite. Figure 1 shows the raw number of nymphs per transect and per month. The number of AQT across all sites present strong spatial and temporal variations: (1) some transects present a more continuous and recurrent shape, whereas others have an erratic tick count (e.g. Gieten vs. Bilthoven); (2) some transects produce very

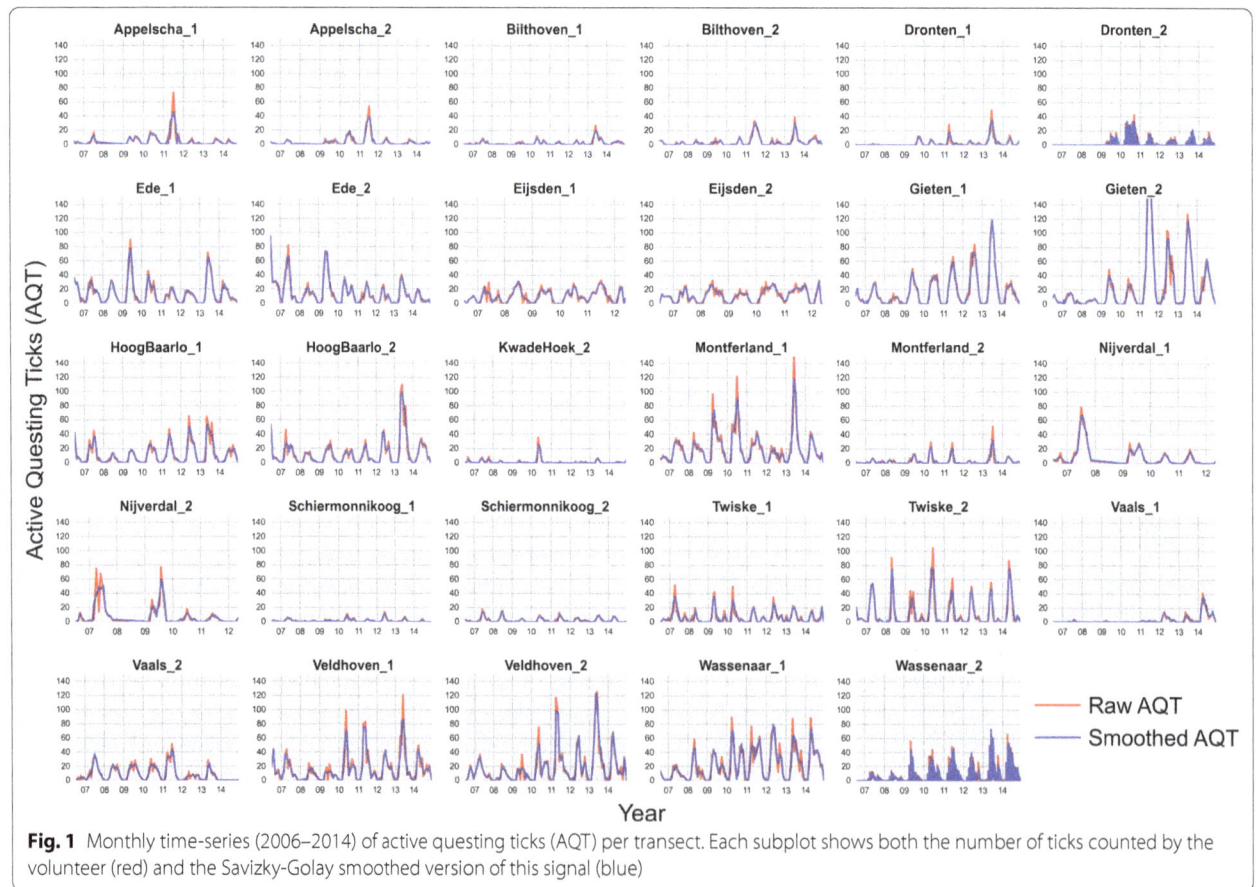

Fig. 1 Monthly time-series (2006–2014) of active questing ticks (AQT) per transect. Each subplot shows both the number of ticks counted by the volunteer (red) and the Savizky-Golay smoothed version of this signal (blue)

different yields, from low tick counts to high peaks (e.g. Veldhoven vs. Eijsden); (3) transects within a sampling site may yield a different number of ticks, even though they are close in space and sampled on the same day (e.g. Montferland). The reasons of these strong local and seasonal variations are still poorly understood, but previous works have found clear links between tick populations and the abundance of small mammals in the area [35], mast years [24] or warming weather conditions [25, 48], which are major influences over tick dynamics, as seen in "Environmental factors" section.

Volunteered projects have proved useful to acquire information at a timely and fine spatial scale, but the quality and the amount of uncertainty of such data collections is difficult to measure [4, 5, 16]. A visual inspection of Fig. 1 shows that the monthly tick counts signal presents an irregular and noisy shape. A closer descriptive analysis of the raw data reveals that out of 3073 records in the dataset, around one-third of the samples are zeros, and a small proportion of samples present high peaks. Zero AQT means that a volunteer visited a site for tick sampling on a particular date and no ticks were caught questing, whereas a peaky AQT means the ticks were very active on that day.

To assess the potential impact that zero and peaky AQT may have in our modelling process, we created four versions of the original dataset, which vary in the amount of zeroes and peaky observations. In two datasets we removed all samples with a zero AQT within the tick season (i.e. 1st March until 31st October) and half of the samples with a zero AQT outside the season. This creates a group with two datasets with a reduced amount of zeros, and a second group with two datasets which are not modified with respect to the original. After this step, we applied a smoothing process to only one of the datasets of each group. We chose a Savitzky–Golay filter to mitigate the effect of peaky AQT in the modelling process, whereas the other dataset was kept with the original AQT signal. In this way, the modelling process accounts for the possible effect of extreme observations to fit the AQT signal, and helps distinguishing whether varying levels of noise is hampering the learning process of the chosen modelling algorithm.

Characterizing the environment

Feature engineering is a common process in the machine learning field to obtain new predictors from original data sources, which incorporate the knowledge of a domain to create predictive models. In our case, we obtained a set of features, based in the theoretical grounds described in "Tick sampling" and "Environmental factors" sections, which aim to that aim to characterize the environmental conditions in each tick sampling site. Thus, this work uses 101 features (Table 1) classified in five types: weather, remote-sensed vegetation, land cover, habitat and mast. Weather and vegetation features contain a value aggregated in a particular time window. Land cover, habitat and mast features contain the value of land cover in a point, the type of tick habitat in the sampling sites, and the strength of a mast year for three tree species, respectively. The remaining of this section describes how the features associated to each type were obtained from the original data sources.

Because of the lack of consensus in the literature on the optimal temporal unit(s) to model AQT, we created a suite of features by aggregating each weather variable (i.e. minimum and maximum temperature, precipitation, evapotranspiration, relative humidity, saturation deficit, and vapour pressure deficit) at multiple temporal scales. These temporal scales are defined by the number of days before the date of the tick sampling. The reason for doing this is straightforward: we assume the tick count produced today, depends on past weather conditions. Therefore, for each tick sampling date we calculated weather features using a range of 1–7 days before the sampling date (i.e. fine temporal units), and of 14, 30, 90 and 365 days (i.e. coarse temporal units). This procedure leads to 11 features per weather variable, adding up a total of 77 features (indices 16–92, type W).

Using GEE, we averaged the 3–4 images available per month to reduce the impact of clouds. Then, using the coordinates of each of the flagging sites, we obtained three (NDVI, EVI and NDWI) time-series summarizing the evolution of vegetation indices since 2005. To remove further noise in these time series, we decomposed each of them into their seasonal, trend and noise components. We kept the seasonal component and obtained the minimum value and range (i.e. width between the minimum and maximum values) per transect and vegetation index. This procedure creates 6 vegetation features (indices 93–98, type V) that condense the general vegetation and moisture conditions in the site over the time-series.

For the land cover, we reduced the number of classes to 12 due to two reasons: (1) the flagging sites are located only in certain types of land cover (e.g. deciduous, grasslands); (2) several land cover types are unrelated to the tick ecology (e.g. sweet water, saltmarshes) or can be aggregated to a coarser level (e.g. types of crop to agricultural land), thus can be unified in a single category. After re-classifying the LGN, the product was resampled to 500 and 1000 m of spatial resolution using a majority filter. This process allows to account for the surroundings of each flagging site, and reduces the chances of the flagging site to be placed in a noisy pixel at 25 m resolution. We obtained the value of the land cover for each of the flagging sites at these three different spatial resolutions

Table 1 List of features involved in the current analysis

ID	Feature name	Short description	Type
1	Litter	Thickness of litter layer (Gassner et al. [15])	H
2	Moss	Coverage on a 1–10 scale of the moss layer	H
3	Herb	Coverage on a 1–10 scale of the herb layer	H
4	Brush	Coverage on a 1–10 scale of the brush layer	H
5	Tree	Coverage on a 1–10 scale of the tree layer	H
6	BioLC	Land cover as described in [15]	H
7	Oak-Y	Strength of mast year in a oak forests	M
8	AOak-Y	Strength of mast year in American oak forests	M
9	Beech-Y	Strength of mast year in European beech forests	M
16	tmin-X	Average minimum temperature in a time window	W
17	tmax-X	Average maximum temperature in a time window	W
18	prec-X	Average precipitation in a time window	W
19	rv-X	Average evapotranspiration in a time window	W
20	rh-X	Average relative humidity in a time window	W
21	sd-X	Average saturation deficit in a time window	W
22	vp-X	Average vapour pressure in a time window	W
93	min_ndvi	Minimum NDVI value for a particular location in a year	V
94	range_ndvi	Range for NDVI value for a particular location in a year	V
95	min_evi	Minimum EVI value for a particular location in a year	V
96	range_evi	Range for EVI value for a particular location in a year	V
97	min_ndwi	Minimum NDWI value for a particular location in a year	V
98	range_ndvi	Range for NDWI value for a particular location in a year	V
99	lc25 m	Land cover type in a particular location at 25 m spatial resolution	L
100	lc500 m	Land cover type in a particular location at 500 m spatial resolution	L
101	lc1 km	Land cover type in a particular location at 1 km spatial resolution	L

The features belong to the following categories: tick habitat (H), mast years (M), weather (W), vegetation (V) and land cover (L). The weather features are calculated at 11 temporal aggregations, so there are 77 weather features in total. The X character is replaced by a number between 1 and 7 for short-term temporal aggregations or by a 14, 30, 90 or 365 in the case of bi-weekly, monthly, seasonal or yearly temporal aggregation, respectively. Mast features have a Y character that will be replaced by a number between 0 and 2 in function of the mast year they are referring to. In total, there are 101 features involved in this work

(indices 99-101, type L). The strength of the mast year of the year of the observation, as well as the strength of the previous 2 years (indices 7–15, Type M) is included in our work, because tick dynamics might have a delayed response to mast years. Finally, the habitat characteristics per transect are described using 5 variables: the thickness of litter layer and the amount of moss, herbal, brush and tree layers, which are encoded in 5 features (indices 1–6, Type H).

Modelling AQT with Random Forest

Random forest (RF) [6] is an ensemble learning method that can be used both for classification and regression problems. Ensemble methods rely on the creation of a committee of experts, which work on solving a real-world problem while minimize the chances of taking a poor decision. In the case of RF, the ensemble is formed by a group of weak learners called decision trees, which are combined to create a robust decision ensemble.

RF is a combination of the bagging growing scheme [7] and the random subspace method [20]. These two sources of randomness contribute to create an ensemble with very different trees that lead to high variance predictions when tested individually [28]. Bagging allows RF to see multiple variations of the input data, whereas the RSM introduces randomness in the samples and features presented to each tree during the learning phase. This process creates an ensemble of trees, which is capable of adapting to the tick dynamics phenomenon, and yield predictions with great robustness and stability [43].

The mechanism used by RF to grow decision trees for regression problems, such as modelling AQT as a function of environmental features, is conceptually simple. For each tree (B), N bootstrap samples (with replacement) are drawn from the available training data. This subsample is used to grow a unique decision tree (T_b) by recursively partitioning the N samples until a stop condition is reached, namely: (1) all the samples within a node have the same target response target; (2) the samples in the node are homogeneous with respect to the selected features; (3) a heuristic, such as the maximum depth of the tree, is reached. If none of these conditions are met, the algorithm grows the tree by selecting the best feature and split point among a given and random subset of training features, where best means that it minimizes the Mean Squared Error (MSE). This process creates two child nodes, and the available samples are assigned to them considering the split criteria (e.g. samples with values for feature m larger than the split point value go to the left child node). This procedure is repeated until a full forest with B trees is grown.

After completing the training phase, RF predicts unseen samples by averaging the predictions of the B trees. This reduce the variance and the generalization error of the predictions. In fact, the generalization error converges as the number of trees increases, thus reducing the chances of overfitting data [6, 43].

A key characteristic of RF is that it provides a measure of the importance of the features involved in the modelling. This is done by averaging the reduction in MSE associated to the use of each variable in each of the nodes/trees that form the ensemble [28]. In our work, we exploit this characteristic to understand the main drivers of tick dynamics. Thus, the ranking of features provided by RF gives an idea about what the most relevant (or irrelevant) features are, regardless of the dimensionality of the problem. This is particularly suitable to understand the complex and non-linear interactions found in biological and environmental systems.

RF, like most data-driven regression methods, are not time-aware models. This means that its standard application to regression problems involving (seasonal) time-series, such as the AQT dataset, can lead to sub-optimal results. The reason for this is that the trees in the RF ensemble are trained with random subsets of the training set, where each data sample belongs to a particular date. Thus, RF is trained to predict single snapshots and remains unaware of the temporal continuity of the time-series.

In this work we overcome this limitation by introducing time-awareness in RF. To do so, we transformed the AQT counts into monthly Z-scores by: (1) grouping the 9 years of observations according to the month when they were collected; (2) calculating monthly means and standard deviations, after removing extreme observations from each group so that the Z-scores are not biased. In this context, extreme observations are those that report AQT counts above the 3rd quartile or below the 1st quartile of the monthly values; (3) creating monthly Z-scores, by subtracting the monthly mean from each observation, and dividing the result by the corresponding monthly standard deviation. In this way, we ensure that samples collected during the same month have a constrained and normalized range of AQT counts.

With this monthly normalization we train RF to understand which factors increase or decrease AQT with respect to the long-term average, instead of modelling the absolute number of ticks recorded in a particular location and month. Moreover, by predicting monthly Z-scores we help RF to understand the temporality of the data and hope to get more realistic seasonal dynamics than by using the classical (single snapshot) RF model.

The general set-up of the RF models was as follows: (1) we reserved 70% of the data for training, and the remaining 30% was used for testing the model. Samples were randomly assigned to the training and test subsets; (2) To account for the randomness of RF (different features and samples used in each tree/run), we executed the models 10 times (keeping the training and test samples constant) and the error metrics and feature importance were averaged; (3) we use two well-known statistical metrics to validate our results, the root mean squared error (RMSE) and the normalized RMSE (NRMSE). Note that the error metrics were obtained after de-normalizing the Z-scored signal. Finally, we used the trained model to prepare maps illustrating its performance in a country-wide scenario.

Experiments

The process described in "Volunteered tick counts reports" section creates four versions of the original dataset with a varying number of zero and peaky AQT, and the process of feature engineering from "Characterizing the environment" section enriches each of the volunteered observations with 101 features. With this set-up, we designed the tree experiments explained in the next sub sections, whose goal is: (1) to assess the impact of noisy observations and selecting the best model capable of capturing AQT dynamics; (2) to evaluate the most important features to model AQT at different time scales; (3) to create AQT map for forested areas in the Netherlands.

Model selection by assessing the impact of noisy AQT

We modelled the four versions of the volunteered AQT dataset with our time-aware version of RF. Figure 2 shows the general performance of the models. To ease the interpretation of these results, three elements are included: (1) a 1:1 line showing the ideal predictions; (2) a grey band showing one standard deviation from the mean of the observations; (3) a grey box containing the selected statistical metrics for this experiment. The visual inspection of the four plots shows that the two experiments using raw data perform poorly when compared to the two

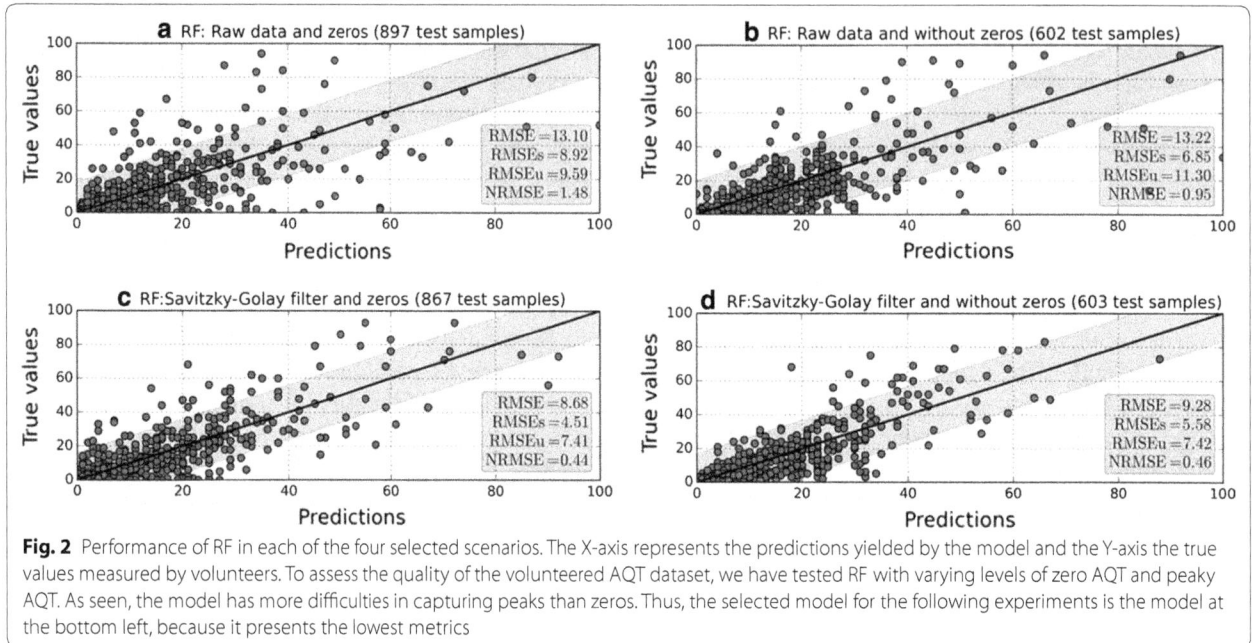

Fig. 2 Performance of RF in each of the four selected scenarios. The X-axis represents the predictions yielded by the model and the Y-axis the true values measured by volunteers. To assess the quality of the volunteered AQT dataset, we have tested RF with varying levels of zero AQT and peaky AQT. As seen, the model has more difficulties in capturing peaks than zeros. Thus, the selected model for the following experiments is the model at the bottom left, because it presents the lowest metrics

experiments using smoothed data. The models built with raw data have the highest errors in terms of RMSE and NRMSE and also present a higher dispersion of the predictions, indicating that these models did not properly capture the peaky AQT observations.

A close inspection of the NRMSE metric reveals that RF models with smoothed data present very similar performances, regardless of the number of zeros left in the AQT dataset. This suggests that smoothed models can capture the conditions yielding low AQT, but peaky AQT may be actually hampering the modelling process. This is clearly visible when inspecting the points falling outside the gray band in the bottom subplots: a certain number of high AQT true observations could not be captured by the model, thus producing a lower prediction than the true value. We selected the model for next experiments based on the lowest RMSE and NRMSE metrics, thus, out of the four models, we picked the one keeping zero AQT and smoothing the peaky AQT with the Savitzky-Golay filter.

Table 2 presents the feature importance of the top 10 features for the selected RF model. To ease the interpretation of results, we restrict the ranking of the feature importance to the top 10 most prominent out of 101. As seen in this table, the modelled phenomenon is driven by a combination of several weather variables and a vegetation one. The two most explanatory features are the annual evapotranspiration (i.e. ev-365) and the monthly relative humidity (i.e. rh-30). Temperature, which has been traditionally spotted in tick modelling studies as a major driver of tick dynamics, only appears

Table 2 Ranking of the top ten most important features (out of 101) for the selected RF model

Position	Feature	Importance
1	ev-365	15
2	rh-30	11
3	tmax-365	7
4	prec-90	4
5	prec-3	4
6	ev-90	3
7	rh-365	3
8	tmin-365	2
9	prec-365	2
10	tmax-90	2

The sum of the feature importance for all features provided by RF equals to 1, but to ease the interpretation of results we multiplied it by a hundred to have natural numbers. As seen, features involving atmospheric water levels (i.e. evapotranspiration and relative humidity) are found to be important to predict tick activity, since they appear several times in the current ranking

once (as tmax-365) and with a relatively low importance. In this experiment, water-related features perform better than temperature. Note that evapotranspiration and relative humidity do appear several times in the ranking (i.e. ev-90, rh-365), suggesting that in a context with multiple atmospheric variables, water-levels are again more important than temperature. It is also important to highlight that variables about mast years or tick habitat do not appear in the top ten. This could be because they are static (i.e. one value for the whole study period) and, hence, unable to explain the temporal and spatial variation in seen in the AQT dataset.

To further evaluate the usefulness of our RF-based model to predict AQT, we split the test samples according to their associated transect (cf. Fig. 3). The goodness of the fitting (R^2) between the predictions and the real smoothed AQT values varies between 0.19 and 0.94, indicating that the performance of the model strongly depends on each transect. In Fig. 4 (left) we sort the R^2 values to provide a better depiction of the performance of the model per transect. Based on these results, we note that the model presents a moderate-to-strong R^2 (i.e. $0.7 < R^2 < 1$) for roughly half of the sites. This means that these transects better respond to weather variables than the remaining transects, in which AQT may be driven by variables, such as wildlife, not included in the current model. Note that for transects within the same site (e.g. Vaals, Montferland) the goodness of fit is very different, revealing the very local nature of AQT. Figure 4 (right) shows the geographic representation of the transects. Symbols in green represent the transects better responding to weather variables, whereas red symbols represent the poorly fitted transects. The visual inspection of this figure shows no strong spatial pattern (e.g. north–south gradient).

Feature importance across multiple time scales

The model structure selected in the previous section is used here to find out the best temporal scale to model AQT. To do so, we train one RF model for each of the 11 time scales described in "Characterizing the environment" section and we execute the model with a subset of features of the input dataset: we keep all the non-weather features (a total of 24 features) and we add the weather features corresponding to that particular time scale (7 features). Thus, we run the modelling process 11 times with 31 features, providing at each iteration the feature importance. In this way, it is possible to get new insights about whether the importance of the features to model AQT change over increasing temporal windows, which might guide the choice of a particular time scale to model AQT optimally.

Table 3 shows the importance of the features at multiple time scales. Each column of the table shows the top five most important features (out of 31) for each of the selected time scales. To ease the description of results at multiple time scales, we restrict the ranking of features to the most relevant top five. This table shows that the most explanatory features for all time scales are

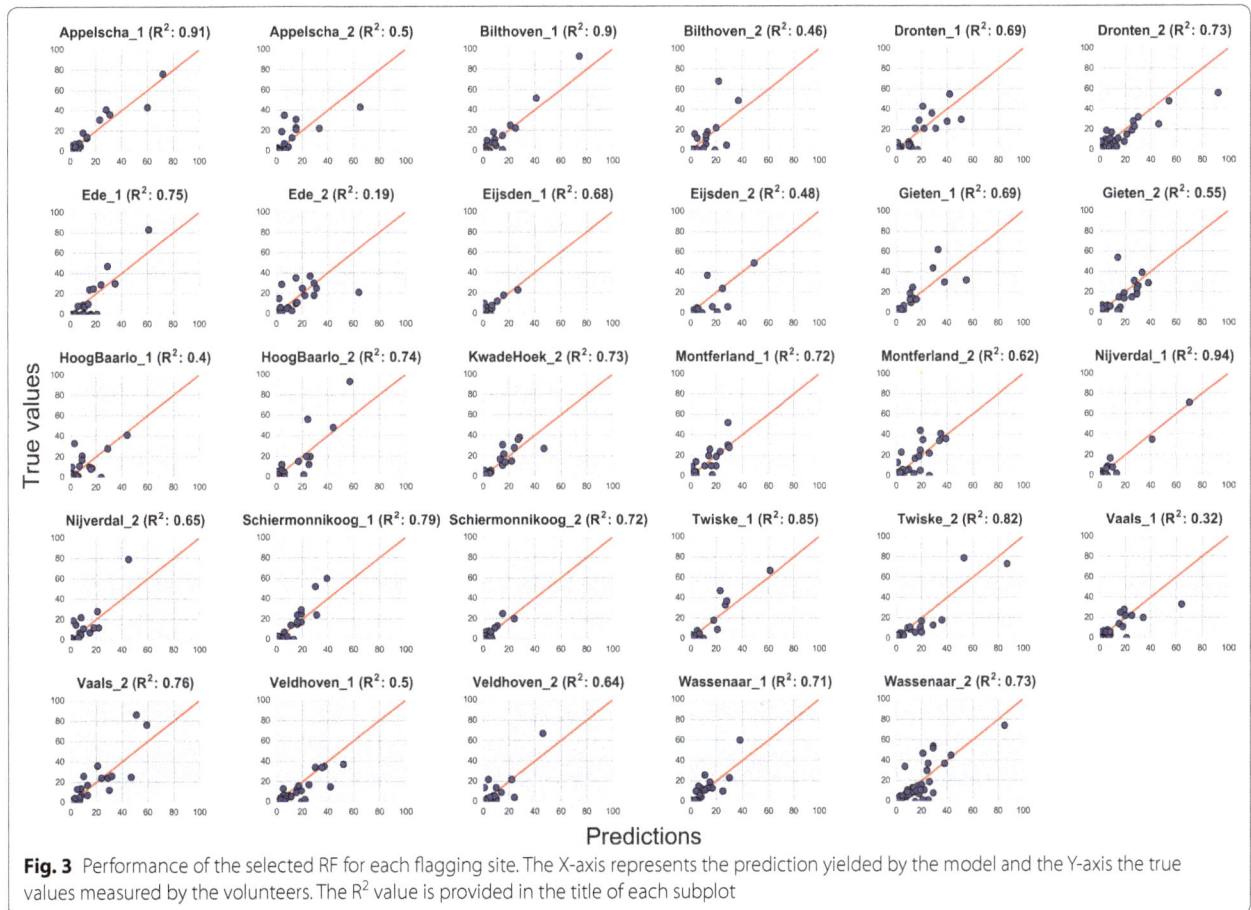

Fig. 3 Performance of the selected RF for each flagging site. The X-axis represents the prediction yielded by the model and the Y-axis the true values measured by the volunteers. The R^2 value is provided in the title of each subplot

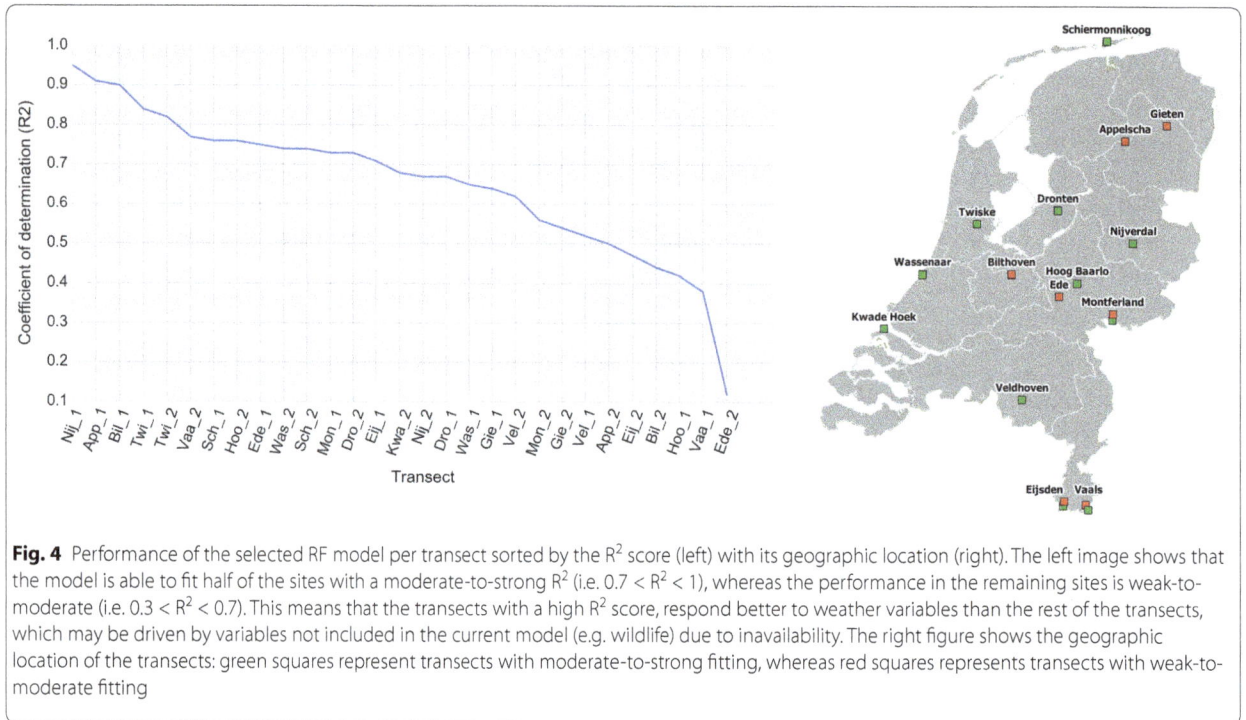

Fig. 4 Performance of the selected RF model per transect sorted by the R^2 score (left) with its geographic location (right). The left image shows that the model is able to fit half of the sites with a moderate-to-strong R^2 (i.e. $0.7 < R^2 < 1$), whereas the performance in the remaining sites is weak-to-moderate (i.e. $0.3 < R^2 < 0.7$). This means that the transects with a high R^2 score, respond better to weather variables than the rest of the transects, which may be driven by variables not included in the current model (e.g. wildlife) due to inavailability. The right figure shows the geographic location of the transects: green squares represent transects with moderate-to-strong fitting, whereas red squares represents transects with weak-to-moderate fitting

Table 3 Ranking of the top five features for the selected RF model across all temporal scales

	Days																							
	1		2		3		4		5		6		7		14		30		90		365	
	F	I	F	I	F	I	F	I	F	I	F	I	F	I	F	I	F	I	F	I	F	I
Ranking																						
1	EV	15	EV	15	EV	15	EV	15	TX	16	TX	14	EV	14	TX	14	TX	15	RH	17	RH	16
2	TX	13	TX	14	TX	14	TX	14	EV	13	EV	13	TX	13	TN	13	PR	14	EV	15	TX	15
3	TN	11	TN	12	PR	13	PR	11	TN	12	P	13	TN	12	EV	12	RH	12	PR	14	PR	13
4	RH	11	RH	11	TN	12	TN	11	PR	11	RH	12	RH	12	PR	12	TN	12	SD	9	EV	13
5	PR	10	PR	9	RH	10	RH	10	RH	10	TN	9	PR	11	RH	11	EV	11	TN	9	TN	12

Each feature is accompanied by its importance, which has been calculated as the mean of 10 runs. Features involving atmospheric water levels (i.e. evapotranspiration and relative humidity) are found to be relevant to model tick activity in all temporal scales. These results are consistent with the ones provided by the general model. Interestingly, evapotranspiration is marked as the most relevant feature in very short-term time scales, whereas relative humidity is a better predictor for long time scales

weather-based ones and that non-weather features (i.e. vegetation, land cover, tick habitat, mast years) do not significantly contribute to model tick dynamics. Evapotranspiration, relative humidity and the maximum temperature appear to be the most important features. EV better performed in the short-term experiments (i.e. temporal aggregation from 1 day to 4 days before the sampling date), whereas RH is the best one in the long-term experiments (i.e. seasonal and annual temporal aggregation). TX appears to be the best predictor in the remaining experiments.

Mapping tick dynamics

The RF model selected in "Model selection by assessing the impact of noisy AQT" section was used in a country-wide exercise to produce three map products: the mean and standard deviation of AQT for the year 2014, and the AQT on a date expected to be close to the peak activity of ticks in nymphal stage. We selected the year 2014 because it is the last of the AQT time-series.

Since the flagging sites are located in forested areas, we identified forested pixels in the land cover map and extracted their locations. Then, to this selection of pixels, we applied the process of feature engineering described in "Characterizing the environment" section for each day of the selected year, thus obtaining 365 country level datasets. The model was retrained with the 86 features available at the country level (i.e. remove tick habitat and mast year features) and tested with the newly created datasets for forested pixels. The predictions yielded by the model were transformed into raster format to obtain three products: first, we obtained the annual mean and standard deviation of AQT based on the daily computed values, which identifies at the country level regions with higher or lower tick activity; second, we obtained the temporal profile of the pixels containing the sites to visualize the daily seasonality of AQT; third, we mapped the AQT for a particular day of the year, which is expected to be close to the peak of tick populations in the nymphal stage.

Figure 5 illustrates the annual mean (left) and standard deviation (right) of predicted AQT. A visual inspection of the mean map shows that there are more AQT in the eastern half of the country (i.e. orange to red regions),

especially within the provinces of Overijssel and Drenthe. The standard deviation map depicts the spatial variability of the predictions: regions in light green and yellow show areas where the predictions oscillated significantly above or below the mean AQT, whereas regions in dark blue show locations where the prediction is stable throughout the year. Figure 6 shows the daily temporal evolution of AQT for the grid cells where the flagging sites are located. This figure also shows three additional elements: the long-term monthly average for all sites obtained from the boxplots, the long-term monthly average for the site, and the 2014 monthly average for the site. Note that there are 15 sub plots, because each grid cell overlaps the two transects. This allows to visually identify sites whose predicted AQT is (dis)similar to the averages. Figure 7 shows the predicted AQT for June 1st, which we expect to be close to this peak population of nymphs. As seen, the highest predictions of AQT are predicted in the east half of the country, but there is another spot of high activity in the southern province of Noord-Brabant.

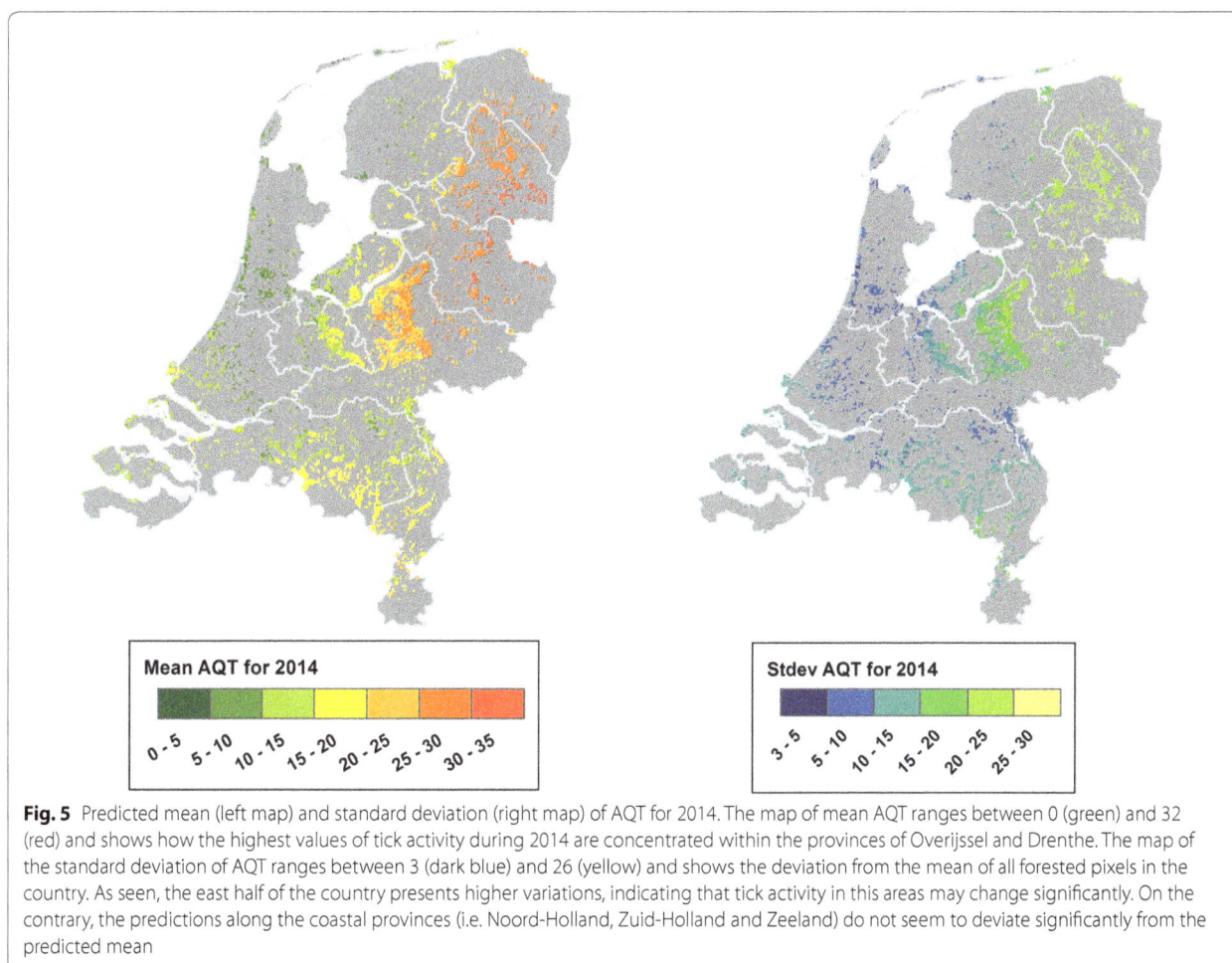

Fig. 5 Predicted mean (left map) and standard deviation (right map) of AQT for 2014. The map of mean AQT ranges between 0 (green) and 32 (red) and shows how the highest values of tick activity during 2014 are concentrated within the provinces of Overijssel and Drenthe. The map of the standard deviation of AQT ranges between 3 (dark blue) and 26 (yellow) and shows the deviation from the mean of all forested pixels in the country. As seen, the east half of the country presents higher variations, indicating that tick activity in this areas may change significantly. On the contrary, the predictions along the coastal provinces (i.e. Noord-Holland, Zuid-Holland and Zeeland) do not seem to deviate significantly from the predicted mean

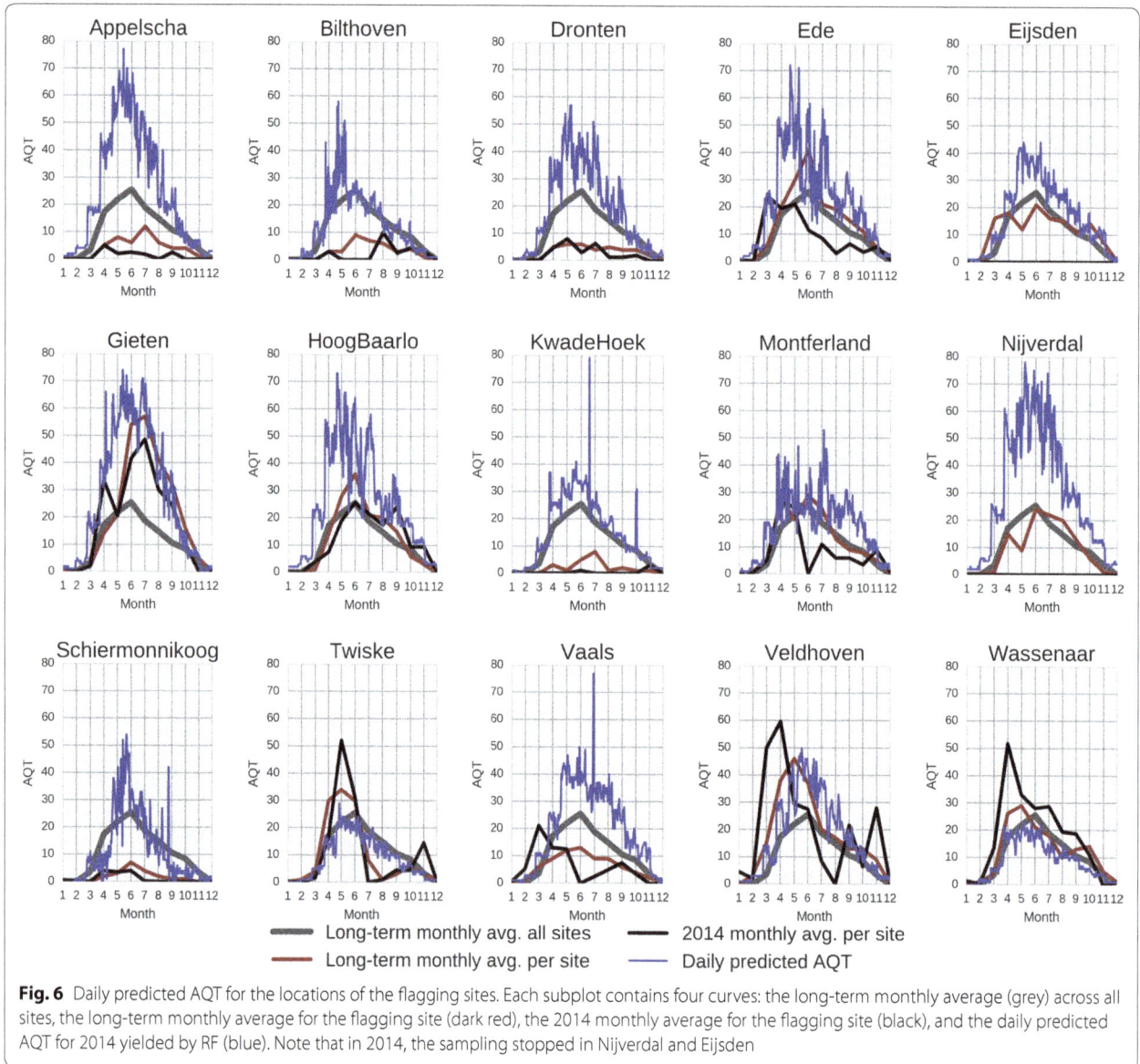

Fig. 6 Daily predicted AQT for the locations of the flagging sites. Each subplot contains four curves: the long-term monthly average (grey) across all sites, the long-term monthly average for the flagging site (dark red), the 2014 monthly average for the flagging site (black), and the daily predicted AQT for 2014 yielded by RF (blue). Note that in 2014, the sampling stopped in Nijverdal and Eijsden

Discussion

Ensemble learning algorithms such as RF can model non-linear relationships in complex natural processes. This data-driven algorithm provides an indication of the relative feature importance of the predictors involved in the analysis. This is particularly useful to model processes in which the main drivers are unknown. RF has a robust and stable behavior when handling potentially noisy data, a condition often occurring in volunteered datasets, like our AQT time-series. However, since RF is not a time-aware method, it performs sub optimally when modelling seasonal phenomena. In this work, we provide a methodological innovation to introduce time-awareness in RF by transforming our target AQT signal into a monthly bounded one, thus helping the trees in the ensemble to distinguish time.

The study on the importance of the features show that water-related features (i.e. evapotranspiration and relative humidity) are better predictors of the tick activity than temperature or vegetation. This suggests that the tick activity may be driven by atmospheric water levels, which are crucial for tick survival. A closer look of the model performances regarding statistical metrics, indicate that the model can fit the AQT signal for half of the transects, but the fitting decays for the other half. A hypothesis that may explain this difference is that the tick activity may be driven by different variable depending on the geographic location: the sites with a higher R^2 score

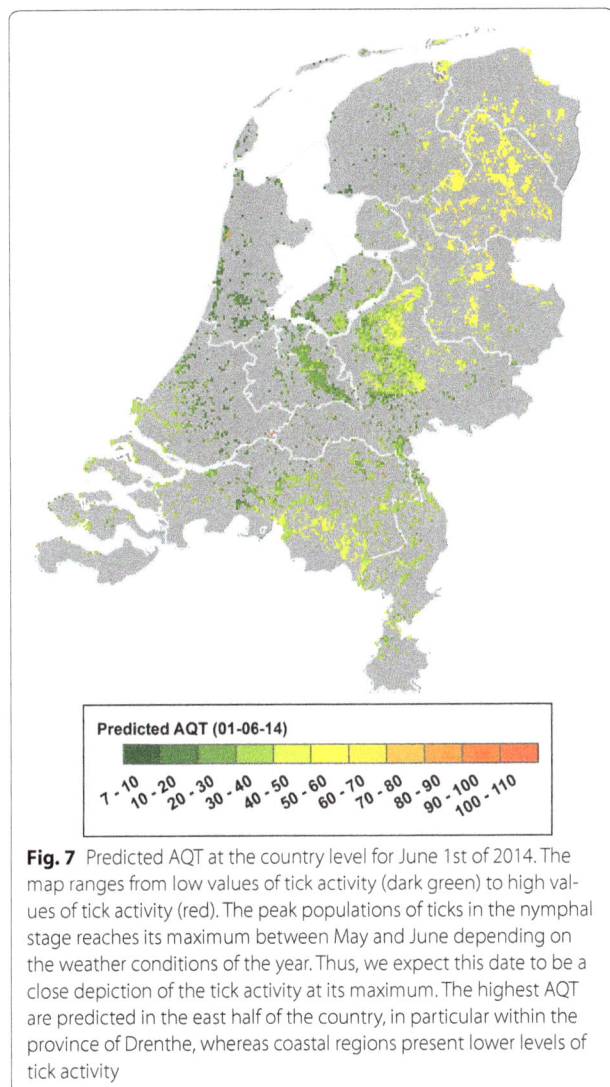

Predicted AQT (01-06-14)

7 - 10 · 10 - 20 · 20 - 30 · 30 - 40 · 40 - 50 · 50 - 60 · 60 - 70 · 70 - 80 · 80 - 90 · 90 - 100 · 100 - 110

Fig. 7 Predicted AQT at the country level for June 1st of 2014. The map ranges from low values of tick activity (dark green) to high values of tick activity (red). The peak populations of ticks in the nymphal stage reaches its maximum between May and June depending on the weather conditions of the year. Thus, we expect this date to be a close depiction of the tick activity at its maximum. The highest AQT are predicted in the east half of the country, in particular within the province of Drenthe, whereas coastal regions present lower levels of tick activity

not discriminative enough to model AQT. Second, the available weather and vegetation datasets have a spatial resolution which is too coarse to model tick dynamics, a phenomenon which was found to be very local as suggested in [14]. This might have an impact when characterizing the AQT with the environmental datasets: different locations with similar weather conditions yield an uncorrelated number of AQT, masking the relationship between weather and ticks and increasing the errors of the model. To mitigate these effects and decrease the average error of the models, we recommend using weather datasets at a finer resolution or involve more volunteers in this long-term citizen science project to get more data.

Conclusion

Citizen science initiatives allow monitoring of environmental phenomena via crowdsourcing, and produce geospatial data collections that can support scientific analysis. The question at the beginning of this work was whether the collective effort carried out by a group of volunteers, would translate into predictive models estimating tick activity in the Netherlands. Results show that combining volunteered AQT data with environmental variables and modelling them with a time-aware version of RF, can capture most of the spatial and temporal variation in the number of active questing ticks in the country.

The combined analysis of volunteered AQT and environmental variables consistently spotted that water-based features, especially evapotranspiration, play a crucial role in predicting AQT. In this sense, further studies in the field of tick ecology should consider adding, besides the classical temperature and vegetation indices, water-based features. Aside identifying the most important variables to model tick dynamics, this study has produced a model that, scaling up from volunteered observations, can map daily tick activity at the country level. The use of this model may open the way to study spatial patterns and seasonal trends at the national level, not only tick activity, but also of other non-linear natural phenomena, such as phenological events or species distributions.

With these new insights, we envision different applications in the field of tick related ecological research, nature management and public health. In ecological research, our tick activity model allows the identification of tick hotspots and of the sampling sites where the model fit was good or bad, which can be used to better select new monitoring sites. With the model we can better analyze the impact of extreme weather events and climate change on tick dynamics and population development. In nature management, these maps can help owners of green areas to be more aware of the variation of tick dynamics in the areas they are responsible for, which can lead to

might be strongly influenced by atmospheric conditions, whereas the sites with a lower R^2 score might be driven by variables currently not included in the model (e.g. wildlife). In addition, the analysis of the feature importance at multiple temporal scales is consistent with the results of the general model, because water-related features are spotted as the most prominent features across all temporal scales.

The two major hurdles encountered during this experiment are related with the weather uniformity in the country and the low spatial resolution of the available environmental datasets. First, the low elevation and the small size of the Netherlands make the country very uniform in terms of weather and vegetation variables (e.g. reduced north–south temperature gradient, high and persistent "greenness"). This means that vegetation indices, often included in previous studies in the field, are a better planning in space and time of different forestry management activities. In tick hotspots with many visitors, nature managers could consider to more frequently mow the grass directly next to walking and cycling trails or picnic areas to try to reduce tick populations. In public health, this model can be used to better inform people that visit natural areas on current tick activity levels. In combination with weather forecasts also detailed forecasts for the coming days can be given. The proposed model predicting tick activity will replace the very basic tick activity forecast currently implemented in the Dutch citizen science website Tekenradar (Tick radar, www.tekenradar.nl). The spatially detailed tick activity forecasts are expected to raise awareness among the general public and many different stakeholders involved in the problem of Lyme disease. Having more detailed information hopefully translates in an increase of protective and preventive measures when visiting forested areas. Overall, we expect that a better understanding of tick dynamics may contribute to design interventions to reduce the incidence of Lyme disease.

Authors' contributions
AvV and WT participated in the tick data collection. IGM and RZM designed the experiment together. IGM performed the data analysis. RZM, AvV, WT, and IGM assessed and interpreted the validity of results. IGM drafted the manuscript, which was critically revised and actively contributed by RZM, AvV, and WT. All authors read and approved the final manuscript.

Author details
[1] Department of Geo-Information Processing (GIP), Faculty of Geo-Information and Earth Observation (ITC), University of Twente, Enschede, The Netherlands. [2] Department of Environmental Sciences, Wageningen University, Wageningen, The Netherlands. [3] Department of Plant Sciences, Wageningen University, Wageningen, The Netherlands.

Acknowledgements
We would like to thank the group of specialized volunteers that consistently sampled the sites for the past decade; thanks to Dr. R. Sluiter for swiftly providing the official KNMI relative humidity datasets on request; thanks to Dr. E. Izquierdo-Verdiguier for her advice in the theory behind machine learning algorithms.

Competing interests
The authors declare that they have no competing interests.

Funding
Not applicable.

References
1. Barrios González JM. Spatio-temporal modelling of the epidemiology of Nephropathia Epidemica and Lyme Borreliosis. Leuven: KU Leuven; 2013.
2. Berger KA, Ginsberg HS, Gonzalez L, Mather TN. Relative humidity and activity patterns of Ixodes scapularis (Acari: Ixodidae). J Med Entomol. 2014;51:769–76.
3. Berger K, Ginsberg H, Dugas K, Hamel L, Mather T. Adverse moisture events predict seasonal abundance of Lyme disease vector ticks (Ixodes scapularis). Parasit Vectors. 2014;7:181. https://doi.org/10.1186/1756-3305-7-181.
4. Boulos MNK. Web GIS in practice III: creating a simple interactive map of England's Strategic Health Authorities using Google Maps API, Google Earth KML, and MSN Virtual Earth Map Control. Int J Health Geogr. 2005;8:1–8. https://doi.org/10.1186/1476-072X-4-22.
5. Boulos MNK, Resch B, Crowley DN, Breslin JG, Sohn G, Burtner R, 2011. Crowdsourcing, citizen sensing and sensor web technologies for public and environmental health surveillance and crisis management : trends, OGC standards and application examples. Int. J. Health Geogr. 10;1–29. https://doi.org/10.1186/1476-072X-10-67.
6. Breiman L. Random forests. Mach Learn. 2001;45:5–32.
7. Breiman LEO. Bagging predictors. Mach Learn. 1996;140:123–40.
8. Brownstein JS, Holford TR, Fish D. A climate-based model predicts the spatial distribution of the Lyme disease vector Ixodes scapularis in the United States. Environ Health Perspect. 2003;111:1152–7. https://doi.org/10.1289/ehp.6052.
9. Cianci D, Hartemink N, Ibáñez-Justicia A, 2015. Modelling the potential spatial distribution of mosquito species using three different techniques. Int. J. Health Geogr. 14;1–10. https://doi.org/10.1186/s12942-015-0001-0.
10. Dantas-Torres F, Otranto D. Species diversity and abundance of ticks in three habitats in southern Italy. Ticks Tick Borne Dis. 2013;4:251–5. https://doi.org/10.1016/j.ttbdis.2012.11.004.
11. Estrada-Peña A. Distribution, abundance, and habitat preferences of Ixodes ricinus (Acari: Ixodidae) in Northern Spain. J Med Entomol. 2001;38:361–70. https://doi.org/10.1603/0022-2585-38.3.361.
12. Estrada-Peña A, de la Fuente J. Species interactions in occurrence data for a community of tick-transmitted pathogens. Nat Sci Data. 2016;3:1–13.
13. Estrada-Peña A, Gray JS, Kahl O, Lane RS, Nijhof AM. Research on the ecology of ticks and tick-borne pathogens–methodological principles and caveats. Front Cell Infect Microbiol. 2013;3:29. https://doi.org/10.3389/fcimb.2013.00029.
14. Estrada-Peña A, Sánchez N, Estrada-Sánchez A. An assessment of the distribution and spread of the tick Hyalomma marginatum in the western Palearctic under different climate scenarios. Vector Borne Zoonotic Dis. 2012;12:758–68. https://doi.org/10.1089/vbz.2011.0771.
15. Gassner F, van Vliet AJH, Burgers SLGE, Jacobs F, Verbaarschot P, Hovius EKE, Mulder S, Verhulst NO, van Overbeek LS, Takken W. Geographic and temporal variations in population dynamics of Ixodes ricinus and associated Borrelia infections in The Netherlands. Vector Borne Zoonotic Dis. 2011;11:523–32. https://doi.org/10.1089/vbz.2010.0026.
16. Goodchild MF, Li L. Assuring the quality of volunteered geographic information. Spat Stat. 2012;1:110–20. https://doi.org/10.1016/j.spasta.2012.03.002.
17. Hartemink N, Takken W. Trends in tick population dynamics and pathogen transmission in emerging tick-borne pathogens in Europe: an introduction. Exp Appl Acarol. 2016;68:269–78. https://doi.org/10.1007/s10493-015-0003-4.
18. Hartemink N, Vanwambeke SO, Purse BV, Gilbert M, Dyck H Van. Towards a resource-based habitat approach for spatial modelling of vector-borne disease risks. Biol Rev. 2015;32:1151–62. https://doi.org/10.1111/brv.12149.
19. Heyman P, Cochez C, Hofhuis A, van der Giessen J, Sprong H, Porter SR, Losson B, Saegerman C, Donoso-Mantke O, Niedrig M, Papa A. A clear and present danger: tick-borne diseases in Europe. Expert Rev Anti Infect Ther. 2010;8:33–50. https://doi.org/10.1586/eri.09.118.
20. Ho TK. The random subspace method for constructing decision forests. IEEE Trans Pattern Anal Mach Intell. 1998;20:832–44.
21. Hofhuis A, Bennema S, Harms M, Vliet AJH Van, Takken W. Decrease in tick bite consultations and stabilization of early Lyme borreliosis in the Netherlands in 2014 after 15 years of continuous increase. BMC Public Health. 2016. https://doi.org/10.1186/s12889-016-3105-y.
22. Hofhuis A, Harms M, van den Wijngaard C, Sprong H, van Pelt W. Continuing increase of tick bites and Lyme disease between 1994 and 2009. Ticks Tick Borne Dis. 2015;6:69–74. https://doi.org/10.1016/j.ttbdis.2014.09.006.

23. Jaenson TGT, Eisen L, Comstedt P, Mejlon HA, Lindgren E, Bergström S, Olsen B. Risk indicators for the tick *Ixodes ricinus* and *Borrelia burgdorferi sensu lato* in Sweden. Med Vet Entomol. 2009;23:226–37. https://doi.org/10.1111/j.1365-2915.2009.00813.x.

24. Jones CG, Ostfeld RS, Richard MP. Mast seeding and Lyme disease. Trends Ecol Evol. 1998;9:5347.

25. Jore S, Vanwambeke SO, Viljugrein H, Isaksen K, Kristoffersen AB, Woldehiwet Z, Johansen B, Brun E, Brun-Hansen H, Westermann S, Larsen I-L, Ytrehus B, Hofshagen M. Climate and environmental change drives *Ixodes ricinus* geographical expansion at the northern range margin. Parasit Vectors. 2014;7:11. https://doi.org/10.1186/1756-3305-7-11.

26. Lambin EF, Tran A, Vanwambeke SO, Linard C, Soti V. Pathogenic landscapes: interactions between land, people, disease vectors, and their animal hosts. Int J. Health Geogr. 2010;9:54. https://doi.org/10.1186/1476-072X-9-54.

27. Li S, Colson V, Lejeune P, Speybroeck N, Vanwambeke SO. Agent-based modelling of the spatial pattern of leisure visitation in forests: a case study in Wallonia, south Belgium. Environ Model Softw. 2015;71:111–25. https://doi.org/10.1016/j.envsoft.2015.06.001.

28. Louppe G, Wehenkel L, Sutera A, Geurts P, 2013. Understanding variable importances in forests of randomized trees. In: Burges CJC, Bottou L, Welling M, Ghahramani Z, Weinberger KQ editors. Proceedings of the 26th International Conference on Neural Information Processing Systems (NIPS). Curran Associates Inc, Lake Tahoe, Nevada, P. 431–439.

29. Medlock JM, Hansford KM, Bormane A, Derdakova M, Estrada-Peña A, George J-C, Golovljova I, Jaenson TGT, Jensen J-K, Jensen PM, Kazimirova M, Oteo JA, Papa A, Pfister K, Plantard O, Randolph SE, Rizzoli A, Santos-Silva MM, Sprong H, Vial L, Hendrickx G, Zeller H, Van Bortel W. Driving forces for changes in geographical distribution of *Ixodes ricinus* ticks in Europe. Parasit Vectors. 2013;6:1. https://doi.org/10.1186/1756-3305-6-1.

30. Murray FW. On the computation of saturation vapour pressure. J Appl Meteorol. 1967;6:203–4. https://doi.org/10.1175/1520-0450(1967)006<0203:OTCOSV>2.0.CO;2.

31. Ogden NH, Koffi JK, Pelcat Y, Lindsay LR. Lyme disease Surveillance Environmental risk from Lyme disease in central and eastern Canada: a summary of recent surveillance information. Rep: Canada Commun Dis; 2014. p. 40.

32. Ogden NH, Maarouf A, Barker IK, Bigras-Poulin M, Lindsay LR, Morshed MG, O'callaghan CJ, Ramay F, Waltner-Toews D, Charron DF. Climate change and the potential for range expansion of the Lyme disease vector *Ixodes scapularis* in Canada. Int J Parasitol. 2006;36:63–70. https://doi.org/10.1016/j.ijpara.2005.08.016.

33. Ostfeld RS. Lyme disease: the ecology of a complex system. Oxford: Oxford University Press; 2012.

34. Ostfeld RS. The Ecology of Lyme-Disease Risk. Am. Sci. 1997;85:338–346.

35. Ostfeld RS, Canham CD, Oggenfuss K, Winchcombe RJ, Keesing F. Climate, deer, rodents, and acorns as determinants of variation in lyme-disease risk. PLoS Biol. 2006;4:e145. https://doi.org/10.1371/journal.pbio.0040145.

36. Ostfeld RS, Jones CG, Wolff JO. Of mice and mast. Bioscience. 1996;46:323–30. https://doi.org/10.2307/1312946.

37. Ozdenerol E. GIS and remote sensing use in the exploration of lyme disease. Epidemiology. 2015. https://doi.org/10.3390/ijerph121214971.

38. Randolph SE. Is expert opinion enough? A critical assessment of the evidence for potential impacts of climate change on tick-borne diseases. Anim Health Res Rev. 2017;14:133–7. https://doi.org/10.1017/S1466252313000091.

39. Randolph SE. Ticks and tick-borne disease systems in space and from space. Adv Parasitol. 2000;47:217–43.

40. Randolph SE, Asokliene L, Avsic-Zupanc T, Bormane A, Burri C, Gern L, Golovljova I, Hubalek Z, Knap N, Kondrusik M, Kupca A, Pejcoch M, Vasilenko V, Zygutiene M. Variable spikes in tick-borne encephalitis incidence in 2006 independent of variable tick abundance but related to weather. Parasit Vectors. 2008;1:44. https://doi.org/10.1186/1756-3305-1-44.

41. Randolph SE, Green RM, Peacy MF, Rogers DJ. Seasonal synchrony: the key to tick-borne encephalitis foci identified by satellite data. Parasitology. 2000;121:15–23.

42. Randolph SE, Storey K. Impact of microclimate on immature tick-rodent host interactions (Acari : Ixodidae): implications for parasite transmission. J Med Entomol. 1999;36(6):741–8.

43. Rodriguez-Galiano V, Chica-Olmo M, Chica-Rivas M. Predictive modelling of gold potential with the integration of multisource information based on random forest: a case study on the Rodalquilar area, Southern Spain. Int J Geogr Inf Sci. 2014;28:1336–54. https://doi.org/10.1080/13658816.2014.885527.

44. Ruiz-Fons F, Fernández-de-Mera IG, Acevedo P, Gortázar C, de la Fuente J. Factors driving the abundance of *Ixodes ricinus* ticks and the prevalence of zoonotic *I. ricinus*—borne pathogens in natural foci. Appl Environ Microbiol. 2012;78:2669–76. https://doi.org/10.1128/AEM.06564-11.

45. Rulison EL, Kuczaj I, Pang G, Hickling GJ, Tsao JI, Ginsberg HS. Flagging versus dragging as sampling methods for nymphal *Ixodes scapularis* (Acari : Ixodidae). J Vector Ecol. 2013;38:163–7.

46. Schnurr JL, Ostfeld RS, Canham CD. Direct and indirect effects of masting on rodent populations and tree seed survival. Oikos. 2002;3:402–10.

47. Sprong H, Hofhuis A, Gassner F, Takken W, Jacobs F, van Vliet AJH, van Ballegooijen M, van der Giessen J, Takumi K. Circumstantial evidence for an increase in the total number and activity of Borrelia-infected *Ixodes ricinus* in the Netherlands. Parasit Vectors. 2012;5:294. https://doi.org/10.1186/1756-3305-5-294.

48. Subak S. Effects of climate on variability in Lyme disease incidence in the northeastern United States. Am J Epidemiol. 2003;157:531–8. https://doi.org/10.1093/aje/kwg014.

49. Tack W. Impact of forest conversion on the abundance of *Ixodes ricinus* ticks. Ghent: Dep. For. Water Manag. Dep. Biomed. Sci, Ghent University; 2013.

50. Tack W, Madder M, Baeten L, De Frenne P, Verheyen K. The abundance of *Ixodes ricinus* ticks depends on tree species composition and shrub cover. Parasitology. 2012;139:1273–81. https://doi.org/10.1017/S0031182012000625.

51. Tran P, Tran L. Validating negative binomial lyme disease regression model with bootstrap resampling. Environ Model Softw. 2016;82:121–7. https://doi.org/10.1016/j.envsoft.2016.04.019.

52. Wu X, Duvvuri VR, Wu J. Modeling dynamical temperature influence on tick *Ixodes scapularis* population. In: International congress on environmental modelling and software, 2010.

53. Zeman P, Benes C. Peri-urbanisation, counter-urbanisation, and an extension of residential exposure to ticks: a clue to the trends in Lyme borreliosis incidence in the Czech Republic? Ticks Tick Borne Dis. 2014;5:907–16. https://doi.org/10.1016/j.ttbdis.2014.07.006·

6

Do the risk factors for type 2 diabetes mellitus vary by location? A spatial analysis of health insurance claims in Northeastern Germany using kernel density estimation and geographically weighted regression

Boris Kauhl[1,2,3*], Jürgen Schweikart[2], Thomas Krafft[3], Andrea Keste[1] and Marita Moskwyn[1]

Abstract

Background: The provision of general practitioners (GPs) in Germany still relies mainly on the ratio of inhabitants to GPs at relatively large scales and barely accounts for an increased prevalence of chronic diseases among the elderly and socially underprivileged populations. Type 2 Diabetes Mellitus (T2DM) is one of the major cost-intensive diseases with high rates of potentially preventable complications. Provision of healthcare and access to preventive measures is necessary to reduce the burden of T2DM. However, current studies on the spatial variation of T2DM in Germany are mostly based on survey data, which do not only underestimate the true prevalence of T2DM, but are also only available on large spatial scales. The aim of this study is therefore to analyse the spatial distribution of T2DM at fine geographic scales and to assess location-specific risk factors based on data of the AOK health insurance.

Methods: To display the spatial heterogeneity of T2DM, a bivariate, adaptive kernel density estimation (KDE) was applied. The spatial scan statistic (SaTScan) was used to detect areas of high risk. Global and local spatial regression models were then constructed to analyze socio-demographic risk factors of T2DM.

Results: T2DM is especially concentrated in rural areas surrounding Berlin. The risk factors for T2DM consist of proportions of 65–79 year olds, 80 + year olds, unemployment rate among the 55–65 year olds, proportion of employees covered by mandatory social security insurance, mean income tax, and proportion of non-married couples. However, the strength of the association between T2DM and the examined socio-demographic variables displayed strong regional variations.

Conclusion: The prevalence of T2DM varies at the very local level. Analyzing point data on T2DM of northeastern Germany's largest health insurance provider thus allows very detailed, location-specific knowledge about increased medical needs. Risk factors associated with T2DM depend largely on the place of residence of the respective person. Future allocation of GPs and current prevention strategies should therefore reflect the location-specific higher healthcare demand among the elderly and socially underprivileged populations.

Keywords: Type 2 diabetes mellitus, Healthcare, Germany, Spatial analysis, Geographically weighted regression, Kernel Density Estimation, SaTScan, Street-level, big data

*Correspondence: boris.kauhl@nordost.aok.de
1 Department of Medical Care, AOK Nordost – Die Gesundheitskasse, Berlin, Germany
Full list of author information is available at the end of the article

Background

The prevalence of chronic diseases and therefore the projectable utilization of healthcare depend strongly on the demographic and socio-economic composition of the respective population [1–3]. International studies suggest a strong relationship between the proportion of elderly, low socio-economic status and a higher prevalence of chronic diseases [2, 4–6]. However, planning of GPs in Germany still relies mainly on the ratio of inhabitants to GPs at fairly large scales [7] and does neither sufficiently reflect the location-specific higher prevalence of chronic diseases among the elderly and population groups with a lower socio-economic status, nor the accessibility of GPs in rural areas [8].

With the ongoing demographic transition and migration processes from rural to urban areas, the gap between demand and supply of health care is already widening in Germany. While the ageing of the population and therefore the prevalence of chronic diseases increases in rural areas, the availability of GPs decreases [9]. To meet the increased demand for healthcare especially in rural areas, it is important to identify locations with higher healthcare demand as spatially precise as possible. Additional knowledge about the population groups, which are most at risk in specific locations is necessary to effectively plan the future provision of GPs and immediate preventive measures where they are needed most.

Type 2 Diabetes Mellitus (T2DM) is a major public health threat with an increasing prevalence among the general population worldwide [4, 10, 11] and especially in Germany [3]. Prevention and access to healthcare are necessary not only to prevent a further increase but also to prevent severe complications such as lower-extremity amputation [12] or stroke [10].

Despite behavioral risk factors such as lack of physical exercise, dietary deficits and smoking [13], a wide range of studies additionally highlights an association between age, lower socioeconomic status and T2DM [4, 14–16].

Geographic information systems (GIS) and spatial regression models at the ecological level have gained increasing attention in recent years as this approach allows an analysis of possible risk factors that are often unavailable on an individual level due to privacy restriction [15, 17]. For T2DM, this approach might help to identify the population groups, which are most in need for the provision of healthcare and access to preventive measures. However, several studies point out that socio-demographic risk factors for T2DM, but also for a wide range of other diseases depend largely on the place of residence of the respective individual [4, 14, 15, 17, 18]. As a consequence, a one-size fits all solution seems therefore inappropriate for effective public health strategies and allocation of healthcare [15].

Analyzing the spatial distribution of T2DM and associated risk factors in Germany is challenging, as epidemiological data on chronic diseases is seldom publicly available [19]. Only few studies have examined the spatial distribution of T2DM in Germany [16, 20–23]. However, the majority of these studies are based upon data from Germany's largest telephone survey of the Robert-Koch-Institute (GEDA) [16, 20, 21]. A spatial analysis of this data source is therefore restricted to fairly large areas such as the counties in Germany [16, 21], or includes only a selection of municipalities [20]. Analyses based on surveys however, tend to underestimate the prevalence of T2DM as persons with a higher socioeconomic status are more likely to respond than persons with a lower socio-economic status [20, 21]. Therefore, such surveys have only limited use for a demand-driven planning and allocation of healthcare and prevention strategies.

Health insurance in Germany is generally mandatory and approximately 86% of the population are covered by one of the statutory health insurance providers, 10% are covered by private health insurance providers and the remaining 4% are covered by the state [24]. However, there are large socio-demographic differences between members of the various statutory health insurances [25]. As the provision and allocation of primary healthcare in Germany is planned and organized by the association of statutory health insurance physicians in accordance with the statutory health insurance providers [7], it is necessary for each health insurance provider to engage in planning of primary healthcare based on an empirical evaluation of the medical demand of their respective insurants.

At the federal level, 1671 inhabitants per 1 GP at the spatial scale of central areas (Mittelbereiche) of the Federal Agency of Building and Urban Development (BBSR) is the target-ratio for the allocation of GPs in Germany [7]. The association of statutory health insurance physicians defines over- or undersupply as deviation from this ratio by 110 and 50%, respectively and has to undertake appropriate measures if over- or undersupply exists [7]. However, this ratio was established in the 1990s [7] and does not recognize an increased prevalence of T2DM and other chronic diseases in location-specific population groups. The association of statutory health insurance physicians has reacted to this criticism by incorporating a demographic factor and allowing deviations from the established inhabitants to GP ratio for areas with increased medical demand in their revised planning guidelines [7]. However, due to the lack of reliable, small-scale public health data on chronic diseases, an increased medical demand of a location-specific population group is still difficult to detect [16, 20–23]. To realistically capture such an increased demand for healthcare, more reliable sources than survey data and spatial analyses at smaller scales are necessary than it is currently possible with survey data in Germany.

In this context, health insurance claims of the AOK Nordost have several advantages over survey data: (a) This data source represents a large sample of northeastern Germany's population, (b) can be analyzed on a fine geographic scale and (c) prevalence estimates of health insurance claims are not depending on the response rate of participants and are therefore a more realistic estimate of the "true" prevalence of chronic conditions than survey data [26]. Ultimately, a spatial analysis of this data source might provide new and inclusive insights on the spatial distribution of chronic diseases and population-based risk factors.

The goal of our paper is therefore to (1) analyze the spatial distribution of T2DM based on health insurance claims of northeastern Germany's largest statutory health insurance provider; (2) to evaluate possible risk factors using global ecological regression models and (3) to examine the spatially varying association between sociodemographic risk factors and T2DM.

Methods
Dependent variable
In this study, we used data from northeastern Germany's largest statutory health insurance provider (AOK Nordost) for 2012, which covers roughly 1.79 million persons (approximately one quarter of the population) of which 361 thousand persons are diagnosed with Type 2 Diabetes.

Persons diagnosed with T2DM were defined in our study as having a confirmed diagnosis of T2DM (ICD-10: E11.-). As long as the insurant is treated for T2DM, this diagnosis will remain in the insurant's personal medical file as the diagnosis is renewed with each GP visit associated with T2DM. To ensure that each insurant and diabetic is included only once in the analysis, the unique insurant number was used to exclude possible double entries within the database from the analysis.

The data was anonymized and was geocoded based on exact street-level data using the ESRI ArcGIS geocoder. The data included only age in broad age categories (0–5, 6–11, 12–17, 18–24, 25–44, 45–64, 65–79 and 80 and older) and the address coordinates. We used a stepwise geocoding process where the data was first geocoded based on the exact street address where possible (90.2%). Of the remaining data, 6.7% were matched to the centroids of the street and 3.1% were matched to the postal code centroids. The address coordinates for Berlin were obtained from the Senatsverwaltung für Stadtverwaltung Berlin; the address coordinates for Brandenburg were obtained from the Landesvermessungsamt und

Geobasisinformation Brandenburg (Geobasisdaten © GeoBasis-DE/LGB 2016, GB-D 13/16) and the coordinates for Mecklenburg-Vorpommern were obtained from the Landesamt für Innere Verwaltung, Amt für Geoinformation, Vermessungs- und Katasterwesen (Geobasisdaten © GeoBasis-DE/M-V 2016).

Explanatory variables
In this study, we assessed a wide range of demographic, socioeconomic and variables related to the physical environment for their association with T2DM. Demographic variables were calculated based on the proportion of AOK insurants per demographic group. Socioeconomic variables included the proportion of unemployed persons in different age groups, information on taxation, land use, household composition and a wide range of other indicators. Variables related to the physical environment included the proportion of green spaces, recreational spaces and built surfaces. The data were obtained for the year 2012 from the INKAR database of the Federal Agency of Building and Urban Development (BBSR). Data on marital status, household and family composition were obtained from the census 2011 for Germany. All data were available on the spatial scale of the association of municipalities. Additionally, we included data on the spatial distribution of GPs in our analysis to examine whether the availability of healthcare influences the prevalence of T2DM. We included two variables: The proportion of inhabitants to GPs and the average distance to GPs. The average distance to GPs was calculated based on the driving distance of each insurant to the closest GP and was then aggregated to match the association of municipalities. The street network dataset was downloaded from OpenStreetMap [27]. The association of municipalities in Germany was chosen as the unit of analysis as this is the smallest spatial scale, for which a wide range of indicators is available without areas being omitted due to privacy protection as it would be the case for municipalities. However, this scale does not allow an analysis of intra-urban differences as the indicators of BBSR are not available for a smaller administrative unit than the association of municipalities.

Statistical analysis
Bivariate kernel density estimation
In this study, we used a bivariate, adaptive kernel density estimation (KDE) to display the spatial heterogeneity of T2DM independent of administrative boundaries. In most epidemiological studies, disease and population data are only available for aggregated data such as postal codes, municipalities, counties or districts [10, 16, 21, 28]. However, problems arise in the detection of local clusters and associations to socio-demographic exposure

factors due to the relatively arbitrary shape and quantity of spatial units, which is often referred to as the "modifiable area unit problem" [29]. This may be especially misleading in rural areas where administrative boundaries are very large. As a consequence, a cartographic visualization of disease risk without the restrictions of artificially created boundaries is favorable.

Bivariate kernel density estimation has been previously applied in small-scale studies for HIV [30, 31], cancer [32, 33], Alzheimer [34] and crime intensity [35] and thus seems useful for a small-scale analysis of T2DM as well.

A major concern when applying a bivariate KDE is the choice of bandwidth. If the bandwidth is too small, rates become highly unstable and spatial patterns are difficult to detect. If the bandwidth is too large, the map appears to be over smoothed and local extremes are smoothed away [33]. Although several statistical models exist to calculate the "optimal" bandwidth, such as the Likelihood Cross Validation [33, 36, 37], Least Squares Cross Validation [33, 38], Biased Cross Validation [33, 39], Smoothed Cross Validation [33, 40], or the direct plug-in method [33, 41], these aforementioned bandwidth selection models are generally only available for fixed bandwidth types [33].

As our study area comprises highly densely populated urban areas such as Berlin, Potsdam or Schwerin while at the same time comprising a large proportion of very sparsely populated rural areas, a KDE employing a fixed bandwidth would deliver no stable results. We therefore favored an adaptive bandwidth, which accounts for the varying population densities within our study area [32, 33].

Although a wide range of selection methods exist for a fixed bandwidth, automated procedures to select an optimal number of points to be included in an adaptive bandwidth for a bivariate KDE are scarce and are not yet fully satisfactory [33]. As there are no definite recommendations to define a bandwidth for a bivariate KDE, we therefore visually evaluated several possible combinations of minimum sample points [42, 43]. Including at least 0.1% of T2DM cases and 0.1% of insurants delivered the most useful results. The T2DM prevalence was therefore calculated as the ratio of at least 361 T2DM cases per km^2 to 1791 insurants per km^2. Given the varying population densities, the kernel was thus smaller in highly populated areas and larger in sparsely populated rural areas. In this study, we used a Gaussian kernel as it tends to produce more robust results than a kernel type with a definite boundary [43].

The calculation of the bivariate KDE was carried out using the CrimeStat IV software [43]. The results were then imported in ESRI ArcGIS 10.3.

Sex- and age-standardization of prevalence rates

The bivariate, adaptive kernel density estimation allows a visualization of T2DM prevalence without the limitations of administrative areas but has the disadvantage of not being able to incorporate sex- and age-standardization.

To further facilitate interpretation of the spatial variations in T2DM prevalence, we directly adjusted for sex and age using the WHO standard population from 1976 [44] based on the five-digits postal codes of our study area. As the number of insurants between the five-digits postal code varies considerably, we applied spatial empirical Bayesian smoothing to borrow strength from neighboring postal codes to estimate more stable prevalence rates [45]. Neighboring areas were defined as postal codes sharing a common edge or boundary [46]. The computation was carried out in GeoDa 1.2.0 and the results were then imported in ESRI ArcGIS 10.3.

Cluster detection

The aim of cluster detection in our study was to evaluate whether a statistically significant elevated risk exists in certain areas. A purely visual inspection of the KDE and the adjusted rates would be misleading, as it is not possible to examine the number of cases behind the estimated rates alone. Applying a local cluster test on health data is important to prioritize areas for future public health interventions [30, 47] and has been previously shown useful to locate new clinics for chronically ill patients for diabetic kidney patients [48].

In this study, we used the spatial scan statistic (SaTScan). The spatial scan statistic is a local cluster test, which determines the location and significance of local clusters. This is achieved by a circular scanning window, which moves over the coordinates of the study area and evaluates all possible cluster locations and cluster sizes up to either a user defined maximum or the default settings of including up to 50% of the population at risk inside a cluster [30, 49]. The statistical significance is calculated using 999 Monte-Carlo replications [50]. We applied a purely spatial Poisson model, where the T2DM cases per coordinate/sex- and age-adjusted number of T2DM cases per postal code were assigned as cases and all insurants per coordinate/postal code were assigned as population [30, 49, 50]. The maximum cluster size was restricted to a maximum radius of 10 km. This was done as (a) the standard setting of including up to 50% of the population at risk often produces results of no practical use [51] and (b), we defined 10 km as the maximum reasonable driving distance to GPs in rural areas of northeastern Germany. For the analysis of the point data, we used the exact street-level coordinates and for the cluster analysis of the sex- and age-adjusted rates we used the centroid coordinates of the postal codes. The analysis was carried out using SaTScan v9.4.2.

Spatial regression modelling
Ordinary least squares regression modelling
To create a meaningful and correct specified geographically weighted regression model (GWR), we first aimed to identify all possible explanatory variables through the global ordinary least squares (OLS) regression model. To achieve this, we first performed a natural log-transformation of the T2DM prevalence to satisfy the assumption of the OLS model that the dependent variable has to be normally distributed [52]. We used the raw rate instead of the age-adjusted T2DM prevalence as we specifically wanted to model the effect of older age groups on the T2DM prevalence.

We then compared the association between each potential explanatory variable and T2DM prevalence through univariate OLS regression models. As a large number of explanatory variables were found to be significantly associated to T2DM, we used a data-mining tool called "exploratory regression" in ESRI ArcGIS 10.3 to determine all possible variable combinations. This tool is comparable to a step-wise regression. It evaluates all possible variable combinations based on four criteria: (1): the coefficients are statistically significant; (2): the explanatory variables are free from multicollinearity; (3): the residuals are normally distributed and (4): the residuals are not spatially autocorrelated [52–54].

We then determined overall model significance, autocorrelation of the residuals, the presence of heteroscedasticity and a wide range of other diagnostics by creating an OLS model in ESRI ArcGIS 10.3. with the same explanatory variables as suggested by the exploratory regression that were found to deliver a plausible explanation of the T2DM prevalence.

Geographically weighted regression modelling
The OLS model is a global model, it therefore estimates only one single coefficient per explanatory variable averaged over the entire study area. However, the socio-demographic composition of the population in northeastern Germany varies strongly at the local level. It is therefore unlikely that the association between socio-demographic explanatory variables and T2DM is realistically reflected by a global regression model. Previous studies applying GWR on Diabetes [4, 15] as well as on a wide range of other diseases [18, 55, 56] pointed out that the correlations between explanatory variables and T2DM vary strongly across space. We therefore hypothesize that this applies to our study area as well. The GWR methodology is an extension to the standard regression models and estimates a wide range of local parameters to

reflect changes over space in the association between an epidemiological outcome and explanatory variables [57].

Similar to the OLS model, we used the log-transformed T2DM prevalence as the dependent variable with the same explanatory variables that were found to be significant in the OLS model.

We used the centroids of the association of municipalities as the input coordinates. Similarly to the KDE, the GWR methodology uses a circular kernel to calculate the local estimates. The GWR model fits for each coordinate a regression equation where the coordinates in the center of the kernel are the regression points. The data points inside the kernel are then weighted with decreasing weights from the center towards the edge of the kernel. The bandwidth of the kernel can be either fixed or adaptive and the shape of the kernel can follow a Gaussian or a bi-square distribution. The optimization of the bandwidth can be based on one of the four available criteria: (1) Akaikes Information Criterion (AIC); (2) Akaikes corrected Information Criterion (AICc); (3) Bayesian Information Criterion (BIC) and (4) Cross Validation (CV) [57, 58]. We thus evaluated all 14 possible combinations of kernel shape, bandwidth type and bandwidth optimization method. The models without clustered residuals were further considered and out of those, the model with the lowest AICc value and highest adjusted R^2 was then chosen as the final model. The calculation of the GWR model was carried out in the GWR4 software. To enhance visualization of the spatially varying coefficients, we used the software's "prediction at non-sample points" function and calculated the predicted values for a grid of northeastern Germany based on a cell size of 100 m × 100 m. The obtained values were then interpolated using ordinary kriging in ESRI ArcGIS 10.3.

Ethics statement
The data and results used in this study were anonymized and do not contain any personal information. The use of anonymized data for research purposes does not require a vote by an ethics committee or an institutional research board.

Results
Spatial distribution of T2DM
The overall raw prevalence of T2DM was 20.0% and the sex- and age-adjusted prevalence was 14.2%. However, the prevalence varied widely within the study area (Fig. 1). Generally, the prevalence was relatively low in the center of larger villages or urban areas and increased towards remote, rural areas. The highest prevalence and clusters with most cases could be observed in a ring in Brandenburg, surrounding Berlin. In Mecklenburg-Vorpommern, the number of clusters as well as the

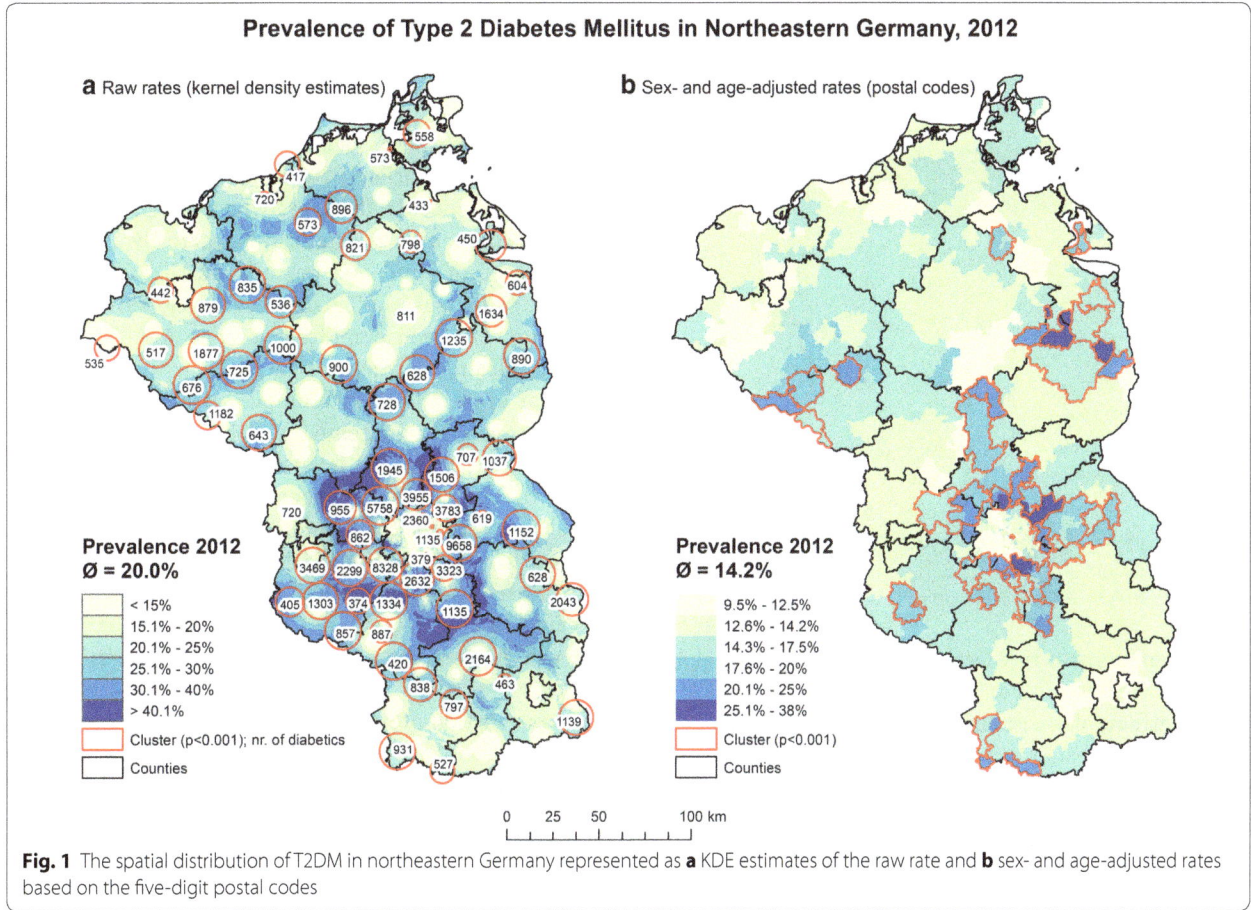

Fig. 1 The spatial distribution of T2DM in northeastern Germany represented as **a** KDE estimates of the raw rate and **b** sex- and age-adjusted rates based on the five-digit postal codes

number of cases inside local clusters was lower than in Brandenburg.

Socio-demographic risk factors of T2DM

Six variables were identified as significant predictors for T2DM in northeastern Germany (Table 1): (1) proportion of persons aged 65–79, (2) proportion of persons aged 80 and older, (3) proportion of unemployed persons aged 55–65; (4) proportion of employed persons which are subject to social insurance contribution, (5) mean income tax and (6) proportion of non-married couples, which live together in the same household. These six variables explained 44% of the variation in T2DM prevalence (Table 1). However, the residuals were clustered, reflecting that a global OLS model is not suitable to model the prevalence of T2DM.

Spatially-varying risk factors of T2DM

By comparing all 14 possible combinations of bandwidth type, kernel shape and optimization methods in terms of their AICc value, adjusted R^2 and Moran's I of the residuals (Table 2), the model using an adaptive bandwidth with a bi-square kernel shape and an AIC optimized

Table 1 Results of the global OLS regression model

Variable	Coefficient	VIF
Intercept	2.259540***	
Persons aged 65–79 (%)	0.027251***	1.656689
Persons aged 80 and older (%)	0.010704**	1.650654
Unemployed persons aged 55–65 (%)	0.013354***	2.593295
Employed persons (%)	−0.006181**	1.602619
Mean income tax	0.000780**	2.272369
Non-married couples (%)	0.014524*	1.452730
Adjusted R^2	0.44	
AICc	−313	
Global Moran's I of residuals	I = 0.264 (p < 0.001)	

Significance levels: * ≤ 0.05; ** ≤ 0.01; *** ≤ 0.001

bandwidth selection method fulfils the requirements of the residuals not being clustered and has the best model fit, both, in terms of the AICc value and adjusted R^2. This model explains 66% of the spatial variations of T2DM prevalence and has a much better fit (AICc: −374) than the global OLS model (AICc: −313). This suggests that a local model is more suitable to model the

Table 2 Comparison of bandwidth types, kernel shapes and bandwidth optimization methods

Modell (bandwidth type, kernel shape, optimization method)	AICc	Adjusted R²	Moran's I of residuals
Adaptive, Gaussian, AICc	−347	0.51	p < 0.001
Adaptive, Gaussian, AIC	−347	0.51	p < 0.001
Adaptive, Gaussian, BIC	−315	0.44	p < 0.001
Adaptive, Gaussian, CV	−347	0.51	p < 0.001
Fixed, Gaussian, AICc	−385	0.62	p < 0.05
Fixed, Gaussian, AIC	−265	0.66	p > 0.05
Fixed, Gaussian, BIC	−316	0.44	p < 0.001
Fixed, Gaussian, CV	−370	0.64	p > 0.05
Adaptive, bi-square, AICc	−394	0.63	p < 0.001
Adaptive, bi-square, AIC	−374	0.66	p > 0.05
Adaptive, bi-square, BIC	−320	0.45	p < 0.001
Fixed, bi-square, AICc	−385	0.62	p < 0.01
Fixed, bi-square, AIC	40	0.68	p > 0.05
Fixed, bi-square, BIC	−316	0.44	p < 0.001

socio-demographic risk factors for T2DM than a global model.

The cartographic visualization of the GWR regression coefficients revealed strong regional differences of the association between the examined socio-demographic variables and T2DM prevalence (Fig. 2).

The impact of proportion of persons aged 65–79 was strongest in the areas north of Berlin in Brandenburg and two districts in the western part of Mecklenburg-Vorpommern. In these areas, 1% increase in persons aged 65–79 will increase the prevalence of T2DM between 3.2 and 5.4%. The association between persons aged 65–79 and T2DM prevalence was not significant in several districts west of Berlin and the northeastern districts in Mecklenburg-Vorpommern.

The association to proportion of persons aged 80 and older was significant in those areas where persons aged 65–79 were not significant with the exception of the islands Rügen and Usedom. The strongest impact could be observed in parts of the districts Vorpommern-Greifswald, Mecklenburgische Seenplatte and Prignitz. In these areas, 1% increase in persons aged 80 and older will increase the T2DM prevalence between 2.3 and 4%.

Unemployment rate among persons aged 55–65 was a significant positive predictor in several districts north of Berlin in Brandenburg and Mecklenburg-Vorpommern. In these areas, 1% increase in unemployment among the 55–65 year olds will increase the prevalence of T2DM between 3.8 and 6.6%. A significant negative association could only be observed in a small part of the districts Oder-Spree and Dahme-Spreewald. 1% decrease of unemployment among the 55–65 year olds will increase the T2DM prevalence between 1.3 and 6.4%.

The association between proportion of employed persons, which are subject to social insurance contribution, and T2DM changed sign across the study area. In the areas, where the proportion of employed persons was significant positively associated, 1% increase in employed persons was associated with 1.5–3.5% increase in T2DM prevalence. In the areas where the proportion of employed persons was significant negatively associated, 1% decrease of employed persons was associated with a 0.5–3.2% increase in T2DM prevalence. However, the association between employed persons and T2DM was only significant in a fraction of areas.

Similar to proportion of employed persons, the association between mean income tax and T2DM changed sign across the study area. In several districts north of Berlin, where the association between income tax and T2DM prevalence was positive, 10 Euro income tax per person per year will increase the T2DM prevalence by 0.1–3.2%. In the areas where the association to income tax was significant negative, 10 Euro less income tax per person per year will increase the T2DM prevalence between 1.6 and 3%.

The proportion of non-married couples sharing a common flat was only significant in several small parts of the districts Dahme-Spreewald and Teltow-Fläming. In these areas, 1% increase in non-married couples will increase the T2DM prevalence between 2.2 and 6.3%.

Discussion

The prevalence of T2DM varies strongly at the very local level and clusters especially in rural areas in Brandenburg and Mecklenburg-Vorpommern. Socio-demographic risk factors consisted of proportion of persons aged 65–79, proportion of persons aged 80 and older, unemployment rate among the 55–65 year olds, proportion of employed persons, which are subject to social insurance contribution, mean income tax and proportion of non-married couples sharing a common flat. However, all associations displayed strong regional differences.

The overall prevalence of T2DM was 20%. After adjusting for sex and age, the prevalence of 14.2% was still higher than national estimates based on data derived from the telephone survey of the Robert-Koch-Institute (GEDA), which estimated the prevalence of known Diabetes to be at 8.8% among adults in Germany [3]. However, estimates derived from surveys such as the GEDA study are rather underestimated as healthy participants are more likely to respond than chronically ill patients [20, 21]. In this study, the estimated prevalence exceeds these previous estimates by far. As our study area comprises the most deprived areas in Germany [28], it is not surprising that our estimates exceed those of the GEDA study. Additionally, the proportion of older inhabitants, persons with

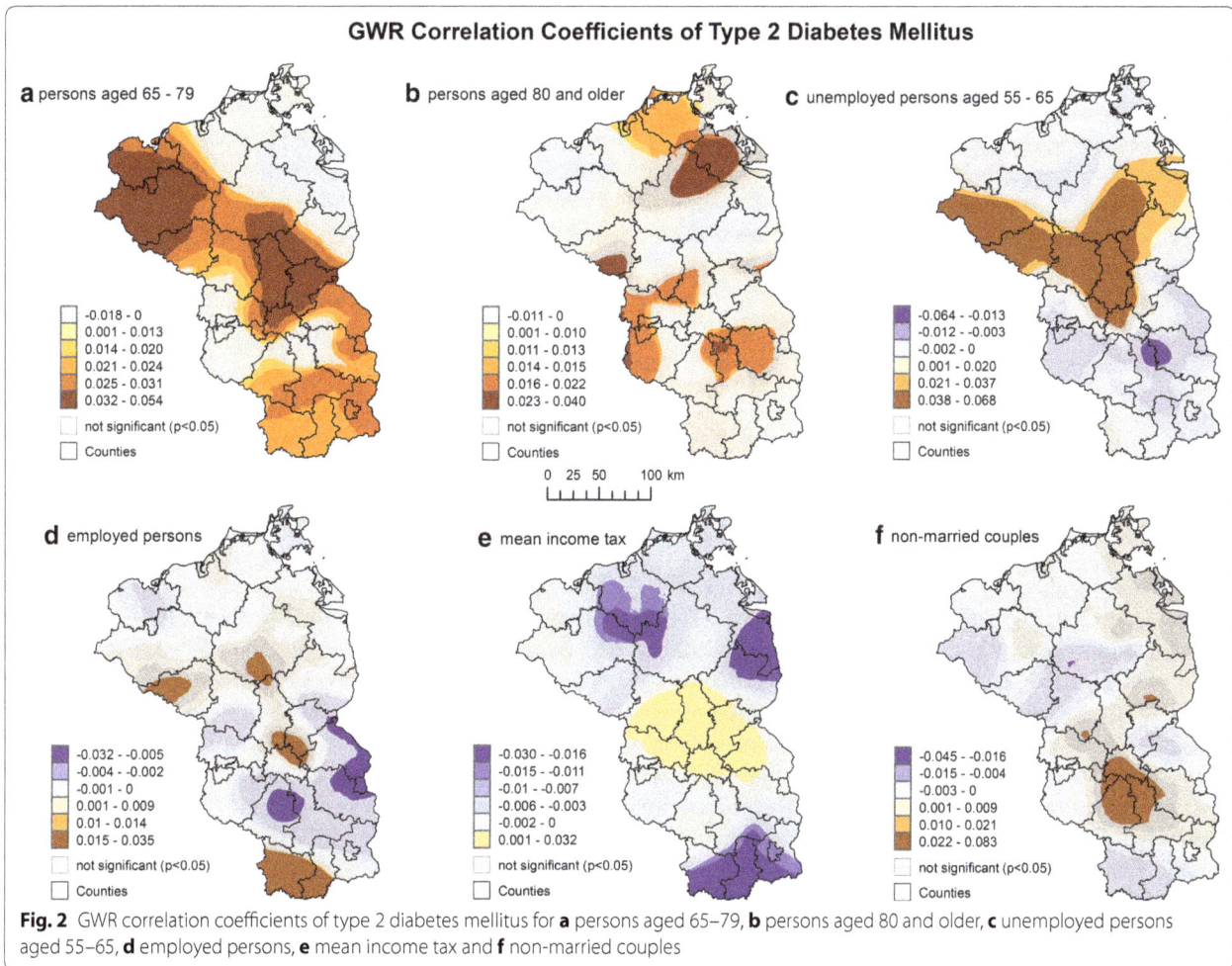

Fig. 2 GWR correlation coefficients of type 2 diabetes mellitus for **a** persons aged 65–79, **b** persons aged 80 and older, **c** unemployed persons aged 55–65, **d** employed persons, **e** mean income tax and **f** non-married couples

low levels of education and unemployed persons among the local AOK health insurances is generally higher than in other statutory health insurances. As a logical consequence, the prevalence of chronic diseases is higher in our population sample than in the rest of the population [25].

The spatial distribution of T2DM varied strongly and formed clusters on small geographic scales. This was reflected by the results of the bivariate kernel density estimation and the results of the spatial scan statistic. Spatial heterogeneity and local clustering is typical for a wide range of chronic diseases [12, 59–62]. Our results are therefore in line with other studies but add an important level of spatial detail to previous research. The combination of the bivariate KDE and the spatial scan statistic complimented each other fairly well using the settings chosen in this study. However, we had to use a very conservative p value for the cluster analysis, as the number of clusters using a p-value of 0.05 was simply too high to allow a detailed investigation.

We identified six risk factors for T2DM in northeastern Germany: (1) proportion of persons aged 65–79, (2)

proportion of persons aged 80 and older, (3) proportion of unemployed persons aged 55–65; (4) proportion of employed persons which are subject to social insurance contribution, (5) income tax and (6) proportion of non-married couples, which live together in the same household.

The association of T2DM to older age groups was expected as T2DM displays a strong association to older age groups [3, 4, 22]. The association of T2DM to the proportion of persons aged 65–79 and persons aged 80 and older is therefore in line with these studies although these associations were not in the entire study area significant.

Several studies pointed out that T2DM is associated with a lower socio-economic status [4, 14–16]. This is reflected by the strong association of unemployed persons aged 55–65 to T2DM. Given the high proportion of older persons among the AOK insurants, it is not surprising that specifically the unemployment rate among persons aged 55–65 was significant, but not unemployment rate in general. Additionally, this reflects the value of stratified socio-economic data as these findings could allow a more targeted prevention strategy among the at-risk population group.

The association to employed persons, which are subject to social insurance contribution, has to be seen in the context of income tax. Employed persons were positively associated in the areas, where income tax was negatively (but not significant) associated with T2DM prevalence. This reflects the association of T2DM to the lower-income groups [4, 15] and thus highlights the importance of determining location-specific association for T2DM. The negative association of employed persons to T2DM in specific areas can in part be explained by the exclusion criteria of employed persons in Germany. Excluded under this definition are for example persons working in marginal employment, soldiers, self-employed persons, non-working family members and government officials [63]. Given the association of T2DM to lower socio-economic status, these results might indicate that in areas where the association to employed persons is negative, persons working in marginally employment and non-working family members are at major risk for T2DM.

Although income tax was overall positively associated to T2DM, the results of GWR point out that income tax was in several areas significant negatively associated, confirming the results of previous studies [4, 15]. The positive association of income tax to T2DM prevalence is very specific to the area surrounding Berlin, which is often referred to as the commuter belt. This positive association reflects that in specific areas, a higher income may pose a risk factor for T2DM as well.

Several studies have shown that marital status has an effect on the overall health of the population. An unmarried status is often associated with a higher prevalence of chronic diseases and premature death [64], although not all studies can confirm this association [65]. The positive association of non-married couples sharing a common flat to T2DM can therefore be considered as very specific to the commuting belt around Berlin. Further research on an individual level is necessary to confirm this association.

Although several studies found an association between land-use, built environment and obesity and T2DM [66, 67], we found only a very moderate association between the proportion of built surfaces and T2DM. After carefully reviewing the results of a GWR model including the proportion of built surfaces as independent variable, we concluded that this association was misleading in our study area as it was only significant in the most sparsely populated area in Brandenburg. This seems implausible as villages in this area are generally very small and green spaces are widely available and accessible in walking distance. We thus excluded the proportion of built areas as independent variable from our analysis. However,

this highlights the value of local regression models over global regression models to question the plausibility of possible associations.

We found no associations between availability of GPs and the prevalence of T2DM. Thus, access to and availability of GPs has no influence on the diagnosis of T2DM in our study area. Since the majority of T2DM is detected among persons in their 40 s and older [68], and diabetics in rural areas consulting GPs less frequently than diabetics in urban areas [69], it seems reasonable to assume that a substantial amount of diabetics in our study area only sought medical attention when symptoms of T2DM persisted as our population sample is older than the rest of northeastern Germany's population. As a consequence, the number of undiagnosed diabetics in rural areas is potentially higher among middle-aged persons, which do not display any symptoms yet.

Strengths and limitations
Strengths
In this study, we used a large database, consisting of 1.8 million insurants. Our results clearly demonstrate that a spatial analysis using "big data" of health insurance providers is feasible and can be used to provide a finer spatial resolution for prevalence estimates of T2DM than it is currently possible with survey data.

Several spatial-epidemiological studies highlight the benefits of performing a cluster test based on point data over administrative data [30, 70, 71]. Detailed cluster detection based on point data could not only enhance prevention strategies [17, 30] but could also be used for a demand-driven allocation of healthcare facilities where they are needed most [48]. In northeastern Germany, this is of particular importance as the population is very unevenly distributed and the smallest administrative unit–municipalities–vary strongly in size and population among the states [72]. Further, Germany's largest city Berlin counts as only one municipality. Five-digit postal codes were thus used for the sex- and age standardization to highlight intra-urban differences. German postal codes have the disadvantage of - specifically in predominantly rural regions - covering very large areas and are thus not very suitable for the allocation of future healthcare. As a consequence, our approach of combining a bivariate KDE with a cluster analysis may serve as an alternative and relative exact prioritization for allocating new GP resources in the near future.

Limitations
First, our study was based on health insurance claims of northeastern Germany's largest statutory health insurance provider. Although the AOK Nordost covers approximately one quarter of the population, the results

cannot be assumed to sufficiently reflect the prevalence of T2DM for the whole population. Large socio-demographic differences exist between the insurants of the various statutory health insurance providers with the AOK having the largest proportion of persons with low income, low educational level and thus the highest prevalence of chronic diseases [25].

Second, we included all persons that were insured in 2012 with the AOK Nordost, irrespective of the length of insurance. We therefore did not exclude persons who died in 2012 from the analysis or persons being insured for short time-periods as these persons still contributed to the overall prevalence of T2DM.

Third, it is clear that the results of the bivariate KDE for T2DM represent the demographic distribution of insurants to a certain extent, given the strong association of T2DM to older age groups [3, 4, 22]. However, age-standardization is currently not available for a bivariate KDE in the CrimeStat IV software. As a consequence, the combined results of the bivariate KDE and the spatial scan statistic are more relevant for immediate allocation of GPs than for long-term planning of future healthcare.

Fourth, although most clusters were concentrated in areas with above-average prevalence estimates of the KDE, a small proportion of clusters was also concentrated in areas with below-average prevalence estimates. This is attributable to the different settings used in this study for the bivariate KDE and the spatial scan statistic. As we used an adaptive kernel for the KDE and a fixed radius of 10 km for the spatial scan statistic, higher prevalences cannot be sufficiently visualized if several hundred cases are concentrated in a very small location. This may occur for example with adjacent multi-story apartment blocks, which still constitute a significant cluster as detected by the spatial scan statistic but are smaller than the resolution offered by the KDE. When using fixed bandwidths of the same size for KDE and the spatial scan statistic simultaneously, this problem becomes less prominent [30].

Fifth, the associations examined in this study are based on aggregated data. Although our results generally reflect the results of other spatial-epidemiological studies on T2DM, it is necessary to review whether the associations revealed in this study at the ecological level are also valid associations on an individual level.

Implications for future planning of healthcare

Our results clearly demonstrate that the prevalence of T2DM varies at very fine geographic scales. The small-scale spatial variability of T2DM thus challenges the applicability of the spatial scale of central areas (Mittelbereiche) at which the allocation of GPs is currently planned [7, 73]. Based on our results, a planning on

smaller scales such as the association of municipalities would be more suitable to reflect the strong spatial variability of T2DM. It has been argued that the current provision of GPs–based on the ratio of 1 GP per 1671 inhabitants [7]—is too simplified and also outdated [8, 74]. The association of T2DM to location-specific socio-demographic population characteristics demands a strong deviation from these ratios and calls for a stronger acknowledgement of increased medical needs among the elderly and socially underprivileged populations. The revised planning guidelines of the federal association of statutory physicians in 2013 would allow deviations from the current ratio for areas with a particular high prevalence of diseases or specific socio-economic characteristics [75]. However, these revised planning guidelines still remain unspecific on how exactly a particular high prevalence or specific socio-economic characteristics can be translated into additional GP positions for a particular area. As a consequence, our analysis can only point out areas with a currently high medical demand and location-specific associations between T2DM and socio-demographic population characteristics.

Given that the spatial variability of T2DM is not only determined by current socio-demographic factors but also by the change of these factors over time [4], the results of our GWR analysis could serve as a first basis in developing approaches to model the expected, long-term future burden of T2DM to assist in allocating future GPs where they will be needed most.

Conclusion

This is to date the largest small-scale spatial-epidemiological study of T2DM in northeastern Germany. Our results clearly show that T2DM varies at the very local level and that a large variation of T2DM prevalence can be explained by location-specific, socio-demographic population characteristics. Future planning of healthcare would greatly benefit from smaller spatial scales and need to deviate from simple inhabitants to GP ratios to reflect the increased prevalence of chronic diseases in older and socially underprivileged population groups. These results are therefore valuable for the future planning of healthcare in northeastern Germany. Our approach of analyzing the spatial distribution of chronic diseases at the very local level and geographically weighted regression is not only useful for northeastern Germany, but could be an effective way of targeting location-specific population groups with increased medical needs as precisely as possible in all countries, where chronic diseases are on the rise.

Abbreviations
AIC: Akaike's information criterion; AICc: Akaike's corrected information criterion; BBSR: Federal Agency of Building and Urban Development; BIC: Bayesian

information criterion; CV: cross validation; GIS: geographic information systems; GP: general practitioner; GWR: geographically weighted regression; ICD-10: international classification of disease, 10th revision; KDE: kernel density estimation; OLS: ordinary least squares; T2DM: type 2 diabetes mellitus.

Authors' contributions

BK developed the design of the study, undertook the statistical analysis and wrote the manuscript. JS, TK, AK and MM, critically reviewed the manuscript and provided helpful feedback. All authors read and approved the final manuscript.

Author details

[1] Department of Medical Care, AOK Nordost – Die Gesundheitskasse, Berlin, Germany. [2] Department III, Civil Engineering and Geoinformatics, Beuth University of Applied Sciences, Berlin, Germany. [3] Department of Health, Ethics and Society, School of Public Health and Primary Care (CAPHRI), Faculty of Health, Medicine and Life Sciences, Maastricht University, Maastricht, The Netherlands.

Competing interests

The authors declare that they have no competing interests.

References

1. Glynn LG, Valderas JM, Healy P, Burke E, Newell J, Gillespie P, et al. The prevalence of multimorbidity in primary care and its effect on health care utilization and cost. Fam Pract. 2011;28(5):516–23.
2. Dalstra JA, Kunst AE, Borrell C, Breeze E, Cambois E, Costa G, et al. Socioeconomic differences in the prevalence of common chronic diseases: an overview of eight European countries. Int J Epidemiol. 2005;34(2):316–26.
3. Heidemann C, Du Y, Scheidt-Nave C. Diabetes mellitus in Deutschland. In: GBE kompakt 3. Berlin, Germany: Robert-Koch-Institute; 2011.
4. Dijkstra A, Janssen F, De Bakker M, Bos J, Lub R, Van Wissen LJ, et al. Using spatial analysis to predict health care use at the local level: a case study of type 2 diabetes medication use and its association with demograpHic change and socioeconomic status. PLoS ONE. 2013;8(8):e72730.
5. Kanjilal S, Gregg EW, Cheng YJ, Zhang P, Nelson DE, Mensah G, et al. Socioeconomic status and trends in disparities in 4 major risk factors for cardiovascular disease among US adults, 1971–2002. Arch Intern Med. 2006;166(21):2348–55.
6. Avendano M, Kunst AE, Huisman M, Lenthe FV, Bopp M, Regidor E, et al. Socioeconomic status and ischaemic heart disease mortality in 10 western European populations during the 1990s. Heart. 2006;92(4):461–7.
7. Bundesausschuss G. Bedarfsplanungs - Richtlinie Stand: 15. Oktober 2015 des Gemeinsamen Bundesausschusses über die Bedarfsplanung sowie die Maßstäbe zur Feststellung von Überversorgung und Unterversorgung in der vertragsärztlichen Versorgung: Gemeinsamer Bundesausschuss; 2012 [cited 2016 17th May]. https://www.g-ba.de/downloads/62-492-1109/BPL-RL_2015-10-15_iK-2016-01-06.pdf.
8. Ozegowski S, Sundmacher L. Wie „bedarfsgerecht"ist die Bedarfsplanung? Eine Analyse der regionalen Verteilung der vertragsärztlichen Versorgung. Gesundheitswesen. 2012;74(10):618–26.
9. Swart E, von Stillfried DG, Koch-Gromus U. Kleinräumige Versorgungsforschung Wo sich Wissenschaft, Praxis und Politik treffen. Bundesgesundheitsbl. 2014;57:161–3.
10. Barker LE, Kirtland KA, Gregg EW, Geiss LS, Thompson TJ. Geographic distribution of diagnosed diabetes in the US: a diabetes belt. Am J Prev Med. 2011;40(4):434–9.
11. Wild S, Roglic G, Green A, Sicree R, King H. Global prevalence of diabetes estimates for the year 2000 and projections for 2030. Diabetes Care. 2004;27(5):1047–53.
12. Margolis DJ, Hoffstad O, Nafash J, Leonard CE, Freeman CP, Hennessy S, et al. Location, location, location: geographic clustering of lower-extremity amputation among Medicare beneficiaries with diabetes. Diabetes Care. 2011;34(11):2363–7.
13. Espeland M. Reduction in weight and cardiovascular disease risk factors in individuals with type 2 diabetes. Diabetes Care. 2007;30(6):1374–83.
14. Siordia C, Saenz J, Tom SE. An introduction to macro-level spatial nonstationarity: a geographically weighted regression analysis of diabetes and poverty. Hum Geogr. 2012;6(2):5.
15. Hipp JA, Chalise N. Peer reviewed: spatial analysis and correlates of county-level diabetes prevalence, 2009–2010. Prevent Chronic Dis. 2015;12:140404.
16. Maier W, Scheidt-Nave C, Holle R, Kroll LE, Lampert T, Du Y, et al. Area level deprivation is an independent determinant of prevalent type 2 diabetes and obesity at the national level in Germany. Results from the National Telephone Health Interview Surveys 'German Health Update'GEDA 2009 and 2010. PLoS ONE. 2014;9(2):e89661.
17. Kauhl B, Heil J, Hoebe CJ, Schweikart J, Krafft T, Dukers-Muijrers NH. The spatial distribution of hepatitis C virus infections and associated determinants—an application of a geographically weighted poisson regression for evidence-based screening interventions in hotspots. PLoS ONE. 2015;10(9):e0135656.
18. Weisent J, Rohrbach B, Dunn JR. Socioeconomic determinants of geographic disparities in campylobacteriosis risk: a comparison of global and local modeling approaches. Int J Health Geogr. 2012;11(1):1.
19. Wittchen H-U, Pieper L, Eichler T, Klotsche J. Prävalenz und Versorgung von Diabetes mellitus und Herz-Kreislauf-Erkrankungen: DETECT—eine bundesweite Versorgungsstudie an über 55.000 Hausarztpatienten. Prävention und Versorgungsforschung: Springer; 2008. p. 315–28.
20. Grundmann N, Mielck A, Siegel M, Maier W. Area deprivation and the prevalence of type 2 diabetes and obesity: analysis at the municipality level in Germany. BMC Public Health. 2014;14(1):1.
21. Kroll LE, Lampert T. Regionale Unterschiede in der Gesundheit am Beispiel von Adipositas und Diabetes mellitus. Robert Koch-Institut, editor Daten und Fakten: Ergebnisse der Studie » Gesundheit in Deutschland aktuell. 2010;51–9.
22. Erhart M, Herring R, Schulz M, Stillfried DV. Morbiditätsatlas Hamburg. Gutachten zum kleinräumigen Versorgungsbedarf in Hamburg– erstellt durch das Zentralinstitut für die kassenärztliche Versorgung in Deutschland, im Auftrag der Behörde für Gesundheit und Verbraucherschutz Hamburg « Hamburg. 2013;7.
23. Schipf S, Werner A, Tamayo T, Holle R, Schunk M, Maier W, et al. Regional differences in the prevalence of known Type 2 diabetes mellitus in 45–74 years old individuals: results from six population-based studies in Germany (DIAB-CORE Consortium). Diabet Med. 2012;29(7):e88–95.
24. Ziegler U, Doblhammer G. Prävalenz und Inzidenz von Demenz in Deutschland-Eine Studie auf Basis von Daten der gesetzlichen Krankenversicherungen von 2002. Das Gesundheitswesen. 2009;71(05):281–90.
25. Schnee M. Sozioökonomische Strukturen und Morbidität in den gesetzlichen Krankenkassen. In: Böcken J, Braun B, Amhof R, editors. Gesundheitsmonitor 2008, Gesundheitsversorgung und Gestaltungsoptionen aus der Perspektive der Bevölkerung. Gütersloh: Verlag Bertelsmann Stiftung; 2008. p. 88–104.
26. Schubert I, Köster I, Küpper-Nybelen J. Ihle P (2008) Versorgungsforschung mit GKV-Routinedaten. Bundesgesundheitsblatt-Gesundheitsforschung-Gesundheitsschutz. 2008;51(10):1095–105.
27. OpenStreetMap. [cited 2016 17. Mai]. https://download.geofabrik.de/.
28. Schäfer T, Pritzkuleit R, Jeszenszky C, Malzahn J, Maier W, Günther K, et al. Trends and geographical variation of primary hip and knee joint replacement in Germany. Osteoarthr Cartil. 2013;21(2):279–88.
29. Fotheringham AS, Wong DW. The modifiable areal unit problem in multivariate statistical analysis. Environ Plan A. 1991;23(7):1025–44.
30. Tanser F, Bärnighausen T, Cooke GS, Newell M-L. Localized spatial clustering of HIV infections in a widely disseminated rural South African epidemic. Int J Epidemiol. 2009:dyp148.
31. Larmarange J, Vallo R, Yaro S, Msellati P, Méda N. Methods for mapping regional trends of HIV prevalence from Demographic and Health Surveys (DHS). CyberGeo. 2011.
32. Shi X. Selection of bandwidth type and adjustment side in kernel density estimation over inhomogeneous backgrounds. Int J Geogr Inf Sci. 2010;24(5):643–60.
33. Lemke D, Mattauch V, Heidinger O, Pebesma E, Hense H-W. Comparing adaptive and fixed bandwidth-based kernel density estimates in spatial cancer epidemiology. Int J Health Geogr. 2015;14(1):1.

34. Almeida MCS, Gomes CMS, Nascimento LFC. Spatial distribution of deaths due to Alzheimer's disease in the state of São Paulo, Brazil. Sao Paulo Med J. 2014;132(4):199–204.

35. Oberwittler D, Wiesenhütter M. The Risk of Violent Incidents Relative to Population Density in Cologne Using the Dual Kernel Density Routine. Levine, N, CrimeStat II: A Spatial Statistics Program for the Analysis of Crime Incident Locations, Program Manual, Washington, district fédéral de Columbia National Institute of Justice. 2002; p. 332.

36. Duin RPW. On the choice of smoothing parameters for Parzen estimators of probability density functions. IEEE Trans Comput. 1976;11:1175–9.

37. Habemma JDF, Hermans J, Van Den Broek K. Stepwise discriminant analysis program using density estimation. In: COMPSTAT 1974, Proceedings in computational statistics. Heidelberg: Physica Verlag; 1974. p. 101-10.

38. Rudemo M. Empirical choice of histograms and kernel density estimators. Scand J Stat. 1982;65–78.

39. Scott DW, Terrell GR. Biased and unbiased cross-validation in density estimation. J Am Stat Assoc. 1987;82(400):1131–46.

40. Sheather SJ, Jones MC. A reliable data-based bandwidth selection method for kernel density estimation. J R Stat Soc Ser B (Methodol). 1991;683–90.

41. Hall P, Sheather SJ, Jones M, Marron JS. On optimal data-based bandwidth selection in kernel density estimation. Biometrika. 1991;78(2):263–9.

42. Lai P-C, So F-M, Chan K-W. Spatial epidemiological approaches in disease mapping and analysis. Boca Raton: CRC Press; 2008.

43. Levine N. CrimeStat III: a spatial statistics program for the analysis of crime incident locations (version 3.0). Houston (TX): Ned Levine & Associates/Washington, DC: National Institute of Justice. 2004.

44. Ahmad OB, Boschi-Pinto C, Lopez AD, Murray CJ, Lozano R, Inoue M. Age standardization of rates: a new WHO standard. Geneva: World Health Organization; 2001. p. 9.

45. Lawson A, Biggeri A, Böhning D, Lesaffre E, Viel J-F, Bertollini R. Disease mapping and risk assessment for public health. London: Wiley; 1999.

46. Anselin L. Exploring spatial data with Geoda: a workbook, Spatial Analysis Laboratory Department of Geography. University of Illinois, Center for Spatially Integrated Social Science. 2006.

47. Coleman M, Coleman M, Mabuza AM, Kok G, Coetzee M, Durrheim DN. Using the SaTScan method to detect local malaria clusters for guiding malaria control programmes. Malar J. 2009;8(1):1–6.

48. Faruque LI, Ayyalasomayajula B, Pelletier R, Klarenbach S, Hemmelgarn BR, Tonelli M. Spatial analysis to locate new clinics for diabetic kidney patients in the underserved communities in Alberta. Nephrol Dial Transplant. 2012;27(11):4102–9.

49. Kulldorff M. SaTScan user guide for version 9.4. 2015. 2016.

50. Kulldorff M. A spatial scan statistic. Commun Stat Theory Methods. 1997;26(6):1481–96.

51. Chen J, Roth RE, Naito AT, Lengerich EJ, MacEachren AM. Geovisual analytics to enhance spatial scan statistic interpretation: an analysis of US cervical cancer mortality. Int J Health Geogr. 2008;7(1):1.

52. Poole MA, O'Farrell PN. The assumptions of the linear regression model. Trans Inst Br Geogr. 1971;145–58.

53. Haque U, Scott LM, Hashizume M, Fisher E, Haque R, Yamamoto T, et al. Modelling malaria treatment practices in Bangladesh using spatial statistics. Malar J. 2012;11(63):101–86.

54. ESRI. How Exploratory Regression works [cited 2016 17. Mai]. http://desktop.arcgis.com/en/arcmap/10.3/tools/spatial-statistics-toolbox/how-exploratory-regression-works.htm.

55. Hu M, Li Z, Wang J, Jia L, Liao Y, Lai S, et al. Determinants of the incidence of hand, foot and mouth disease in China using geographically weighted regression models. PLoS ONE. 2012;7(6):e38978.

56. Gebreab SY, Roux AVD. Exploring racial disparities in CHD mortality between blacks and whites across the United States: a geographically weighted regression approach. Health Place. 2012;18(5):1006–14.

57. Fotheringham AS, Brunsdon C, Charlton M. Geographically weighted regression. London: Wiley; 2003.

58. Nakaya T. GWR4 user manual. WWW document, http://www.st-andrews.ac.uk/geoinformatics/wp-content/uploads/GWR4manual_201311.pdf. 2012.

59. Curtis AJ, Lee WAA. Lee W-AA. Spatial patterns of diabetes related health problems for vulnerable populations in Los Angeles. Int J Health Geogr. 2010;9(1):1.

60. Fukuda Y, Umezaki M, Nakamura K, Takano T. Variations in societal characteristics of spatial disease clusters: examples of colon, lung and breast cancer in Japan. Int J Health Geogr. 2005;4(1):1.

61. Schmiedel S, Jacquez GM, Blettner M, Schüz J. Spatial clustering of leukemia and type 1 diabetes in children in Denmark. Cancer Causes Control. 2011;22(6):849–57.

62. Schlundt DG, Hargreaves MK, McClellan L. Geographic clustering of obesity, diabetes, and hypertension in Nashville, Tennessee. J Ambul Care Manag. 2006;29(2):125–32.

63. Arbeit Bf. Methodische Hinweise zu sozialversicherungspflichtig und geringfügig Beschäftigten 2013 [cited 2016 May 17th]. https://statistik.arbeitsagentur.de/nn_280848/Statischer-Content/Grundlagen/Methodische-Hinweise/BST-MethHinweise/SvB-und-GB-meth-Hinweise.html.

64. Kaplan RM, Kronick RG. Marital status and longevity in the United States population. J Epidemiol Community Health. 2006;60(9):760–5.

65. Azimi-Nezhad M, Ghayour-Mobarhan M, Parizadeh M, Safarian M, Esmaeili H, Parizadeh S, et al. Prevalence of type 2 diabetes mellitus in Iran and its relationship with gender, urbanisation, education, marital status and occupation. Singapore Med J. 2008;49(7):571.

66. Salois MJ. Obesity and diabetes, the built environment, and the 'local' food economy in the United States, 2007. Econ Hum Biol. 2012;10(1):35–42.

67. Papas MA, Alberg AJ, Ewing R, Helzlsouer KJ, Gary TL, Klassen AC. The built environment and obesity. Epidemiol Rev. 2007;29(1):129–43.

68. Koopman RJ, Mainous AG, Diaz VA, Geesey ME. Changes in age at diagnosis of type 2 diabetes mellitus in the United States, 1988 to 2000. Ann Fam Med. 2005;3(1):60–3.

69. Dansky KH, Dirani R. The use of health care services by people with diabetes in rural areas. J Rural Health. 1998;14(2):129–37.

70. Warden CR. Comparison of Poisson and Bernoulli spatial cluster analyses of pediatric injuries in a fire district. Int J Health Geogr. 2008;7(1):1.

71. Olson KL, Grannis SJ, Mandl KD. Privacy protection versus cluster detection in spatial epidemiology. Am J Public Health. 2006;96(11):2002–8.

72. Maier W, Fairburn J, Mielck A. Regional deprivation and mortality in Bavaria Development of a community-based index of multiple deprivation. Gesundheitswesen. 2012;74(7):416–25.

73. Gerlach F, Greiner W, Haubitz M. Bedarfsgerechte Versorgung-Perspektiven für ländliche Regionen und ausgewählte Leistungsbereiche. Gutachten; 2014.

74. Kucharska W, Pieper J, Schweikart J. Zugang zur Kindergesundheit in Brandenburg–eine Untersuchung auf der Grundlage freier Geodaten. Angewandte Geoinformatik. 2014;282–91.

75. Bundesvereinigung K. Die neue Bedarfsplanung Grundlagen, Instrumente und regionale Möglichkeiten: Kassenärztliche Bundesvereinigung. Cited 2016 May 17th. http://www.kbv.de/media/sp/Instrumente_Bedarfsplanung_Broschuere.pdf.

7

Differences in physical environmental characteristics between adolescents' actual and shortest cycling routes: a study using a Google Street View-based audit

Hannah Verhoeven[1,2,3]* ⓘ, Linde Van Hecke[1,2,3], Delfien Van Dyck[3,4], Tim Baert[5], Nico Van de Weghe[5], Peter Clarys[2], Benedicte Deforche[1,2] and Jelle Van Cauwenberg[1,3]

Abstract

Background: The objective evaluation of the physical environmental characteristics (e.g. speed limit, cycling infrastructure) along adolescents' actual cycling routes remains understudied, although it may provide important insights into why adolescents prefer one cycling route over another. The present study aims to gain insight into the physical environmental characteristics determining the route choice of adolescent cyclists by comparing differences in physical environmental characteristics between their actual cycling routes and the shortest possible cycling routes.

Methods: Adolescents (n = 204; 46.5% boys; 14.4 ± 1.2 years) recruited at secondary schools in and around Ghent (city in Flanders, northern part of Belgium) were instructed to wear a Global Positioning System device in order to identify cycling trips. For all identified cycling trips, the shortest possible route that could have been taken was calculated. Actual cycling routes that were not the shortest possible cycling routes were divided into street segments. Segments were audited with a Google Street View-based tool to assess physical environmental characteristics along actual and shortest cycling routes.

Results: Out of 160 actual cycling trips, 73.1% did not differ from the shortest possible cycling route. For actual cycling routes that were not the shortest cycling route, a speed limit of 30 km/h, roads having few buildings with windows on the street side and roads without cycle lane were more frequently present compared to the shortest possible cycling routes. A mixed land use, roads with commercial destinations, arterial roads, cycle lanes separated from traffic by white lines, small cycle lanes and cycle lanes covered by lighting were less frequently present along actual cycling routes compared to the shortest possible cycling routes.

Conclusions: Results showed that distance mainly determines the route along which adolescents cycle. In addition, adolescents cycled more along residential streets (even if no cycle lane was present) and less along busy, arterial roads. Local authorities should provide shortcuts free from motorised traffic to meet adolescents' preference to cycle along the shortest route and to avoid cycling along arterial roads.

Keywords: Active transport, Cycling, Route choice, Physical environment, Audit, Youth

*Correspondence: hannah.verhoeven@ugent.be
[1] Department of Public Health, Faculty of Medicine and Health Sciences, Ghent University, Corneel Heymanslaan 10, 9000 Ghent, Belgium
Full list of author information is available at the end of the article

Background

Air pollution, which is partially caused by vehicle emissions, is consistently related to acute respiratory infections among young children, cardiopulmonary disease and lung cancer [1]. By replacing private car use (passive transport) by active modes of transport such as cycling, carbon dioxide emissions can be reduced substantially [2]. Although the risk of a higher intake of carbon dioxide can be considered as a negative aspect of active transport [3], a growing body of evidence emphasizes the potential benefits of cycling for transport for public health [2, 4]. Since adolescence is characterised by a steep decrease in physical activity levels [5], increasing cycling for transport is also a promising strategy to meet the recommended 60 min of daily physical activity among adolescents [4, 6]. Cycling for transport has been associated with higher levels of cardiorespiratory fitness [7] and lower levels of overweight [8] among adolescents and it can easily be incorporated into their daily lives once the skills for cycling have been acquired [9].

The role of the physical environment for health behaviours such as cycling for transport has been acknowledged by socio-ecological models and previous research [10–12]. However, the majority of previous studies investigating physical environmental correlates of cycling for transport focused on the neighbourhood environment close to home, although cycling for transport does not necessarily take place in the immediate neighbourhood environment. Nevertheless, the evaluation of physical environmental characteristics along adolescents' actual cycling routes remains understudied, although it is important to find out why individuals chose a specific cycling route. In addition, although previous studies emphasized the importance of distance for adolescents' cycling for transport [12–14], it is likely that adolescents do not always take the shortest cycling route. By comparing adolescents' actual cycling routes with the shortest possible cycling routes, important information regarding which physical environmental characteristics determine the route choice of adolescent cyclists may be obtained. Among adults, two recent studies compared physical environmental characteristics of actual and shortest cycling routes [15, 16]. Winters et al. [16] found that actual cycling routes of Canadian adults had significantly more traffic calming facilities (e.g. traffic circles or median barriers to slow or block motorized traffic) and participants cycled less along arterial (busy) roads and more along local roads, off-street paths and roads with cycling facilities. Krenn et al. [15] also found that Austrian cyclists avoid busy roads and prefer roads with cycle lanes. Actual cycling routes included more green and aquatic areas and had fewer traffic lights, fewer crossings and less hilly roads compared to the shortest routes.

Compared to the shortest routes, land use mix (i.e. the extent to which several types of land use, such as residential and industrial areas, shops, services, are included in an area) was significantly higher along actual cycling routes. A study among children in the Netherlands (8–12 years) found that there were significantly fewer trees, zebra crossings and sidewalks along actual cycling routes compared to the shortest routes [17]. In addition, actual cycling routes had significantly more traffic lights, junctions and a higher chance of being on residential streets compared to the shortest routes. Safety showed thus to be an important factor among children in this study. According to Dessing et al. [17], most of the zebra crossings in the Netherlands are located on or near busy streets, that were avoided by the children. Furthermore, when main roads have to be crossed children preferred signalized intersections. Because of some inconsistent results across these previous studies, similar studies among adolescents may provide additional insights into which physical environmental factors are related to an individuals' route choice.

Methodologies to assess the physical environment include both subjective and objective measurements. Subjective measurements, such as self-reported questionnaires, encounter limitations such as recall bias [18] and may not accurately assess the effect of the actual physical environmental factors on cycling for transport [11]. Therefore, observational field audits are frequently applied as an objective tool for measuring the physical environment related to physical activity [19–21]. Vanwolleghem et al. [22] developed EGA-Cycling (Environmental Google Street View Based Audit-Cycling) to virtually assess physical micro- and macro-environmental characteristics along cycling routes using Google Street View. EGA-Cycling was based on existing audit instruments (e.g. Pikora-SPACES instruments [20], Audit Tool Checklist version [21], Irvine-Minnesota Inventory [23]), but was adapted to the Flemish street infrastructure. In the last decade, using virtual technologies, such as Google Street View, to assess the physical environment is gaining attention [24–29]. Auditors are able to virtually walk through a street which is time- and cost-saving [24, 28] and they are not exposed to unsafe (traffic) situations compared to field audits. Previous studies showed good agreement between virtual and field audit tools [24, 26, 29]. However, virtual audit tools showed to be less accurate when measuring micro-environmental characteristics (e.g. litter, sidewalk condition) [24, 26, 28]. Nevertheless, Ben-Joseph et al. [28] concluded that Google Street View was more accurate in measuring small features compared to Google Maps and MS Visual Oblique.

The aim of the present study is to gain insight into the physical environmental characteristics determining the

route choice of adolescent cyclists by comparing differences in physical environmental characteristics between
their actual cycling routes and the shortest possible
cycling routes using a Google Street View-based audit
(EGA-Cycling).

Methods

Participants

A convenience sample of 12 secondary schools in and
around Ghent was contacted to participate in the study.
Ghent is a city in Flanders, northern part of Belgium,
that has 253,266 inhabitants and comprises an area of
156.2 km^2 (population density: 1622 h/km^2) [30, 31]. In
the six schools that agreed to participate, school prin-
cipals or staff members randomly selected at least two
classes from the first to fourth grade (12–16 years). A
total of 18 classes was selected and 283 adolescents were
invited to participate in the study. Only participants who
were present at school when measurement materials
were handed out, could be included in the study. Passive informed consent was obtained from adolescents'
parents. If parents did not agree to let their child participate in the study, they had to sign a form. Furthermore,
researchers also obtained active informed consent from
adolescents. This procedure resulted in a group of 238

adolescents (response rate = 84.1%) participating in the
study.

Study protocol

The study protocol consisted of two parts (see Fig. 1 for a
flow chart). In the first part of the study, each participating school was visited three times by the research team
between September and December 2015. During a first
visit, the purpose of the study was explained to the adolescents and informed consent was obtained. Each participant received a unique ID number in order to be able
to link data of all measurements. Participants completed
a questionnaire assessing socio-demographics. Furthermore, participants received a Global Positioning System
(GPS) device and a charger for the device together with
verbal and written instructions on how and when to wear
the device. All participants were instructed to wear the
GPS device, which was attached to their waist with an
elastic belt, during waking hours until the research team
returned to the school to collect the devices (4–5 days
later). During activities that could damage the GPS
device or during which it could be uncomfortable to
wear it (e.g. showering, swimming or rugby), the adolescents were asked to temporarily remove the GPS device.
They were also instructed not to turn off the GPS device
during data collection. Participants were asked for their

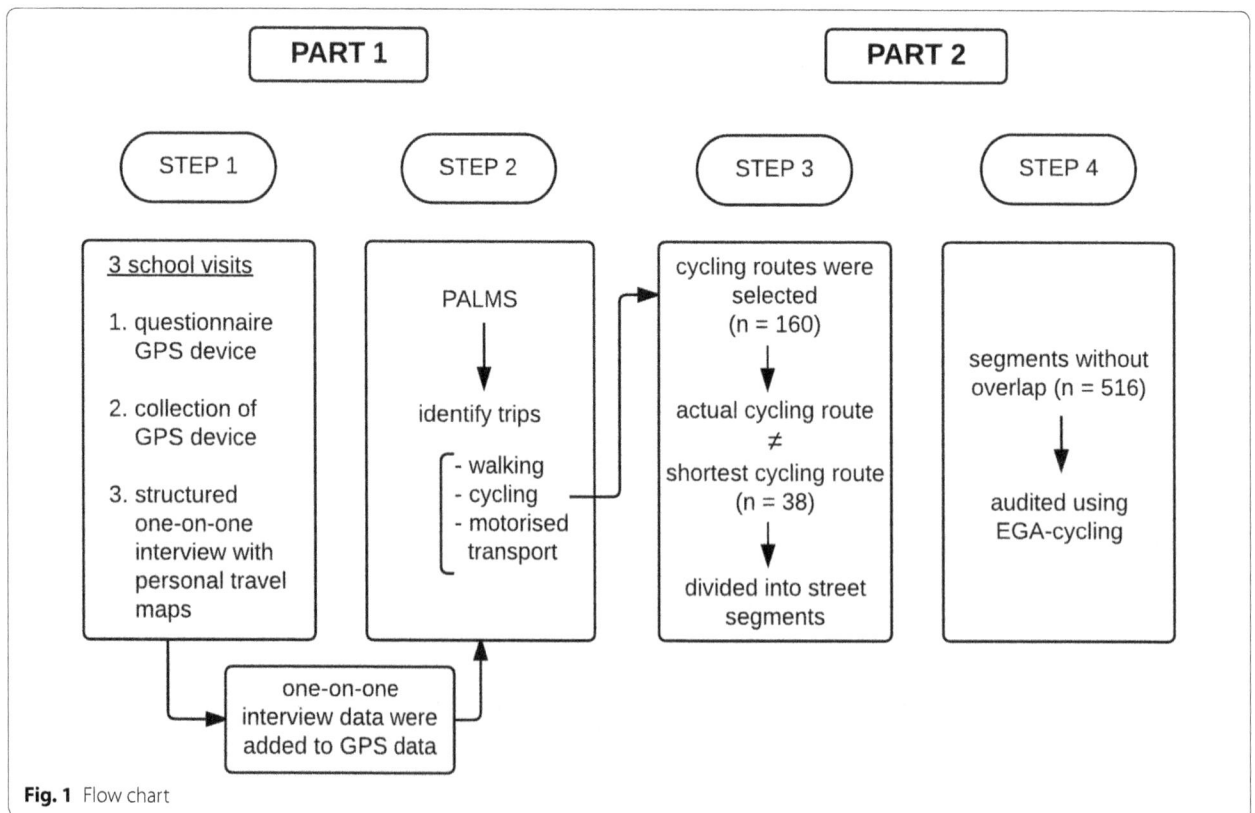

Fig. 1 Flow chart

mobile phone number. Two text messages per day (in the morning and evening) were sent to the participants willing to give their number in order to remind them to wear the GPS devices and to charge it. During a second visit, researchers returned to the schools to collect the devices. Afterwards, the GPS data were downloaded and a web application was created in order to visualize the data on a personal travel map. During the last visit, which took place within the first week after collection of the GPS devices, researchers conducted a structured one-on-one interview (Additional file 1) during which a researcher chronologically discussed the personal travel maps. Per trip travelled, participants were asked about their transport mode and why they took a particular route. Participants who completed all measurements and returned the GPS device received an incentive (i.e. movie ticket).

In the second part of the study, adolescents' cycling routes were selected, and for each actual cycling route the shortest cycling route was calculated using Google Maps. For each cycling route which was not the shortest cycling route, an adapted version of EGA-Cycling was used to obtain information about physical environmental characteristics along adolescents' actual cycling routes and along the corresponding shortest routes using Google Street View.

The study protocol was approved by the Ethics Committee of the University Hospital of Ghent University (EC 2015/0317).

Measurements and data processing
Questionnaire
Participants completed a paper-and-pencil questionnaire assessing following socio-demographics: home address, gender, date of birth, grade (first to fourth year), educational type (general, technical or vocational) and highest education of parents (primary education, secondary education, tertiary education-non university, tertiary education-university, I don't know). Education of parents was used to as a proxy for socio-economic status (SES). Adolescents were identified as being 'of a higher SES family' when at least one parent completed tertiary education [32].

GPS device
The geographical position of participants was recorded by the QStarz BT-Q1000X GPS device. In addition, the GPS device recorded participants' speed which was used to define their transport mode [33]. The GPS devices were set to collect data every 30 s using Q-travel software. Furthermore, the devices were set to stop logging when the memory was full (this did not occur during data collection). Q-travel software was used to download the collected GPS data.

Structured one-on-one interview with personal travel maps
GPS data were stored in a PostgreSQL database with PostGIS in order to generate a personal travel map per day in the web application. This web application showed the geographical position of participants for every 30-second-interval. Figure 2 shows an example of a personal travel map. These personal travel maps were used as a guide to conduct a structured one-on-one interview discussing routes on two selected days. The first week- and weekend day with complete data (excluding the day the devices were handed out) were selected for the interview. When no weekdays with complete data were available, two weekend days were selected and vice versa. When only 1 day with complete data was available, the structured interview was completed for 1 day. During these interviews, a researcher chronologically identified, together with the participants, the trips they made during a day. For each identified trip, the participant was asked which transport mode was used. For active trips (walking or cycling/skateboard/...) the participant was also asked why he/she chose that particular route to reach his/her destination.

GPS data processing
Data processing was executed using the Personal Activity and Location Measurement System (PALMS©) [34, 35]. PALMS filtered invalid GPS data when extreme speed (> 150 km/h) or extreme changes in distance (> 1000 m) or elevation (> 100 m) between two consecutive data points were identified. The programming software Python was used to combine the PALMS dataset with information on school schedules of each participating class, school addresses and home addresses of participants. PALMS categorised data into location (home, school, leisure) or transport. Data were categorised in the domain 'transport' when a trip was detected. A trip was defined as a period of at least 3 min of movement with the same transport mode, allowing for stationary periods of maximum 3 min. PALMS classified all trips into walking, cycling or motorised transport based on speed. A trip was classified as walking when speed was between 1 and 9 km/h, cycling between 10 and 24 km/h and motorised transport starting from 25 km/h [33, 36].

Subsequently, all data from the structured one-on-one interviews were inserted into the database. For trips or locations that were misclassified by PALMS [e.g. when a car trip was classified as a bicycle trip due to traffic congestion (speed < 25 km/h)], corrections were made based on the data of the structured interviews. The number of corrections due to misclassification by PALMS was rather limited.

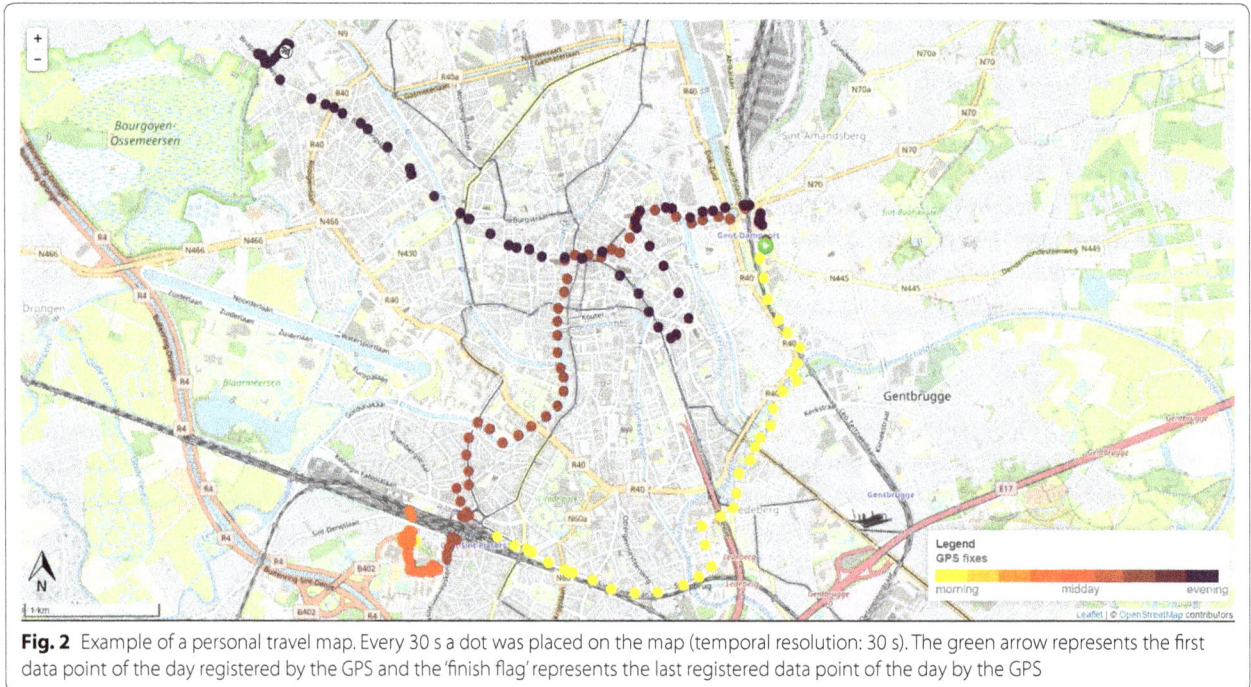

Fig. 2 Example of a personal travel map. Every 30 s a dot was placed on the map (temporal resolution: 30 s). The green arrow represents the first data point of the day registered by the GPS and the 'finish flag' represents the last registered data point of the day by the GPS

EGA-cycling

EGA-Cycling (Additional file 2) consists of five subscales and includes 37 items: (1) land use (8 items; e.g. commercial destinations, heavy industry and public destinations), (2) general characteristics of the street segment (12 items; e.g. road type and speed limit), (3) cycling facilities (7 items; e.g. type and width of cycle lane), (4) pedestrian facilities (3 items; e.g. presence and maintenance of the sidewalk) and (5) aesthetics (7 items; e.g. trees and front yards). EGA-Cycling shows acceptable reliability and validity [22]. However, since measures about (safety at) intersections are very limited from this tool, three additional items regarding this topic were added (i.e. amount of side streets, amount of intersections and visibility at the corners). The item regarding visibility at the corners is part of the Microscale Audit of Pedestrian Streetscape (MAPS) Global tool [37]. Furthermore, another item was included that assessed whether or not the street segment concerned a walking/cycling road (i.e. a separate road only accessible for non-motorised traffic). Data on differences in pedestrian facilities between actual cycling routes and the shortest possible cycling routes are not shown since they are not relevant for cycling.

Auditing of actual and shortest cycling routes

For all cycling trips that could be identified in the previous steps, the shortest cycling route was calculated using Google Maps. Only actual cycling routes that were not the shortest possible cycling routes were selected to be used in subsequent analyses. All routes for which the actual cycling route was not the shortest possible cycling route were included, even if only one segment differed between the actual and the shortest cycling route. Differences in distance between actual cycling routes and the shortest possible cycling routes were calculated absolutely in meters as well as relatively in percentage of the shortest cycling route (reported as 'detour'). Google My Maps (a Google Maps application) was used to visualize actual cycling routes and the corresponding shortest cycling routes. Each cycling route was manually divided into several street segments (average distance: 342 ± 468 m), a new street segment started when participants turned into another street or when the street name changed. For each street segment, EGA-Cycling was filled out by one out of three trained observers (the first author and two independent observers). Google Street View was used to perform the audits, which took approximately 2 weeks per observer (6 weeks in total). Google Street View images ranged from March 2009 till April 2015. The majority (53.0%) of images were taken between August 2014 and October 2014. Prior to auditing the pre-defined routes, two independent observers were trained by the first author. The training included specific instructions; all items of the EGA-Cycling tool were explained and illustrated with photographs if necessary. Subsequently, the observers audited three random street segments which enabled them to raise questions. Thereafter, five test routes (i.e. no routes that were part of the study) were rated by the first author and the two independent observers. Prior to auditing the pre-defined routes, 95% agreement with the first author's scores was required. For the actual audits, only street segments for which there was no overlap between the actual cycling route and the shortest cycling route were audited (516 segments). Distances of segments were measured in Google My Maps. Figure 3 shows examples of actual versus shortest cycling routes.

Data analyses

Data were analysed using IBM SPSS Statistics 24. A paired samples t-test was used to calculate the difference in distance between actual and shortest cycling routes. Because EGA-Cycling was developed to assess physical environmental characteristics along entire cycling routes instead of individual segments [22], a total score per cycling route was calculated for each item. Per item, the score for a particular segment was multiplied by the distance of that segment. These weighted item scores of several segments of a route were summed to obtain one total score per route for that item. Subsequently, item scores were expressed in m/km in order to be able to compare the actual cycling route with the shortest cycling route (for which the route length differed). Univariate multilevel logistic regression analyses were used to investigate differences in physical environmental characteristics between actual and shortest cycling routes (three levels: participant, route and street segment). Statistical significance was set at $p < 0.05$.

Results

Sample characteristics

From the 238 adolescents participating, adolescents older than 17 years (n = 4) and participants who did not wear/charge the material properly (n = 13) were removed from the dataset as were participants who were absent when the structured interviews were completed (n = 17). A final sample of 204 adolescents (85.7%) was used for data analyses (46.5% boys, 14.4 ± 1.2 years). Table 1 presents descriptive characteristics of the sample. Within this sample, a total of 1126 trips was identified. Passive transport (car, as a passenger) was used most frequently (34.6% of trips), followed by public transport (33.9% of trips). Active transport such as walking and cycling was used for 17.2 and 14.2% of trips, respectively. The purpose of a trip and the transport mode used showed to be related to each other ($Chi^2 = 257.1$; $p < 0.001$). For trips to and/or from school, the majority (57.2%) was done by public transport, 18.4% was done by bicycle, 12.6% by foot and 11.8% by passive transport. For leisure-related

Table 1 Descriptive characteristics of the sample (n = 204)

Socio-demographic characteristics	
Gender (% boys)	46.5
Age (years; mean ± SD)	14.4 ± 1.2
Socio-economic status (SES) parents (%)	
Lower SES (% no parent completed tertiary education)	28.4
Higher SES (% at least one parent completed tertiary education)	71.6
Grade (%)	
1st year of secondary school	8.3
2nd year of secondary school	7.4
3rd year of secondary school	46.1
4th year of secondary school	38.2
Educational type (%)	
General education	65.2
Technical education	10.3
Vocational education	24.5

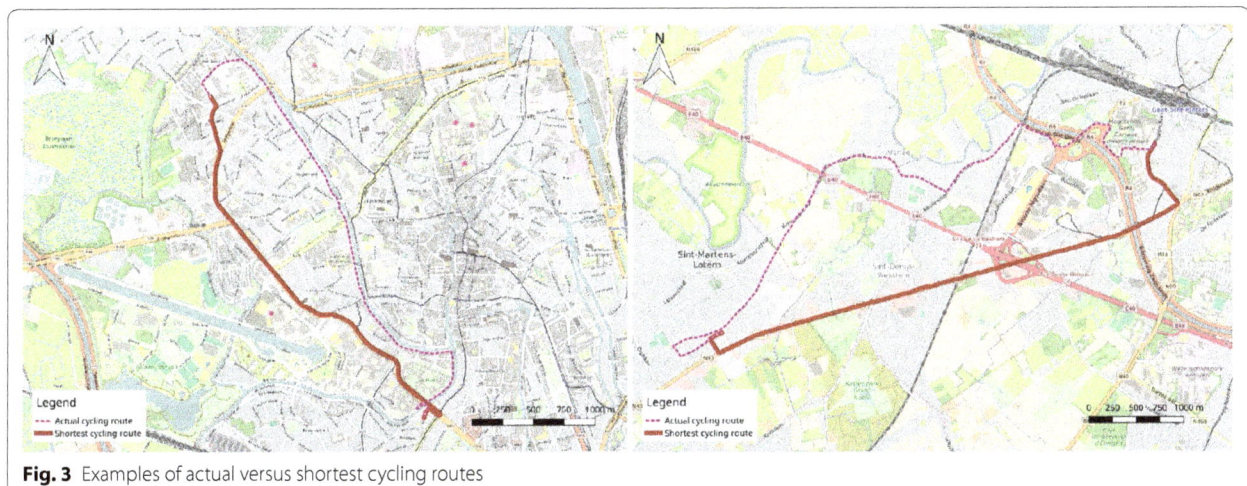

Fig. 3 Examples of actual versus shortest cycling routes

trips, nearly half (49.6%) was done by passive transport, 20.1% was done by foot, 17.8% by public transport and 12.5% by bicycle. The median distance for car trips was 6312 m and for public transport a median distance of 4934 m was found. Walking trips had a median distance of 710 m, whereas for cycling trips a median distance of 2633 m was found.

Out of 160 actual cycling trips, 73.1% did not differ from the shortest possible cycling routes. Thirty-eight unique cycling routes for which the actual route differed from the shortest possible cycling route could be identified (see Fig. 4). The 38 routes were spread over 22 adolescents, with a range of 1 to maximum 4 routes per person. A significant difference in distance between actual and shortest possible cycling routes was found (t = 8.606; p < 0.001). Actual cycling routes had a mean distance of 4505 ± 2201 m (med = 4100 m; min = 1000 m; max = 8800 m), whereas for the shortest possible cycling routes a mean distance of 3989 ± 2048 m (med = 3600 m; min = 700 m; max = 8100 m) was found. The mean difference between actual cycling routes

and the shortest possible cycling routes (detour) was 516 ± 369 m (med = 400 m; min = 100 m; max = 1600 m). The average detour was 15.6% (med = 12.1%; min = 2.0%; max = 45.7%) in comparison to the shortest possible cycling route.

Table 2 presents results on differences in physical environmental characteristics concerning land use between actual cycling routes and the shortest possible cycling routes. An increase in 100 m/km of mixed land use along the actual cycling route, resulted in 16% lower odds that the actual cycling route was chosen over the shortest cycling route. In addition, an increase in 100 m/km where commercial destinations are present along the actual cycling route, resulted in 17% lower odds that the actual cycling route was chosen over the shortest cycling route.

Table 3 presents results on differences in general characteristics between actual cycling routes and the shortest possible cycling routes. An increase in 100 m/km of a road type which consists of two roads divided in two lanes each direction (i.e. arterial road) along the actual

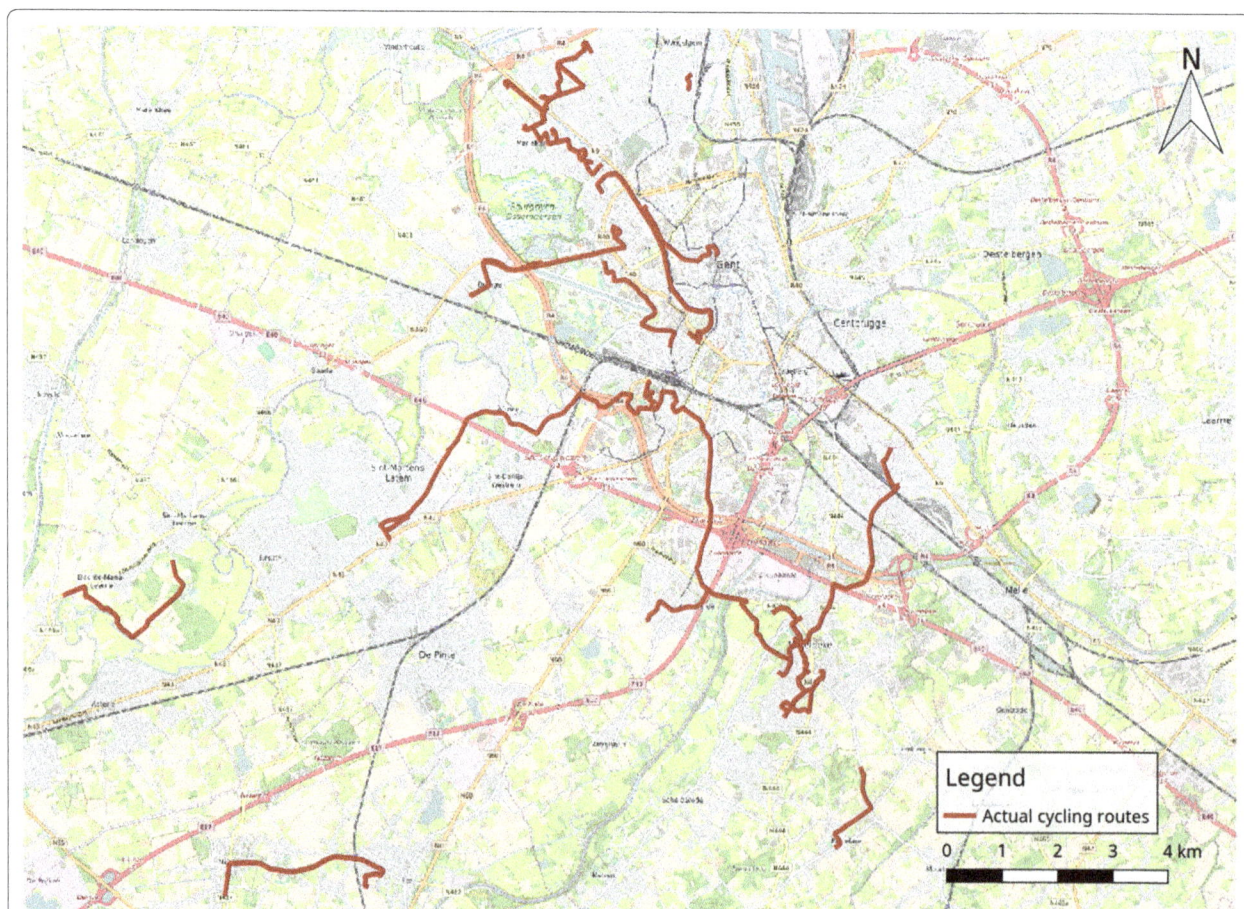

Fig. 4 Overview of the 38 actual cycling routes that differed from the shortest possible cycling route

Table 2 Presence of items on land use along actual cycling routes compared to shortest cycling routes

Item	Actual cycling route (m/km; M ± SD)	Shortest cycling route (m/km; M ± SD)	OR (95% CI)
Mixed land use	256 ± 226	386 ± 317	0.84 (0.71; 1.00)*
Types of buildings			
Single buildings	155 ± 247	153 ± 256	1.00 (0.83; 1.21)
Closed/semi-detached buildings	225 ± 190	139 ± 182	1.30 (0.99; 1.70)^t
Apartment buildings	111 ± 200	161 ± 244	0.90 (0.73; (1.12)
Commercial destinations	233 ± 229	367 ± 304	0.83 (0.69; 0.99)*
Heavy industry	9 ± 39	17 ± 63	0.74 (0.29; 1.91)
Public destinations	248 ± 196	355 ± 300	0.84 (0.70; 1.02)^t
Recreational destinations	85 ± 105	121 ± 212	0.87 (0.65; 1.17)
Natural features	315 ± 314	257 ± 286	1.07 (0.91; 1.25)
Openness view			
Open view	65 ± 174	24 ± 81	1.29 (0.85; 1.96)
Not open/closed view	354 ± 229	370 ± 271	0.98 (0.81; 1.17)
Closed view	166 ± 168	146 ± 185	1.07 (0.82; 1.39)

Reference = shortest cycling route. For ease of interpretation of OR, distances were converted to hectometres (100 m/km)

OR odds ratio, *CI* confidence interval

*p ≤ 0.05; **p ≤ 0.01; ^{t}p ≤ 0.1

cycling route, resulted in 47% lower odds that the actual cycling route was chosen over the shortest cycling route. An increase in 100 m/km with a speed limit of 30 km/h along the actual cycling route, resulted in 50% higher odds that the actual cycling route was chosen over the shortest cycling route. Furthermore, an increase in 100 m/km for roads where few buildings with windows on the street are present along the actual cycling route, resulted in 192% higher odds that the actual cycling route was chosen over the shortest cycling route. This last item refers to crime safety/social control (i.e. if few buildings with windows on the street (or few buildings in general) are present, few people have a clear view on the street and there is thus less social control) [22].

Table 4 presents results on differences in cycling facilities between actual cycling routes and the shortest possible cycling routes. For an increase in 100 m/km of a cycle lane which is part of the road (cycle lane separated from traffic by white lines) along the actual cycling route, 36% lower odds that the actual cycling route was chosen over the shortest cycling route was found. For an increase in 100 m/km road with no cycle lane along the actual cycling route, 25% higher odds that the actual cycling route was chosen over the shortest cycling route was found. In addition, an increase in 100 m/km of a small cycle lane along the actual cycling route, resulted in 32% lower odds that the actual

cycling route was chosen over the shortest cycling route. Finally, for an increase in 100 m/km of a cycle lane that is covered by lighting along the actual cycling route, 25% lower odds that the actual cycling route was chosen over the shortest cycling route was found.

Table 5 presents results on differences in aesthetics between actual cycling routes and the shortest possible cycling routes. For none of the included variables, a significant result was found.

Subjective results of the structured one-on-one interviews showed that, for the 38 actual cycling routes that differed from the shortest possible cycling route, adolescents still indicated for 35.1% (n = 13) of the trips that they chose that route because it was the shortest/fastest route. For 16.2% (n = 6) of these cycling trips, participants indicated they chose that particular route to cycle together with friends/siblings/.... For another 16.2% (n = 6) of the trips, they chose that particular route because of lower traffic density. Furthermore, for 13.5% (n = 5) of the trips participants indicated that route choice was determined by their parents and for 5.4% (n = 2) of the trips they indicated to choose that particular route because of the presence of few/safe crossings. For another 5.4% (n = 2) of the trips, participants indicated they chose that particular route because of a commercial destination they wanted to visit.

Table 3 Presence of items on general characteristics along actual cycling routes compared to shortest cycling routes

Item	Actual cycling route (m/km; M ± SD)	Shortest cycling route (m/km; M ± SD)	OR (95% CI)
Road type			
Walking/cycling road	89 ± 99	62 ± 111	1.29 (0.82; 2.03)
One road for one-direction traffic	120 ± 168	56 ± 107	1.43 (0.97; 2.11)^t
One road not divided into lanes	259 ± 232	160 ± 195	1.25 (0.99; 1.57)^t
One road divided in one lane each direction	82 ± 125	123 ± 199	0.86 (0.64; 1.15)
Two roads divided in one lane each direction	21 ± 58	7 ± 24	2.44 (0.63; 9.41)
Two roads divided in two lanes each direction	14 ± 46	130 ± 245	0.53 (0.28; 0.99)*
Speed limit			
30 km/h	145 ± 185	58 ± 131	1.50 (1.02; 2.21)*
50 km/h	309 ± 261	316 ± 255	0.99 (0.83; 1.18)
70 km/h or more	43 ± 87	106 ± 225	0.78 (0.57; 1.08)
Traffic calming measures	248 ± 222	344 ± 304	0.87 (0.73; 1.04)
Amount of side streets	13 ± 11	11 ± 10	1.02 (0.98; 1.07)
Amount of intersections	2 ± 2	3 ± 3	0.90 (0.75; 1.09)
Crossing aids	372 ± 247	414 ± 310	0.95 (0.80; 1.12)
Poor visibility when crossing a street	23 ± 54	4 ± 16	4.85 (0.80; 29.52)^t
Well-maintained street segment	548 ± 267	531 ± 282	1.02 (0.86; 1.21)
Streetlights	522 ± 265	536 ± 290	0.98 (0.83; 1.16)
Parking facilities			
On street parking facilities	180 ± 173	122 ± 156	1.25 (0.93; 1.68)
Parking facilities next to the street	210 ± 206	321 ± 297	0.84 (0.69; 1.02)^t
Parking facilities on adjacent parking	18 ± 62	3 ± 15	2.98 (0.44; 20.35)
No parking facilities	88 ± 193	33 ± 55	1.45 (0.86; 2.44)
Slope			
Flat	546 ± 266	499 ± 297	1.06 (0.90; 1.25)
Gentle to moderate slope	39 ± 62	41 ± 105	0.97 (0.56; 1.66)
Swerving alternatives	407 ± 254	353 ± 266	1.08 (0.91; 1.30)
Buildings			
No buildings with windows on street side	47 ± 182	30 ± 82	1.10 (0.78; 1.55)
Few buildings with windows on street side	58 ± 78	22 ± 45	2.92 (1.12; 7.63)*
Many buildings with windows on street side	391 ± 248	427 ± 293	0.95 (0.80; 1.13)
Driveways			
No driveways	54 ± 136	65 ± 105	0.93 (0.63; 1.37)
Approx. 25% of buildings have one driveway	181 ± 207	167 ± 238	1.03 (0.84; 1.27)
Approx. 50% of buildings have one driveway	17 ± 29	35 ± 88	0.61 (0.25; 1.51)
Most buildings have one driveway	244 ± 247	213 ± 259	1.05 (0.88; 1.26)
Garages			
No garages	228 ± 240	187 ± 175	1.10 (0.88; 1.38)
Approx. 25% of buildings have one garage	252 ± 228	270 ± 273	0.97 (0.81; 1.17)
Approx. 50% of buildings or more have one garage	17 ± 32	22 ± 47	0.72 (0.22; 2.32)

Reference = shortest cycling route. Results regarding 'one road divided in two lanes each direction' (road type) are not shown since this road type did not appear along the routes. For ease of interpretation of OR, distances were converted to hectometres (100 m/km)

OR odds ratio, *CI* confidence interval

*p ≤ 0.05; **p ≤ 0.01; ^{t}p ≤ 0.1

Table 4 Presence of items on cycling facilities along actual cycling routes compared to shortest cycling routes

Item	Actual cycling route (m/km; M ± SD)	Shortest cycling route (m/km; M ± SD)	OR (95% CI)
Type of cycle lane			
Cycle lane separated from the road	74 ± 133	45 ± 75	1.30 (0.82; 2.08)
Adjoining cycle lane (slightly increased)	76 ± 105	89 ± 141	0.91 (0.63; 1.33)
Cycle lane is part of the road (white lines)	52 ± 84	180 ± 252	0.64 (0.44; 0.92)*
Non-compulsory cycle lane or of a different colour	24 ± 101	7 ± 29	1.45 (0.65; 3.25)
No cycle lane	271 ± 243	159 ± 209	1.25 (1.01; 1.56)*
Width cycle lane			
Small	72 ± 106	166 ± 206	0.68 (0.48; 0.96)*
Wide	242 ± 260	237 ± 276	1.01 (0.85; 1.20)
Two-way cycle lane	224 ± 254	121 ± 203	1.23 (0.98; 1.54)[t]
Well-maintained cycle lane	294 ± 240	376 ± 286	0.89 (0.74; 1.06)
Lighting covering cycle lane	174 ± 182	332 ± 284	0.75 (0.61; 0.94)**
Surface cycle lane			
Bitumen	273 ± 177	260 ± 237	1.03 (0.83; 1.29)
Continuous concrete	8 ± 37	5 ± 17	1.50 (0.27; 8.41)
Paving bricks	181 ± 199	126 ± 131	1.22 (0.91; 1.63)
Concrete slabs	80 ± 112	109 ± 181	0.73 (0.64; 1.20)
Cobblestones	12 ± 30	16 ± 44	0.71 (0.20; 2.48)
Gravel	32 ± 77	23 ± 92	1.13 (0.65; 1.98)
Condition cycle lane			
Poor	28 ± 58	18 ± 78	1.25 (0.61; 2.58)
Moderate	223 ± 182	257 ± 258	0.93 (0.76; 1.15)
Good	335 ± 226	264 ± 229	1.15 (0.93; 1.41)

Reference = shortest cycling route. For ease of interpretation of OR, distances were converted to hectometres (100 m/km)

OR odds ratio, CI confidence interval

*p ≤ 0.05; **p ≤ 0.01; [t]p ≤ 0.1

Table 5 Presence of items on aesthetics along actual cycling routes compared to shortest cycling routes

Item	Actual cycling route (m/km; M ± SD)	Shortest cycling route (m/km; M ± SD)	OR (95% CI)
Trees	459 ± 241	428 ± 294	1.04 (0.88; 1.24)
Attractive buildings	60 ± 111	70 ± 134	0.94 (0.65; 1.37)
Well-maintained buildings	501 ± 240	500 ± 287	1.00 (0.84; 1.19)
Front yards	297 ± 257	328 ± 294	0.96 (0.81; 1.13)
Well-maintained front yards	315 ± 247	398 ± 274	0.88 (0.73; 1.07)
Attractive natural features	250 ± 310	163 ± 243	1.12 (0.95; 1.33)
Graffiti and litter	120 ± 201	93 ± 205	1.07 (0.85; 1.35)

Reference = shortest cycling route. For ease of interpretation of OR, distances were converted to hectometres (100 m/km)

OR odds ratio, CI confidence interval

*p ≤ 0.05; **p ≤ 0.01; [t]p ≤ 0.1

Discussion

The present study aimed to investigate differences in physical environmental characteristics between adolescents' actual cycling routes and the shortest possible cycling routes using a Google Street View-based audit. A mixed land use, roads with commercial destinations, arterial roads, cycle lanes separated from traffic by white lines, small cycle lanes and cycle lanes covered by lighting were less frequently present along adolescents' actual cycling routes in comparison to the shortest possible cycling routes. Besides, a speed limit of 30 km/h, roads having few buildings with windows on street side and roads without cycle lane were more frequently present along actual cycling routes compared to the shortest possible cycling routes.

In line with previous studies [12–14], the present study showed that a short cycling distance is one of the most important factors determining the route choice of adolescent cyclists, as for 73.1% of the cycling trips participants took the shortest possible route. In addition, for 35.1% of the cycling trips which were not the shortest possible, adolescents still indicated that they chose that route because they perceived it as the shortest/fastest route. Thus, even if a route is not actually the shortest, adolescents may choose this route because they perceive it as the shortest route. For all cycling trips that were not the shortest possible, a mean difference of 516 m (15.6%) between the actual and the shortest cycling route was found. When only looking at those routes which were not the shortest but adolescents perceived as the shortest/fastest route, a mean difference of 431 m between the actual and the shortest cycling route was found, and thus, the detour showed to be smaller. It is possible that adolescents do not notice the difference in cycling time between their actual cycling route they perceive as the shortest and the shortest possible cycling route.

Although some findings of the present study seem to be in contradiction with results of previous cross-sectional studies [12], the findings generally have a clear explanation. The present study showed that adolescents avoid routes with a mixed land use where commercial destinations are present. In contradiction, a US study showed that children and adolescents (5–18 years) were more likely to walk or cycle to school if their parents reported having stores in the neighbourhood environment [38]. However, in accordance with the present study, shops and services were also less present along the actual cycling routes of adults in Austria [15]. Dessing et al. [17] found that children in The Netherlands mainly cycled to school along residential areas to avoid busy streets. These findings are similar to results in our study since residential areas are, in general, characterised by a lower land use mix and less commercial destinations. In the study by Dessing et al. [17], it was suggested that residential streets may be perceived as safe, quiet streets to cycle for transport, even if separate cycle lanes are absent. This could be confirmed by the results of the present study which showed that adolescents mainly cycled along local roads, such as roads for one-direction traffic and roads which were not divided into lanes (trends towards significance), where speed limits of 30 km/h apply. Furthermore, our study also showed that actual cycling routes included more m/km road where no cycle lane was present which is typical for residential streets in Flanders. In addition, the present study found that actual cycling routes included a larger part of the route where only few buildings with windows on the street were present, which is also an attribute of local roads. As already mentioned above, the presence of buildings with windows on the street refers to social control from people living in the area [22]. Another study among 5-to-18-year-old youth found similar results, participants in that study agreeing that 'walkers and bikers on the streets in my neighbourhood can easily be seen by people in their homes' were less likely to use active transport to school [39]. These findings could be explained by the fact that adolescents perceive cycling along local roads with lower speed limits as more important than potential social control from residents. Among adults, Winters et al. [16] also found that cyclists spent most of their travel distance along local roads. In the present study, arterial roads, such as road types which consist of two separate roads each divided in two lanes each direction, were avoided. A number of previous studies also found that cyclists avoid busy, arterial roads [15, 16, 40] and roads with high traffic speed [41]. In Flanders, if any type of cycle path is available along these busy roads it is typically a small cycle path separated from traffic by white lines, which explains why the present study found that this type of cycle path is less present along actual cycling routes.

With regard to walking/cycling roads that are not accessible for motorised traffic, no significant difference in presence along actual and shortest cycling routes was found. Nevertheless, a previous study among adults found that cyclists spent more time on off-street paths [16]. In addition, among 10-to-15-year-old US girls, it was found that the presence of walking/cycling trails in the neighbourhood was associated with higher levels of active transport to school [39]. Although, in the present study, these walking/cycling roads occurred relatively frequently along actual cycling routes (on average for 89 m/km), shortest cycling routes also included some amount of walking/cycling roads (62 m/km) since the city of Ghent already provides an extensive network of walking/cycling roads. These walking/cycling roads often serve as shortcuts for pedestrians and cyclists. This could explain why no significant difference between actual and shortest cycling routes was found for walking/cycling roads in this study.

Practical implications
Based on the findings of the present study, some recommendations for policy and practice can be formulated. The present study showed that adolescents mainly choose the (perceived) shortest route to cycle for transport and that adolescents frequently use walking/cycling roads that are not accessible for motorised traffic. It might thus be important for local authorities to provide

walking/cycling roads that are not accessible for motorised traffic and could serve as shortcuts for cyclists [42]. These shortcuts free from motorised traffic also meet the preference of adolescents to avoid cycling along arterial roads. However, since it is not always possible for an individual to avoid to cycle along busy, arterial roads, these roads should be made more bike-friendly by providing adequate cycling infrastructure.

Strengths and limitations

A first strength of the present study was that the evaluated routes were actual cycling routes which were objectively recorded using a GPS device. Using objective GPS data limits recall bias related to route choice. Particularly for young people such as adolescents it may be difficult to recall and indicate on a map which route they took at a particular moment. Second, information obtained by the structured one-on-one interviews enabled to correct trip mode when this was misclassified by PALMS (e.g. when a car trip was classified as a bicycle trip due to traffic congestion). Furthermore, this was the first study to collect subjective information regarding route choice via one-on-one interviews, and combine this with audits. This allowed participants to indicate their actual reason for choosing a particular route. Third, the presence of physical environmental characteristics along the routes was measured objectively using a tool (EGA-Cycling) that showed acceptable reliability and validity [22], which limits the bias of results compared to self-reported questionnaires. Nevertheless, some limitations should be acknowledged. First, virtual audit tools showed to be less accurate for measuring micro-environmental features. However, Google Street View showed to be more accurate in measuring micro-environmental features compared to other virtual audit tools [28]. Nevertheless, a discrepancy in physical environmental factors may exist between the Google Street View images and the period in which GPS data were collected. The Google Street View images ranged from March 2009 till April 2015, whereas participants' GPS data were collected between September and December 2015. Second, the sample size was relatively small as only 38 actual cycling routes (spread over 22 adolescents) that were not the shortest cycling route could be identified and were evaluated. A small sample size increases the likelihood of a type II error and, thus, the chance that an effect was not detected when there was one to be detected. Third, some characteristics (i.e. poor visibility when crossing a street, parking facilities on adjacent parking) were only present along a few street segments. This resulted in wide 95% confidence intervals due to insufficient variability. Fourth, as data collection took place among adolescents attending secondary schools in the city of Ghent, the majority of cycling trips

were performed in a (sub)urban area. Thus, results cannot be generalized to rural areas where less alternative routes are available because of a less dense street network. Fifth, because of the limited time window of the study (i.e. 2 days of data per participant), it is difficult to draw generalizable conclusions regarding the impact of the physical environment on adolescents' route choice while cycling. Sixth, the majority of adolescents was of a higher SES family, which could have influenced the results. Previous research showed that children and adolescents living in lower SES neighbourhoods perceive the neighbourhood environment as less attractive and safe, and more often report heavy traffic in their neighbourhood compared to those living in higher SES neighbourhoods [43, 44]. It is thus possible that adolescents from lower SES families attach importance to other factors on their cycling route compared to adolescents from higher SES families. Thus, caution is needed when generalizing results to the overall adolescent population. Seventh, data were collected during autumn/winter which may have influenced the results. Bad weather and less hours of daylight may influence adolescents' choice of transport mode and route choice. Finally, results of the present study do not enable to draw conclusions regarding non-cyclists.

Recommendations for future research

Since data collection was very time-consuming and the burden on participants was rather high, future studies should consider to make use of dedicated smartphone applications to identify adolescents' actual cycling routes. Adolescents generally carry their smartphones with them during the day, thus running dedicated mobile apps may be less considered as a burden compared to wearing portable GPS-devices. The use of dedicated smartphone applications would enable to include a larger sample and would allow to track adolescents' mobility patterns over a longer time period [45]. Thus, this method has the advantage that much more actual cycling routes can be identified in more diverse areas. The introduction of smartphones with a longer battery life and a higher storage space and memory capacity should be able to facilitate this type of data collection. Nevertheless, this would imply a huge burden on the researchers to audit such a large set of cycling routes. Geographic Information Systems (GIS) could be used instead, since GIS makes use of existing data sources (e.g. governmental data sources) to measure physical environmental characteristics that have some spatial reference [46]. However, since for some locations (i.e. rural or suburban areas) GIS data may not be available [46] and micro-environmental factors are also not commonly available in GIS databases [46, 47], virtual or on-street audits may be used to complement GIS data where needed. In addition, future studies should consider to investigate potential moderators (e.g. individual and social environmental factors) of the relationships between the presence of physical environmental factors and adolescents' route choice while cycling for transport. It may be interesting to investigate whether the relationship between the presence of certain physical environmental factors and adolescents' preference for a certain cycling route is moderated by, for example, psychosocial factors. It could be that adolescents with lower self-efficacy or less social models for active transport attach importance to other physical environmental factors when choosing a cycle route compared to adolescents with higher self-efficacy or more social models for active transport. Results of the present study only enable to draw conclusions for the general adolescent population, no specific conclusions for subgroups of adolescents (e.g. those with a low psychosocial profile towards cycling for transport or the least regular cyclists) can be drawn. Since this study was one of the first exploring the factors associated with route choice among adolescent cyclists, results are valuable. However, future studies may consider to conduct moderation analyses among larger samples in order to be able to formulate recommendations to target specific subgroups of adolescents. More research investigating adolescents' route choice for cycling is needed. In order to be able to formulate recommendations regarding which factors may stimulate adolescents to cycle for transport, future studies should also investigate which factors along a route are important among non-cyclists. An experimental study which aimed to investigate adolescents' preferences towards cycling for transport using manipulated photographs, showed that the least regular cyclists in that study attached most importance to cycling distance when indicating which route they preferred to cycle along [48]. The most regular cyclists in that study attached most importance to being able to cycle together with a friend. However, no associations with actual participation in cycling for transport were investigated in that study.

Conclusions

For 73.1% of the cycling trips, participants took the shortest route possible which confirmed the importance of cycling distance for adolescents. When not taking the shortest cycling route, adolescents avoided to cycle for transport along arterial roads with a small cycle lane

separated from traffic by white lines. Local roads with a speed limit of 30 km/h in an area with a low land use mix where few commercial destinations are located were more frequently used, even when no cycle lane was available. In general, the ability to cycle along quiet, local roads overruled the importance of all other physical environmental factors besides distance. Local authorities should provide shortcuts free from motorised traffic in order to meet the preference of adolescents to cycle along the shortest route and to avoid cycling along busy, arterial roads. In addition, it may also be important to provide adequate cycling infrastructure along busy, arterial roads since these roads cannot always be avoided.

Authors' contributions
HV, LVH, DVD, NVDW, BD and JVC designed the protocol for this study. HV and LVH collected the data and coordinated the data collection. HV, LVH and TB contributed to the data processing. HV performed the statistical analyses and drafted the manuscript. HV, LVH, DVD, NVDW, PC, BD, JVC critically revised and helped to draft the manuscript. All authors read and approved the final manuscript.

Author details
[1] Department of Public Health, Faculty of Medicine and Health Sciences, Ghent University, Corneel Heymanslaan 10, 9000 Ghent, Belgium. [2] Physical Activity, Nutrition and Health Research Unit, Faculty of Physical Education and Physical Therapy, Vrije Universiteit Brussel, Pleinlaan 2, 1050 Brussels, Belgium. [3] Research Foundation - Flanders (FWO), Brussels, Belgium. [4] Department of Movement and Sport Sciences, Faculty of Medicine and Health Sciences, Ghent University, Watersportlaan 2, 9000 Ghent, Belgium. [5] Department of Geography – CartoGIS, Faculty of Sciences, Ghent University, Krijgslaan 281, 9000 Ghent, Belgium.

Acknowledgements
We would like to thank the schools and the adolescents who participated in the study. Furthermore, we would like to thank master's students for assisting with the data collection and processing. We would also like to thank R. Colman for her help with the data analyses.

Competing interests
The authors declare that they have no competing interests.

Funding
HV and LVH are supported by the Research Foundation Flanders (FWO, http://www.fwo.be/en, 3GOA8514). JVC is supported by a FWO postdoctoral fellowship (FWO - 12I1117N). DVD is supported by a FWO postdoctoral fellowship (FWO12/PDO/158).

References
1. Cohen AJ, Ross Anderson H, Ostro B, Pandey KD, Krzyzanowski M, Kunzli N, Gutschmidt K, Pope A, Romieu I, Samet JM, Smith K. The global burden of disease due to outdoor air pollution. J Toxicol Environ Health A. 2005;68:1301–7.

2. Woodcock J, Edwards P, Tonne C, Armstrong BG, Ashiru O, Banister D, Beevers S, Chalabi Z, Chowdhury Z, Cohen A, et al. Public health benefits of strategies to reduce greenhouse-gas emissions: urban land transport. Lancet. 2009;374:1930–43.

3. Int Panis L, de Geus B, Vandenbulcke G, Willems H, Degraeuwe B, Bleux N, Mishra V, Thomas I, Meeusen R. Exposure to particulate matter in traffic: a comparison of cyclists and car passangers. Atmos Environ. 2010;44:2263–70.

4. Oja P, Titze S, Bauman A, de Geus B, Krenn P, Reger-Nash B, Kohlberger T. Health benefits of cycling: a systematic review. Scand J Med Sci Sports. 2011;21:496–509.

5. Ortega FB, Konstabel K, Pasquali E, Ruiz JR, Hurtig-Wennlof A, Maestu J, Lof M, Harro J, Bellocco R, Labayen I, et al. Objectively measured physical activity and sedentary time during childhood, adolescence and young adulthood: a cohort study. PloS ONE. 2013;8:e60871.

6. Chillon P, Ortega FB, Ruiz JR, De Bourdeaudhuij I, Martinez-Gomez D, Vicente-Rodriguez G, Widhalm K, Molnar D, Gottrand F, Gonzalez-Gross M, et al. Active commuting and physical activity in adolescents from Europe: results from the HELENA study. Pediatr Exerc Sci. 2011;23:207–17.

7. Chillon P, Ortega FB, Ruiz JR, Veidebaum T, Oja L, Maestu J, Sjostrom M. Active commuting to school in children and adolescents: an opportunity to increase physical activity and fitness. Scand J Public Health. 2010;38:873–9.

8. Bere E, Seiler S, Eikemo TA, Oenema A, Brug J. The association between cycling to school and being overweight in Rotterdam (The Netherlands) and Kristiansand (Norway). Scand J Med Sci Sports. 2011;21:48–53.

9. Nettleton S, Green J. Thinking about changing mobility practices: how a social practice approach can help. Sociol Health Illn. 2014;36:239–51.

10. Sallis JF, Cervero RB, Ascher W, Henderson KA, Kraft MK, Kerr J. An ecological approach to creating active living communities. Annu Rev Public Health. 2006;27:297–322.

11. Wong BY, Faulkner G, Buliung R. GIS measured environmental correlates of active school transport: a systematic review of 14 studies. Int J Behav Nutr Phys Act. 2011;8:39.

12. Panter JR, Jones AP, van Sluijs EM. Environmental determinants of active travel in youth: a review and framework for future research. Int J Behav Nutr Phys Act. 2008;5:34.

13. Nelson NM, Foley E, O'Gorman DJ, Moyna NM, Woods CB. Active commuting to school: how far is too far? Int J Behav Nutr Phys Act. 2008;5:1.

14. Verhoeven H, Ghekiere A, Van Cauwenberg J, Van Dyck D, De Bourdeaudhuij I, Clarys P, Deforche B. Which physical and social environmental factors are most important for adolescents' cycling for transport? An experimental study using manipulated photographs. Int J Behav Nutr Phys Act. 2017;14:108.

15. Krenn PJ, Oja P, Titze S. Route choices of transport bicyclists: a comparison of actually used and shortest routes. Int J Behav Nutr Phys Act. 2014;11:31.

16. Winters M, Teschke K, Grant M, Setton E, Brauer M. How far out of the way will we travel? Built environment influences on route selection for bicycle and car travel. Transp Res Rec J Transp Res Board. 2010;2190:1–10.

17. Dessing D, de Vries SI, Hegeman G, Verhagen E, van Mechelen W, Pierik FH. Children's route choice during active transportation to school: difference between shortest and actual route. Int J Behav Nutr Phys Act. 2016;13:48.

18. Carpiano RM. Come take a walk with me: the "go-along" interview as a novel method for studying the implications of place for health and well-being. Health Place. 2009;15:263–72.

19. Clifton KJ, Livi Smith ADL, Rodriguez D. The development and testing of an audit for the pedestrian environment. Landsc Urban Plan. 2007;80:95–110.

20. Pikora TJ, Bull FC, Jamrozik K, Knuiman M, Giles-Corti B, Donovan RJ. Developing a reliable audit instrument to measure the physical environment for physical activity. Am J Prev Med. 2002;23:187–94.

21. Day K, Boarnet B, Alfonzo M, Forsyth A. The Irvine-Minnesota inventory to measure built environments: development. Am J Prev Med. 2006;30:144–52.

21. Day K, Boarnet M, Alfonzo M, Forsyth A. The Irvine-Minnesota inventory to measure built environments: development. Am J Prev Med. 2006;30:144–52.

22. Vanwolleghem G, Van Dyck D, Ducheyne F, De Bourdeaudhuij I, Cardon G. Assessing the environmental characteristics of cycling routes to school: a study on the reliability and validity of a Google Street View-based audit. Int J Health Geogr. 2014;13:19.

23. Brownson RC, Hoehner CM, Brennan LK, Cook RA, Elliot MB, McMullen KM. Reliability of 2 Instruments for Auditing the Environment for Physical Activity. J Phys Act Health. 2004;1:189–207.

24. Badland HM, Opit S, Witten K, Kearns RA, Mavoa S. Can virtual streetscape audits reliably replace physical streetscape audits? J Urban Health. 2010;87:1007–16.

25. Taylor BT, Fernando P, Bauman AE, Williamson A, Craig JC, Redman S. Measuring the quality of public open space using Google Earth. Am J Prev Med. 2011;40:105–12.

26. Rundle AG, Bader MD, Richards CA, Neckerman KM, Teitler JO. Using Google Street View to audit neighborhood environments. Am J Prev Med. 2011;40:94–100.

27. Kelly CM, Wilson JS, Baker EA, Miller DK, Schootman M. Using Google Street View to audit the built environment: inter-rater reliability results. Ann Behav Med. 2013;45(Suppl 1):S108–12.

28. Ben-Joseph E, Lee JS, Cromley EK, Laden F, Troped PJ. Virtual and actual: relative accuracy of on-site and web-based instruments in auditing the environment for physical activity. Health Place. 2013;19:138–50.

29. Gullon P, Badland HM, Alfayate S, Bilal U, Escobar F, Cebrecos A, Diez J, Franco M. Assessing walking and cycling environments in the streets of Madrid: comparing On-field and virtual audits. J Urban Health. 2015;92:923–39.

30. Statistics Belgium: Bodemgebruik in België 1834–2017. 2015.

31. Structuur van de bevolking volgens woonplaats: grootste gemeenten. http://statbel.fgov.be/nl/statistieken/cijfers/bevolking/structuur/woonplaats/groot/.

32. Lien N, Friestad C, Klepp KI. Adolescents' proxy reports of parents' socioeconomic status: how valid are they? J Epidemiol Community Health. 2001;55:731–7.

33. Kerr J, Normam G, Godbole S, Raab F, Demchak B, Patrick K. Validating GPS data with the PALMS system to detect different active transportation modes. Med Sci Sports Exerc. 2012;44:647.

34. The Personal Activity and Location Measurement System (PALMS). https://ucsd-palms-project.wikispaces.com/.

35. Demchak B, Kerr J, Raab F, Patrick K, Krüger IH. PALMS: a modern coevolution of community and computing using policy driven development. In 45th Hawaii international conference on system sciences; 2012.

36. Carlson JA, Jankowska MM, Meseck K, Godbole S, Natarajan L, Raab F, Demchak B, Patrick K, Kerr J. Validity of PALMS GPS scoring of active and passive travel compared with SenseCam. Med Sci Sports Exerc. 2015;47:662–7.

37. MAPS GLOBAL audit tool. http://sallis.ucsd.edu/measure_maps.html.

38. Kerr J, Rosenberg D, Sallis JF, Saelens BE, Frank LD, Conway TL. Active commuting to school: associations with environment and parental concerns. Med Sci Sports Exerc. 2006;38:787–94.

39. Evenson KR, Birnbaum AS, Bedimo-Rung AL, Sallis JF, Voorhees CC, Ring K, Elder JP. Girls' perception of physical environmental factors and transportation: reliability and association with physical activity and active transport to school. Int J Behav Nutr Phys Act. 2006;3:28.

40. Timperio A, Ball K, Salmon J, Roberts R, Giles-Corti B, Simmons D, Baur LA, Crawford D. Personal, family, social, and environmental correlates of active commuting to school. Am J Prev Med. 2006;30:45–51.

41. McMillan TE. The relative influence of urban form on a child's travel mode to school. Transp Res Part A. 2007;41:69–79.

42. Pucher J, Buehler R. Making cycling irresistible: lesson from Europe. Transp Rev. 2008;28:495–528.

43. Giles-Corti B, Donovan RJ. Socioeconomic status differences in recreational physical activity levels and real and perceived access to a supportive physical environment. Prev Med. 2002;35:601–11.

44. Timperio A, Crawford D, Telford A, Salmon J. Perceptions about the local neighborhood and walking and cycling among children. Prev Med. 2004;38:39–47.
45. Vlassenroot S, Gillis D, Bellens R, Gautama S. The use of smartphone applications in the collection of travel behaviour data. Int J Intell Transp Syst Res. 2015;13:17–27.
46. Brownson RC, Hoehner CM, Day K, Forsyth A, Sallis JF. Measuring the built environment for physical activity: state of the science. Am J Prev Med. 2009;36(S99–123):e112.

47. Adams MA, Ryan S, Kerr J, Sallis JF, Patrick K, Frank LD, Norman GJ. Validation of the Neighborhood Environment Walkability Scale (NEWS) items using geographic information systems. J Phys Act Health. 2009;6(Suppl 1):S113–23.
48. Verhoeven H, Ghekiere A, Van Cauwenberg J, Van Dyck D, De Bourdeaudhuij I, Clarys P, Deforche B. Subgroups of adolescents differing in physical and social environmental preferences towards cycling for transport: a latent class analysis. Prev Med. 2018;112:70–5.

8

Mapping child maltreatment risk: a 12-year spatio-temporal analysis of neighborhood influences

Enrique Gracia[1]* , Antonio López-Quílez[2], Miriam Marco[1] and Marisol Lila[1]

Abstract

Background: 'Place' matters in understanding prevalence variations and inequalities in child maltreatment risk. However, most studies examining ecological variations in child maltreatment risk fail to take into account the implications of the spatial and temporal dimensions of neighborhoods. In this study, we conduct a high-resolution small-area study to analyze the influence of neighborhood characteristics on the spatio-temporal epidemiology of child maltreatment risk.

Methods: We conducted a 12-year (2004–2015) small-area Bayesian spatio-temporal epidemiological study with all families with child maltreatment protection measures in the city of Valencia, Spain. As neighborhood units, we used 552 census block groups. Cases were geocoded using the family address. Neighborhood-level characteristics analyzed included three indicators of neighborhood disadvantage—neighborhood economic status, neighborhood education level, and levels of policing activity—, immigrant concentration, and residential instability. Bayesian spatio-temporal modelling and disease mapping methods were used to provide area-specific risk estimations.

Results: Results from a spatio-temporal autoregressive model showed that neighborhoods with low levels of economic and educational status, with high levels of policing activity, and high immigrant concentration had higher levels of substantiated child maltreatment risk. Disease mapping methods were used to analyze areas of excess risk. Results showed chronic spatial patterns of high child maltreatment risk during the years analyzed, as well as stability over time in areas of low risk. Areas with increased or decreased child maltreatment risk over the years were also observed.

Conclusions: A spatio-temporal epidemiological approach to study the geographical patterns, trends over time, and the contextual determinants of child maltreatment risk can provide a useful method to inform policy and action. This method can offer a more accurate description of the problem, and help to inform more localized prevention and intervention strategies. This new approach can also contribute to an improved epidemiological surveillance system to detect ecological variations in risk, and to assess the effectiveness of the initiatives to reduce this risk.

Keywords: Child maltreatment, Neighborhood influences, Bayesian spatio-temporal modeling, Disease mapping, Spatial inequality, Small-area study, Area-specific risk estimation

Background

Child maltreatment is a major social, public health, and human rights problem, with severe, far-reaching, and long-lasting consequences. Its impact on victims'

*Correspondence: Enrique.Gracia@uv.es
[1] Department of Social Psychology, University of Valencia, Av. Blasco Ibáñez, 21, 46010 Valencia, Spain
Full list of author information is available at the end of the article

physical, mental, and reproductive health, behavioral problems, or education attainment; its role in the intergenerational transmission of violence; and its elevated costs for the criminal, health, and social welfare systems, poses a high burden on society [1–4]. Child maltreatment is a global phenomenon, and its prevalence in high-income countries remains high and is considered a leading cause of health inequality and social injustice

[4–7]. From a public health perspective, child maltreatment is, however, a preventable problem as potentially risk-modifying factors can be identified and targeted in preventive interventions.

Child maltreatment research has typically focused on individual or family risk factors, but 'place' also matters in understanding prevalence variations and inequalities in child maltreatment risk [8–12]. A growing body of research is increasingly recognizing the importance of the context in which families live, linking neighborhood characteristics and processes—such as poverty, disorder and crime, immigrant concentration, social impoverishment, or diminished social control—to child maltreatment [13–32]. However, studying neighborhood influences on child maltreatment presents important challenges, and there are still some shortcomings in the available literature, which we address in the present study.

Child maltreatment and neighborhood risk factors are not equally distributed spatially, and it is to some extent surprising that the use of spatial analysis techniques and disease mapping methods to analyze geographical patterns of child maltreatment risk, and whether these patterns are associated with neighborhood-level explanatory variables, has been almost non-existing. In this regard, and despite the substantial body of research showing an association between neighborhood characteristics and child maltreatment, most studies examining neighborhood influences fail to take into account the implications of the spatial dynamics of neighborhoods. For example, important issues such as the similarity and influence between neighboring areas, are not appropriately addressed in most studies analyzing neighborhood influences on child maltreatment [10, 11, 25]. Neighborhood risk factors that have been associated with child maltreatment are usually clustered in space, and therefore a spatial analytical approach is particularly appropriate for the study of their influences on the spatial variations of child maltreatment. Furthermore, when analyzing neighborhood influences on ecological variations in child maltreatment risk, the temporal dimension must also be taken into account. Neighborhoods characteristics may change over time and, therefore, their influence on child maltreatment risk can also change over time [10]. In this regard, adding the temporal dimension is a key in identifying and tracking trends in child maltreatment risk—for example, stable high or low risk areas, or areas of increasing or decreasing risk over time. Finally, most studies exploring neighborhood influences on child maltreatment do not provide small-area-specific risk estimations, which limits their relevance to inform more localized intervention and prevention strategies. A new generation of ecological studies needs to take into account the

spatial and temporal dimensions to better understand small-area variations in child maltreatment risk.

Bayesian spatio-temporal modeling provides an adequate methodological framework to overcome the above limitations in studying neighborhood influences on child maltreatment risk variations. This analytical approach, allows to incorporate geographical and temporal information to provide more reliable area-specific risk estimates than other non-Bayesian methods, by addressing important methodological issues such as modeling small area counts, spatial auto-correlation, or overdispersion, that can bias estimates if ignored [33–39]. Although Bayesian spatio-temporal disease mapping is common in other public health and epidemiological areas, this approach is relatively new in the area of family violence [40–44]. So far, only a handful of studies conducted in the US have addressed the spatial and temporal dimensions to study neighborhood influences on child maltreatment with appropriate methodologies [40, 42, 44]. However, these studies are usually low-resolution ones, using larger geographical areas, such as counties, zip codes, or census track, which somehow limits their potential to inform more localized interventions. On the other hand, high-resolution studies using small-area geographical units offer a finer neighborhood characterization, and provide specific risk estimations for small areas, which increases their potential to inform highly localized policies targeting high-risk areas [36, 38, 39].

Based on a social disorganization theoretical framework [43, 45–48] in this study we analyze the influence of a set of neighborhood characteristics on local patterns of substantiated child maltreatment over a 12-year period at the small-area level. Neighborhood-level characteristics analyzed include three indicators of neighborhood concentrated disadvantage—neighborhood economic status, neighborhood education level, and levels of policing activity—, immigrant concentration, and residential instability. As far as we are aware, the present study is the first to conduct a high-resolution small-area study on the spatio-temporal epidemiology of child maltreatment risk using Bayesian spatio-temporal modeling and disease mapping methods. Our study is conducted in a European city which also provides a ground for comparison to US cities where most of the research on neighborhood influences on child maltreatment has been conducted.

Methods
Variables
The study was conducted in the city of Valencia, the third largest city of Spain with a population of 736,580. As neighborhood proxies, we used the 552 census block groups into which the city is divided. This was the minimum administrative unit available, with an average of

1334 residents, and ranging from 630 to 2845. To capture temporal trends, data for 12 years were used, from 2004 to 2015. Data for cases of substantiated child maltreatment were provided by Valencia Child Protection Services. Covariates for each census block group were provided by the Valencia Statistics Office and the Valencia Police Department.

Outcome variable
Number of families with child maltreatment protection measures. Data of all families with child protection measures from 2004 to 2015 were collected—no computerized and systematized data were available before 2004. The data we used correspond to all official cases of substantiated child maltreatment in the city of Valencia during the period of the study, to which a child protection measure is associated after the maltreatment and the risk for the child is established. Child maltreatment refer to any type of child maltreatment, including physical, psychological, or sexual abuse, as well as neglect. Perpetrators were parents or legal tutors–child abuse by other parties, such as non-related adults, are dealt by other agencies and are not considered in this study. The data provided by the Child Protection Services did not allow to distinguish between child maltreatment types or perpetrators. Protection measures are issued by the Child Protection Services for all substantiated cases of child maltreatment, and may include a range of measures such as home visiting, family support programs, family or residential foster care, or adoption. Data for this study were 1799 families with child maltreatment protection measures. To avoid data dependency, cases were 'unique' families, meaning that a family was only included the first time they received a child maltreatment protection measure. Data were geocoded using the family address, and we counted the cases in each census block group for each of the 12 years in the study period.

Covariates
Neighborhood concentrated disadvantage. Economic status: Neighborhood economic status was measured using the average cadastral property value. This value is set by the City Hall and is used to establish local taxes. *Education level*: The average education level of neighborhood residents in each census block group was measured on a 4-point scale, where $1 = $ less than primary education, $2 = $ primary education, $3 = $ secondary education, $4 = $ college education. *Policing activity*: An indirect measure of public disorder and crime was measured through police officers' assessments of their policing activity. Senior police officers provided an index of policing activity that included interventions in drug-related crime, public disorder such as drunkenness and fights,

vandalism, homeless people and truancy. The index was structured as a 5-item scale, and each item ranged from 0—very low level of interventions—to 4—very high level of interventions. This measure of policing activity has been associated in previous studies with other types of family violence such as intimate partner violence [43], as well as with a number of neighborhood-level characteristics, such as neighborhood disorder, low socioeconomic status, and high immigrant concentration [49, 50]. Cronbach's alpha was .74.

Immigrant concentration: Using census data, immigrant concentration was measured as the percentage of immigrant population in each census block group.

Residential instability: An index of residential mobility, based on census data, was used as the proportion—rate per 1000 inhabitants—of the population who had moved into or out of each census block group during the previous year—for example, residential instability for 2015 captures all population movements occurred in 2014.

Statistical analysis
The outcome variable was the number of families with child maltreatment protection measures, corresponding to all substantiated cases of child maltreatment in the city during the period of the study. We use, therefore, a conditionally independent Poisson distribution based on the count of families in each census block group in the 12 years of the study:

$$y_{it}|\eta_{it} \sim Po(E_{it}\exp(\eta_{it})), \quad i=1,\ldots,552 \quad t=1,\ldots,12$$

where E_{it} is a fixed quantity that accounts for the expected number of families with child maltreatment protection measures, in proportion to the total number of families, in census block group i in year t; η_{it} is the log-relative risk for every area and year.

We used different models for η_{it} with an increasing level of complexity, from a Poisson regression model to a spatio-temporal autoregressive model. First, model 1 only included all covariates—that is, economic status, education level, policing activity, residential instability, and immigrant concentration.

$$\eta_{it} = \mu + X_{it}\beta$$

where μ is the intercept, X_{it} is the vector of covariates, and β is a vector of regression coefficients.

Model 2 was specified as a spatial model; it included all covariates and added unstructured and structured random effects. The unstructured random effect accounted for spatial heterogeneity or overdispersion, while the structured random effect accounted for the spatial effect:

$$\eta_{it} = \mu + X_{it}\beta + \phi_i + \theta_i$$

where ϕ_i represents the spatially structured term, and θ_i the spatially unstructured term.

Model 3 included the previous terms and incorporated an unstructured temporal effect:

$$\eta_{it} = \mu + X_{it}\beta + \phi_i + \theta_i + \alpha_t$$

where α_t accounts for the temporal heterogeneity. This model, however, does not account for past cases of child maltreatment—that is, temporal dependency.

Finally, model 4 included a spatio-temporal effect. To this end, we followed an autoregressive approach [51], combining autoregressive time series and spatial modeling. We defined a spatio-temporal structure in which the relative risks are both spatially and temporally dependent.

$$\eta_{i1} = \mu + X_{it}\beta + \alpha_1 + \left(1 - \rho^2\right)^{-1/2} \cdot (\phi_{i1} + \theta_{i1})$$

$$\eta_{it} = \mu + X_{it}\beta + \alpha_t + \rho \cdot \left(\eta_{i(t-1)} - \mu - \alpha_{t-1}\right) + \phi_{it} + \theta_{it}$$

The first equation defines the log-relative risk for the first year observed (2004) and the second equation defines the log-relative risk for the following years. In both, α_t is the mean deviation of the risk in the year t, ρ represents the temporal correlation between years, and ϕ_{it} and θ_{it} refer to structured and unstructured spatial random effects, respectively.

Models were specified following a Bayesian approach. Therefore, we assigned appropriate prior distributions for all parameters. We assigned vague Gaussian distributions for the fixed effects β; μ was specified as an improper uniform distribution; unstructured effects were modeled as a normal distribution $N\left(0, \sigma^2\right)$ in the different models (θ and α). Structured effects (ϕ) were specified by a conditional spatial autoregressive (CAR) model [52] defined as follows:

$$\phi_i | \phi_{-i} \sim N\left(\frac{1}{n_i}\sum_{j \sim i}\phi_j, \frac{\sigma_\phi^2}{n_i}\right)$$

where n_i is the number of neighboring areas of each census block group i, ϕ_{-i} represents the values of the ϕ vector except the component i, σ_ϕ is the standard deviation parameter, and $j \sim i$ indicates all units j that are neighboring areas of census block group i. Finally, and following the structure of the hierarchical Bayesian models, hyperparameters σ were specified by uniform distributions $U(0, 1)$ in the models.

Bayesian estimations were performed using Markov Chain Monte Carlo simulation techniques with the software R and the WinBUGS package. 100,000 iterations were generated, discarding the first 10,000 as a burn-in period. Models were compared by the Deviance

Information Criterion (DIC) [53]. This measure of fit assumes that models with smaller DIC should be preferred to models with larger DIC. Following this criterion, the model with smaller DIC was chosen. Differences in DIC between 5 and 10 are considered substantial; whereas differences of more than 10 units clearly indicate that the model with the higher DIC should be ruled out.

To ensure robustness of the results, we checked convergence with the convergence diagnosis $\hat{R}$ [54] which was near to 1.0 for all parameters. A sensitivity analysis was also performed on prior distributions of hyperparameters, with consistent results.

Results

Table 1 summarizes the descriptive statistics of the variables in the study. The neighborhood-level economic status, based on the average cadastral property value, had a mean of 26,320 € [standard deviation (SD) = 13,046], with wide variation across neighborhoods, ranging from 7943€ to 98,560€. The average neighborhood education level, corresponded to secondary education (Mean = 3; SD = .33). Policing activity had a mean of 7.16 (SD = 3.99), again with wide variations across neighborhoods ranging from 0 to 19. The mean of neighborhood residential instability was 200 (SD = 65.96) meaning that, in average, 200 people moved into or out of a census block group in a specific year. Neighborhood immigrant concentration had a mean of 13.3%, ranging from just 1 to 51%, which means that in some neighborhoods over half of the population were immigrant. Finally, the outcome variable, families with child protection measures, ranged from 0 cases of substantiated child maltreatment in some neighborhoods to a maximum of 7 families per census block group in a single year with child protection measures after child maltreatment was substantiated.

After conducting the four Bayesian Poisson regression models, we analyzed the DIC values (Table 2). Model 1, which included only the covariates, showed the worst fit (DIC = 8517.9). Once we introduced both structured and unstructured spatial random effects in model 2, the DIC decreased significantly (DIC = 8164.9). In model 3,

Table 1 Variables (mean, standard deviation, minimum and maximum values) at the census block group and year level

Variable	Mean (SD)	Min	Max
Economic status (€)	26,320 (13,046)	7943	98,560
Education level	3.155 (.33)	2.39	3.86
Policing activity	7.16 (3.99)	0	19
Residential instability	200 (65.96)	4.2	771.3
Immigrant concentration (%)	13.28 (6.92)	1.03	51.47
Child protection records	0.26 (.57)	0	7

Table 2 Results of different spatial and spatio-temporal regression Bayesian models for child maltreatment risk. Posterior mean, standard deviation (SD) and the 95% credible interval (CI) of all parameters

	Model 1 (β)			Model 2 (β + spatial heterogeneity + spatial effect)			Model 3 (β + spatial heterogeneity + spatial effect + temporal heterogeneity)			Model 4 (spatio-temporal autoregressive model)		
	Mean	SD	95% CI	Mean	SD	95% CI	Mean	SD	95% CI	Mean	SD	95% CI
Intercept	4.055	.289	3.500, 4.615	4.335	.516	3.320, 5.328	4.284	.520	3.916, 5.304	4.135	.500	3.274, 5.127
Economic status[a]	−.021	.003	−.027, −.015	−.016	.004	−.024, −.009	−.016	.004	−.023, −.009	−.016	.004	−.023, −.008
Education level	−1.261	.091	−1.431, −1.083	−1.464	.161	−1.745, −1.123	−1.418	.164	−1.746, −1.096	−1.391	.157	−1.690, −1.122
Policing activity	.026	.006	.014, .038	.036	.011	.012, .053	.035	.012	.012, .057	.031	.011	.009, .053
Residential instability	.000	.001	−.001, .001	.000	.001	−.001, .001	.000	.001	−.001, .001	.000	.001	−.001, .001
Immigrant concentration	.003	.005	−.006, .013	.005	.006	−.005, .016	.005	.005	−.005, .016	.009	.006	−.003, .020
σ_θ				.329	.084	.136, .468	.320	.095	.063, .456	.234	.045	.162, .333
σ_φ				.781	.115	.541, .979	.787	.118	.552, .976	.257	.062	.149, .391
σ_α							.023	.019	.001, .070	.021	.019	.001, .070
ρ										.903	.031	.827, .946
DIC	8517.9			8164.9			8166.8			8126.1		

SD standard deviation, *CrI* credible interval, *DIC* deviance information criterion

σ_θ standard deviation unstructured term

σ_φ standard deviation spatially structured term

σ_α Standard deviation temporally unstructured term

[a] This variable was included as the cadastral value divided by 1000 to solve computational problems with the prior distributions assigned to fixed effects

which included an unstructured temporal effect, the DIC slightly increased to 8166.8. Finally, model 4, an autoregressive model, despite being the most complex had the lowest DIC value (8126.1), 38 units lower than model 2, and was therefore chosen as the final model. The sign of the covariate estimations (positive or negative) remains invariant in the different models, ensuring the stability of the effects.

For model relevance, we consider posterior probability distributions of the regression coefficients (β) of being different from zero. The probability of being positive was higher than 90% for policing activity and immigrant concentration. The probability of being negative was higher than 90% for economic status and education level. These results indicate that the risk of substantiated child maltreatment was particularly high in neighborhoods with low economic status and education level, and with high levels of policing activity and immigrant concentration. Residential instability, however, did not show a relevant association with substantiated child maltreatment.

To know the relative influence of the four neighborhood variables that were relevant for the final model, our results can be interpreted in terms of odds ratios expressed as $\exp(\beta \cdot \Delta X)$. For example a 10,000€ increase in economic status decreases the relative risk of substantiated child maltreatment by 17%; a 0.1 increase in education level decreases the relative risk by 15%; a 5 unit increase in policing activity increases the relative risk by 17%; finally, a 10% increase in immigrant concentration increases the relative risk by 9%.

Bayesian spatio-temporal modeling allows area-specific risks of substantiated child maltreatment to be mapped and differences analyzed over the years. Figure 1 shows the relative risk for each year of the study. These maps show areas with higher (> 1) or lower (< 1) than average risk. In some areas, the relative risk is more than twice the average, which reflects very high-risk levels of substantiated child maltreatment.

These maps also reveal common patterns over the years, showing areas with higher levels of relative risk at the periphery, especially in the eastern part of the city. The parameter ρ ($\rho = .90$) indicated a high temporal correlation between a particular year and the previous one.

Autoregressive models can be used to represent temporal paths of relative risk in different census block groups, thus identifying areas with stable risks and areas with changes in risk over time. Figure 2 shows the most stable areas. Results showed both chronic spatial patterns of high risk of substantiated child maltreatment during the years analyzed, as well as stability over time in areas of low risk. The most stable low risks are located in the city center, while peripheral areas present more stable high

risks. Figure 3 shows areas with increased or decreased substantiated child maltreatment risk over the years.

Discussion

This study showed that the neighborhoods where the families live matter in understanding spatial and temporal variations in child maltreatment risk [8–12]. Our results showed that neighborhoods with low levels of economic and educational status, with high levels of policing activity, and high immigrant concentration had higher risk of substantiated child maltreatment. This study illustrates how the unequal distribution of neighborhood risk factors in an urban area is linked to the unequal spatial distribution of substantiated child maltreatment risk in the city. These results support the view that 'place' matters in relation to child maltreatment, as these ecological variations reflect important inequalities in substantiated child maltreatment risk [10–12]. Among the explanatory mechanisms that have been proposed to explain this link are: social impoverishment—that is, lack of trust and support networks in the neighborhood—, and diminished social control; social isolation from mainstream values regarding what is acceptable in parent–child relationships; and high levels of parental stress [8, 10–12, 19, 27].

Previous studies have linked these neighborhoods characteristics—that is, neighborhood socioeconomic disadvantage, disorder and crime, and immigrant concentration—indicative of social disorganization to child maltreatment rates [10, 11, 27, 29]. However, the present study is, as far as we are aware, the first to analyze this link using a high-resolution Bayesian spatio-temporal approach to study the influence of neighborhood characteristics on small-area variations in substantiated child maltreatment risk. Using this approach, we were able to analyze small-area variations in substantiated child maltreatment risk over a 12-year period, which provided the possibility to identify and track risk trends. Our results, in addition, show that 'time' is also a key element to analyze variations in child maltreatment risk. Studies that do not take into account the temporal dimension may misinterpret risk estimations due to data aggregation—for example increasing or decreasing risks in certain neighborhoods would not be detected. In our study, introducing a spatio-temporal autoregressive structure clearly improved the model fit, and provided more reliable area-specific risk estimates. Thus, our results showed chronic spatial patterns of high risk of substantiated child maltreatment during the years analyzed. We found areas where risks were over five-times higher than the city average, and this high risk was stable over the years. Results suggest that in certain city areas substantiated child maltreatment risk can become 'endemic'. On the

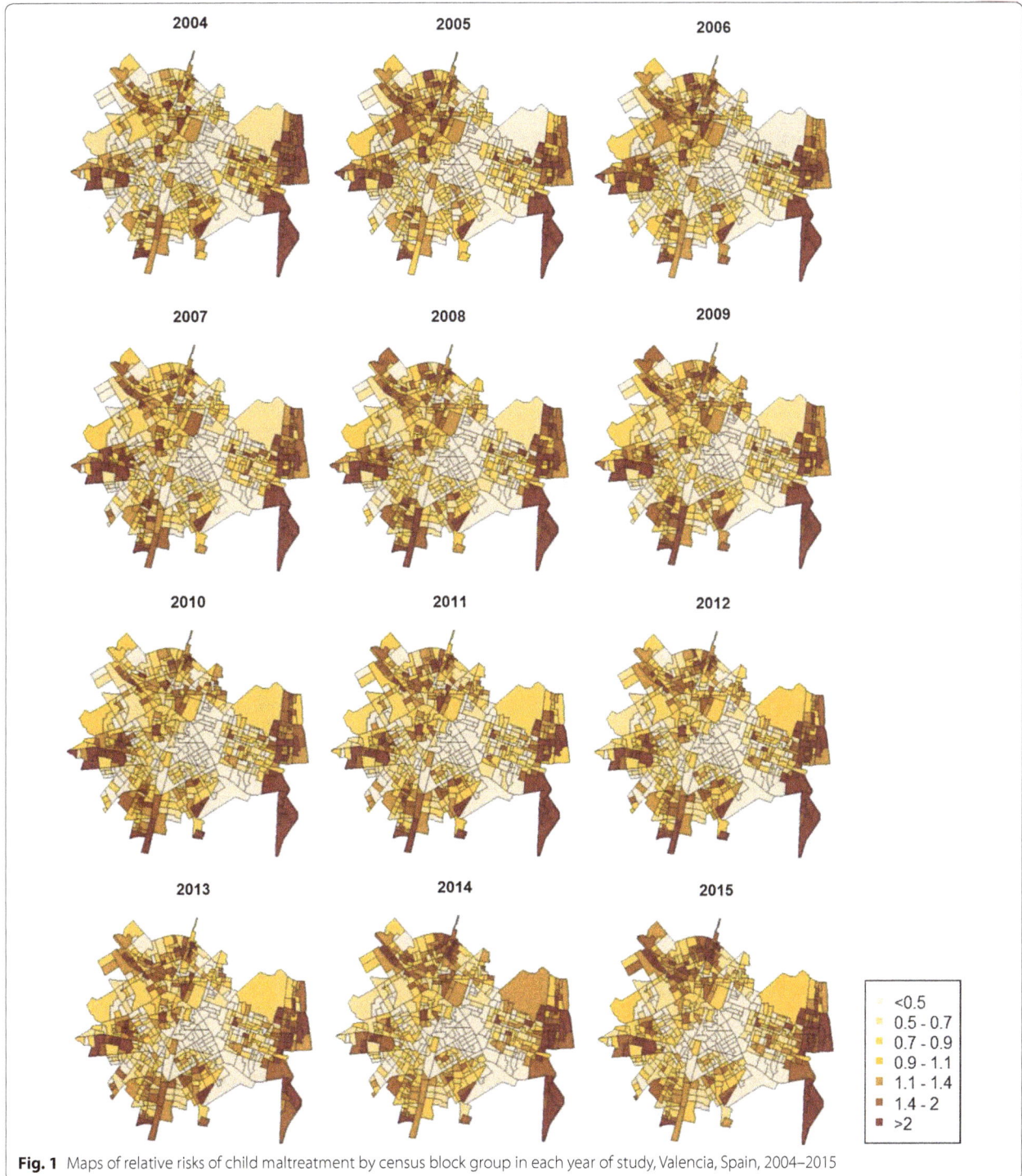

Fig. 1 Maps of relative risks of child maltreatment by census block group in each year of study, Valencia, Spain, 2004–2015

other hand, risks in other areas were between two and four times lower than the city average, and these lower risks were also stable over the years. In this regard, low-risk city areas could be considered to be providing a more protective social environment for the well-being of children, as opposed to the very high-risk ones—for example,

differences in risk between some of the low risk areas and some of the high-risk ones are nearly tenfold. Finally, spatio-temporal analyses allowed us to identify areas where substantiated child maltreatment risk increased or decreased over the years analyzed.

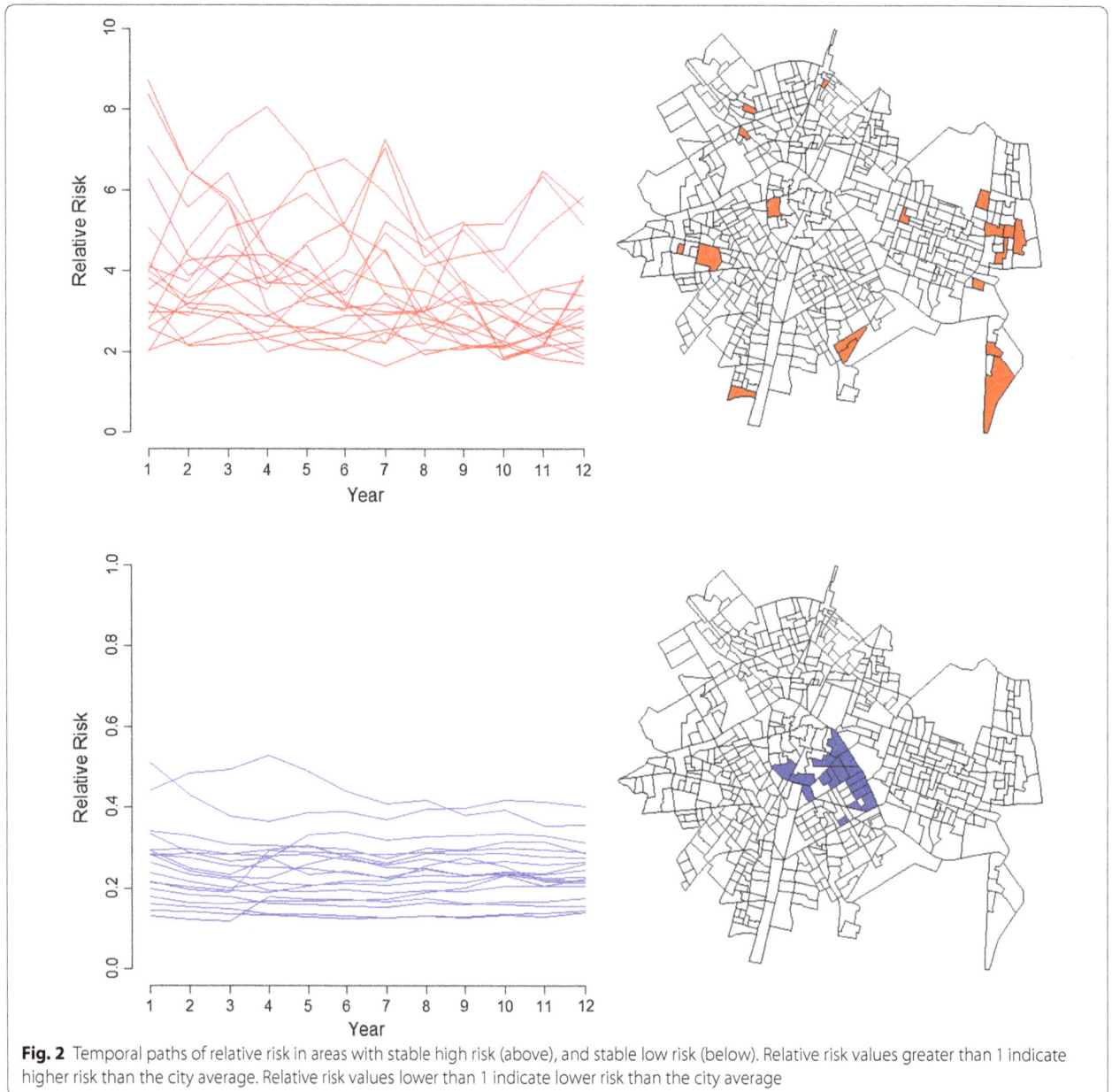

Fig. 2 Temporal paths of relative risk in areas with stable high risk (above), and stable low risk (below). Relative risk values greater than 1 indicate higher risk than the city average. Relative risk values lower than 1 indicate lower risk than the city average

Detecting and tracking these inequalities in substantiated child maltreatment risk is important for better-informed prevention and intervention strategies. One of the advantages of the high-resolution approach used in the present study is that it provides small-area-specific risk estimates pointing to areas of stable excess risk, as well as to areas of increasing or decreasing substantiated child maltreatment risk. Identifying and tracking these risk trends at the small-area level can provide a more useful method to inform policy and action, as compared to other low-resolution approaches—for example, counties or large census tracks. Interventions targeting areas of

excess risk of child maltreatment—for example, increasing or chronic high-risk areas—can have an important preventive potential. Neighborhood-level interventions, as opposed to a person-centered approach, can reach a larger number of families, providing a more cost-effective strategy, as not only the individuals are the subject of the intervention, but also the context where these families live [10, 55, 56]. The spatio-temporal epidemiological approach used in this study not only provides a powerful method to map and track variations in risk, but it can also contribute to a surveillance system to assess the effectiveness of intervention and prevention strategies by

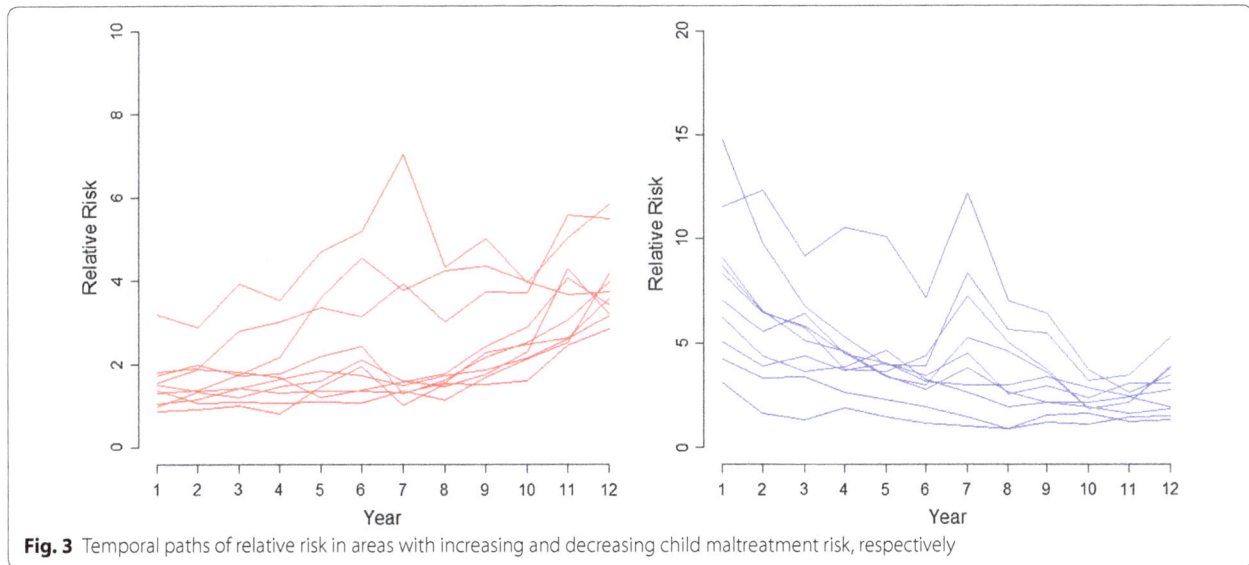

Fig. 3 Temporal paths of relative risk in areas with increasing and decreasing child maltreatment risk, respectively

monitoring changes in risk over time across different city areas [6, 12].

Limitations to our study include the type of data used, namely, only officially reported and substantiated cases of child maltreatment under the supervision of Child Protection Services. Child maltreatment is, however, still largely underreported and underestimated, as many cases do not come to the attention of these services, or are unsubstantiated after reporting [4, 44]. On the other hand, it is important to note that families living in high risk neighborhoods may be more visible to authorities and therefore can be more susceptible to be reported and substantiated, as these residential areas may lead to a higher surveillance by social welfare or law enforcement agencies, as compared to other residential areas [10, 11, 42, 44]. A related issue is the potential problem of neighborhood selection bias, whereby families with higher risk of being investigated by child protection services, either choose or are forced to live in these high-risk neighborhoods [10]. The question here is to which extent the higher risk of substantiated child maltreatment is the result of the influence of neighborhood-level factors or the self-selection of families with certain characteristics in certain neighborhoods. Although this line of criticism tends to give more preeminence to individual-based explanations, than to other higher-order explanations such as neighborhood mechanisms, a substantial body of research supports the link between neighborhood concentrated disadvantage and the spatial inequality in a wide variety of outcomes, including violence, crime, or health. This body of literature led Sampson to conclude that "spatially inscribed social differences, ..., constitute a family of neighborhood effects that are pervasive, strong,

cross-cutting, and paradoxically stable even as they are changing in manifest form" [55, p. 6].

Regarding the covariates used in our study, the measurement of policing activity could be biased by self-report. However, this measure has adequate psychometric characteristics [49, 50] and previous studies have shown that police perceptions capture their valuable experience, are correlated with police records, and can provide important information to identify high crime areas [50, 57–59]. Nevertheless, clearly, future studies would benefit from using more objective crime reports. Another limitation in our study is that a number of potentially relevant neighborhood-level measures were not available for a 12-year spatio-temporal analysis. For example, socioeconomic measures such as people living below the poverty line, rates of unemployment, or income, or other covariates tapping potentially relevant neighborhood processes—such as collective efficacy, social networks, neighborhood disorder, neighborhood social norms, or alcohol outlets—, were not available [29–31, 60–66]. The modifiable areal unit problem is also a potential limitation. We are confident, however, that the high-resolution approach in this study, using the smallest geographical administrative unit available—census block groups are walkable areas with a small number of city blocks—, was particularly adequate to capture neighborhood influences on small-area variations in risk [7].

Regarding the implications for policy and action, the neighborhood conditions linked to substantiated child maltreatment in the present study are risk factors that cluster in space and, therefore, can be targeted in more focused preventive interventions. Although potentially modifiable, some of these factors, such as poor housing, or high levels of crime, or high levels of immigrant concentration are clearly difficult to change. However, other type of focused neighborhood-level interventions can address indirectly these factors. For example, urban planning and environmental approaches such as urban redevelopment and revitalization—for instance, providing new infrastructures, greening vacant lots, improving access to services, or increasing community programs—, have been shown to improve the quality of life of residents, and reduce crime, drug use, and violence in disadvantage communities [67–70].

Finally, this study was conducted in a medium-sized European city. Although similar neighborhood effects in relation to other type of offenses have been observed in European and American cities despite their differences in culture and organization [43, 55, 71, 72], future cross-national research with a similar approach would help to strengthen and generalize our results.

Conclusion

Our 12-year study showed that there are important spatial inequalities in substantiated child maltreatment risk across the city areas and over the years. Our study illustrates that a spatio-temporal epidemiological approach to study the geographical patterns, trends over time, and the contextual determinants of substantiated child maltreatment risk, can provide a useful method that can be of help to better inform policy and action. This methodological approach—that uses data that can be routinely collected—, can offer a more accurate description of the problem, and help to design new local prevention and intervention strategies. A spatio-temporal approach can also contribute to an improved epidemiological surveillance system to detect ecological variations in risk, and to assess the effectiveness of the initiatives to reduce this risk.

Authors' contributions
EG conceptualized the study, drafted the initial manuscript, and approved the final manuscript as submitted. AL-Q designed the analytic strategy and supervised the statistical analysis, drafted the initial manuscript, and approved the final manuscript as submitted. MM conducted statistical analysis, drafted the initial manuscript, and approved the final manuscript as submitted. ML designed and coordinated the data collection, and critically reviewed the manuscript. All authors read and approved the final manuscript.

Author details
[1] Department of Social Psychology, University of Valencia, Av. Blasco Ibáñez, 21, 46010 Valencia, Spain. [2] Department of Statistics and Operations Research, University of Valencia, C/Doctor Moliner, 50, 46100 Burjassot, Valencia, Spain.

Acknowledgements
We would like to thank the Child Protective Services, the Statistics Office, and the Police Department of the city of Valencia, for their support and assistance in collecting the data for this study.

Competing interests
The authors declare that they have no competing interests.

Funding
This study was supported by the Spanish Ministry of Economy and Competitiveness [PSI2014-54561-P, and MTM2016-77501-P] and the Spanish Ministry of Education, Culture and Sports [FPU2013/00164].

References
1. Gilbert R, Kemp A, Thoburn J, Sidebotham P, Radford L, Glaser D, Macmillan HL. Recognising and responding to child maltreatment. Lancet. 2009;373:167–80.
2. Reading R, Bissell S, Goldhagen J, Harwin J, Masson J, Moynihan S, Parton N, Pais MS, Thoburn J, Webb E. Promotion of children's rights and prevention of child maltreatment. Lancet. 2009;373:332–43.
3. Fang X, Brown DS, Florence CS, Mercy JA. The economic burden of child maltreatment in the United States and implications for prevention. Child Abuse Negl. 2012;36:156–65.
4. World Health Organization. European report on preventing child maltreatment. Copenhagen: Regional Office for Europe, World Health Organization; 2013.
5. Finkelhor D, Turner HA, Shattuck A, Hamby SL. Violence, crime, and abuse exposure in a national sample of children and youth: an update. JAMA Pediatr. 2013;167:614–21.
6. Finkelhor D, Turner HA, Shattuck A, Hamby SL. Prevalence of childhood exposure to violence, crime, and abuse: results from the National Survey of Children's Exposure to Violence. JAMA Pediatr. 2015;169:746–54.
7. Stoltenborgh M, Bakermans-Kranenburg MJ, Alink LR, IJzendoorn MH. The prevalence of child maltreatment across the globe: review of a series of meta-analyses. Child Abuse Rev. 2015;24:37–50.
8. Garbarino J, Sherman D. High-risk neighbourhoods and high-risk families: the human ecology of child maltreatment. Child Dev. 1980;51:188–98.
9. Zuravin SJ. The ecology of child abuse and neglect: review of the literature and presentation of data. Violence Vict. 1989;4:101–20.
10. Freisthler B, Merritt DH, LaScala EA. Understanding the ecology of child maltreatment: a review of the literature and directions for future research. Child Maltreat. 2006;11:263–80.
11. Coulton CJ, Crampton DS, Irwin M, Spilsbury JC, Korbin JE. How neighborhoods influence child maltreatment: a review of the literature and alternative pathways. Child Abuse Negl. 2007;31:1117–42.
12. Petersen AC, Joseph J, Feit M. New directions in child abuse and neglect research. Washington, DC: National Academics Press; 2014.
13. Coulton C, Korbin J, Su M, Chow J. Community level factors and child maltreatment rates. Child Dev. 1995;66:1262–76.
14. Korbin JE, Coulton CJ, Chard S, Platt-Houston C, Su M. Impoverishment and child maltreatment in African American and European American neighborhoods. Dev Psychopathol. 1998;10:215–33.
15. Drake B, Pandey S. Understanding the relationship between neighborhood poverty and specific types of child maltreatment. Child Abuse Negl. 1996;20:1003–18.
16. Coulton CJ, Korbin JE, Su M. Neighborhoods and child maltreatment: a multilevel study. Child Abuse Negl. 1999;23:1019–40.
17. Ernst JS. Community-level factors and child maltreatment in a suburban county. Soc Work Res. 2001;25:133–42.
18. Gracia E, Musitu G. Social isolation from communities and child maltreatment: a cross-cultural comparison. Child Abuse Negl. 2003;27:153–68.
19. Molnar BE, Buka SL, Brennan RT, Holton JK, Earls F. A multilevel study of neighborhoods and parent-to-child physical aggression: results from

the Project on Human Development in Chicago Neighborhoods. Child Maltreat. 2003;8:84–97.

20. Paulsen DJ. No safe place: Assessing spatial patterns of child maltreatment victimization. J Aggress Maltreat Trauma. 2003;8:63–85.

21. Freisthler B. A spatial analysis of social disorganization, alcohol access, and rates of child maltreatment in neighborhoods. Child Youth Serv Rev. 2004;26:803–19.

22. Gracia E, Herrero J. Perceived neighborhood social disorder and residents' attitudes toward reporting child physical abuse. Child Abuse Negl. 2006;30:357–65.

23. Freisthler B, Gruenewald PJ, Ring L, LaScala EA. An ecological assessment of the population and environmental correlates of childhood accident, assault and child abuse injuries. Alcohol Clin Exp Res. 2008;32:1969–75.

24. Freisthler B, Bruce E, Needell B. Understanding the geospatial relationship of neighborhood characteristics and rates of maltreatment for black, hispanic, and white children. Soc Work. 2007;52:7–16.

25. Klein S. The availability of neighborhood early care and education resources and the maltreatment of young children. Child Maltreat. 2011;16:300–11.

26. Maguire-Jack K. Multilevel investigation into the community context of child maltreatment. J Aggress Maltreat Trauma. 2014;23:229–48.

27. Freisthler B, Maguire-Jack K. Understanding the interplay between neighborhood structural factors, social processes, and alcohol outlets on child physical abuse. Child Maltreat. 2015;20:268–77.

28. Kim B, Maguire-Jack K. Community interaction and child maltreatment. Child Abuse Negl. 2015;41:146–57.

29. Molnar BE, Goerge RM, Gilsanz P, Gilsanz P, Hill A, Subramanian SV, Holton JK, Duncan DT, Beatriz ED, Beardslee WR. Neighborhood-level social processes and substantiated cases of child maltreatment. Child Abuse Negl. 2016;51:41–53.

30. Maguire-Jack K, Showalter K. The protective effect of neighborhood social cohesion in child abuse and neglect. Child Abuse Negl. 2016;52:29–37.

31. Fujiwara T, Yamaoka Y, Kawachi I. Neighborhood social capital and infant physical abuse: a population-based study in Japan. Int J Ment Health Syst. 2016;10:13.

32. Maguire-Jack K, Font SA. Intersections of individual and neighborhood disadvantage: implications for child. Child Youth Serv Rev. 2016;72:44–51.

33. Bernardinelli L, Clayton D, Pascutto C, Montomoli C, Ghislandi M, Songini M. Bayesian analysis of space-time variation in disease risk. Stat Med. 1995;14:2433–43.

34. Waller LA, Gotway CA. Applied spatial statistics for public health data. Hoboken: John Wiley and Sons; 2004.

35. Haining R, Law J, Griffith D. Modelling small area counts in the presence of overdispersion and spatial autocorrelation. Comput Stat Data Anal. 2009;53:2923–37.

36. Jonker MF, Congdon PD, van Lenthe FJ, Donkers B, Burdorf A, Mackenbach JP. Small-area health comparisons using health-adjusted life expectancies: a Bayesian random-effects approach. Health Place. 2013;29:70–8.

37. Congdon P. Applied Bayesian modelling. West Sussex: Wiley; 2014.

38. Law J, Quick M, Chan P. Bayesian spatio-temporal modeling for analysing local patterns of crime over time at the small-area level. J Quant Criminol. 2014;30:57–78.

39. Quick M, Law J, Luan H. The influence of on-premise and off-premise alcohol outlets on reported violent crime in the region of Waterloo, Ontario: applying Bayesian spatial modeling to inform land use planning and policy. Appl Spat Anal Policy. 2017;10:435–54.

40. Freisthler B, Weiss RE. Using Bayesian space-time models to understand the substance use environment and risk for being referred to child protective services. Subst Use Misuse. 2008;43:239–51.

41. Cunradi CB, Mair C, Ponicki W, Remer L. Alcohol outlets, neighborhood characteristics, and intimate partner violence: ecological analysis of a California city. J Urban Health. 2011;88:191–200.

42. Freisthler B, Kepple NJ, Holmes MR. The geography of drug market activities and child maltreatment. Child Maltreat. 2012;17:144–52.

43. Gracia E, López-Quílez A, Marco M, Lladosa S, Lila M. The spatial epidemiology of intimate partner violence: do neighborhoods matter? Am J Epidemiol. 2015;182:58–66.

44. Thurston H, Freisthler B, Bell J, Tancredi D, Romano PS, Miyamoto S, Joseph JG. The temporal-spatial distribution of seriously maltreated children. Spat Spatiotemporal Epidemiol. 2017;20:1–8.

45. Shaw CR, McKay HD. Juvenile delinquency and urban areas. Chicago: University of Chicago Press; 1942.

46. Bursik RJ, Grasmick HG. Neighborhood and crime. New York: Lexington Books; 1993.

47. Sampson RJ, Groves WB. Community structure and crime: testing social disorganization theory. AJS. 1989;94:774–802.

48. Sampson RJ, Morenoff JD, Gannon-Rowley T. Assessing, "neighborhood effects": social processes and new directions in research. Annu Rev Sociol. 2002;28:443–78.

49. Marco M, Gracia E, Martín-Fernández M, López-Quílez A. Validation of a Google Street View-based neighborhood disorder observational scale. J Urban Health. 2017;94:190–8.

50. Marco M, Gracia E, López-Quílez A. Linking neighborhood characteristics and drug-related police interventions: a Bayesian spatial analysis. ISPRS Int J Geo-Inf. 2017;6:65–77.

51. Martínez-Beneito MA, López-Quilez A, Botella-Rocamora P. An autoregressive approach to spatio-temporal disease mapping. Stat Med. 2008;27:2874–89.

52. Besag J, York J, Mollié A. Bayesian image restoration, with two applications in spatial statistics. Ann Inst Stat Math. 1991;43:1–20.

53. Spiegelhalter DJ, Best NG, Carlin BP, Van der Linde A. Bayesian measures of model complexity and fit. J R Stat Soc Ser B Stat Methodol. 2002;64:583–639.

54. Gelman A, Carlin JB, Stern HS, Rubin DB. Bayesian data analysis. 2nd ed. Boca Raton: CRC Press; 1990.

55. Sampson RJ. Great American city: Chicago and the enduring neighborhood effect. Chicago: University of Chicago Press; 2012.

56. Díez-Roux AV, Mair C. Neighborhoods and health. Ann NY Acad Sci. 2010;1186:125–45.

57. Ratcliffe JH, McCullagh MJ. Chasing ghosts? Police perception of high crime areas. Br J Criminol. 2001;41:330–41.

58. Haining R, Law J. Combining police perceptions with police records of serious crime areas: a modelling approach. J R Stat Soc Ser A Stat Soc. 2007;170:1019–34.

59. Rengert GF, Pelfrey WV. Cognitive mapping of the city center: comparative perceptions of dangerous places. In: Weisburd D, McEwen JT, editors. Crime mapping and crime prevention. Monsey: Criminal Justice Press; 1997. p. 193–218.

60. Gracia E, López-Quílez A, Marco M, Lladosa S, Lila M. Exploring neighborhood influences on small-area variation in intimate partner violence risk: a Bayesian random-effect modeling approach. Int J Environ Res Public Health. 2014;11:866–82.

61. Sampson RJ, Raudenbush SW, Earls F. Neighborhoods and violent crime: a multilevel study of collective efficacy. Science. 1997;277:918–24.

62. Freisthler B, Midanik LT, Gruenewald PJ. Alcohol outlets and child physical abuse and neglect: applying routine activities theory to the study of child maltreatment. J Stud Alcohol. 2004;65:586–92.

63. Freisthler B, Needell B, Gruenewald PJ. Is the physical availability of alcohol and illicit drugs related to neighborhood rates of child maltreatment? Child Abuse Negl. 2005;29:1049–60.

64. Freisthler B, Gruenewald PJ, Remer LG, Lery B, Needell B. Exploring the spatial dynamics of alcohol outlets and child protective services referrals, substantiations, and foster care entries. Child Maltreat. 2007;12:114–24.

65. Morton CM, Simmel C, Peterson NA. Neighborhood alcohol outlet density and rates of child abuse and neglect: moderating effects of access to substance abuse services. Child Abuse Negl. 2014;38:952–61.

66. Daley D, Bachmann M, Bachmann BA, Pedigo C, Bui M, Coffman J. Risk terrain modeling predicts child maltreatment. Child Abuse Negl. 2016;62:29–38.

67. Kelaher M, Warr DJ, Tacticos T. Evaluating health impacts: results from the neighbourhood renewal stratgey in Victoria, Australia. Health Place. 2010;16:861–7.

68. Garvin EC, Cannuscio CC, Branas CC. Greening vacant lots to reduce violent crime: a randomised controlled trial. Inj Prev. 2013;19:198–203.

69. Mehdipanah R, Malmusi D, Muntaner C, Borrell C. An evaluation of an urban renewal program and its effects on neighborhood resident's overall wellbeing using concept mapping. Health Place. 2013;23:9–17.

70. Linton SL, Jennings JM, Latkin CA, Kirk GD, Mehta SH. The association between neighborhood residential rehabilitation and injection drug use in Baltimore, Maryland, 2000–2011. Health Place. 2014;28:142–9.

71. Le Galès P, Zagrodzki M. Cities are back in town: The US/Europe comparison. Paris: Cahier Européen, Centre d'Etudes Européennes de Sciences Po; 2006.

72. Summers AA, Cheshire PC, Senn L. Urban Change in the United States and Western Europe: comparative analysis and policy. Washington, DC: The Urban Institute Press; 1999.

9

Ambient air quality and spatio-temporal patterns of cardiovascular emergency department visits

Eun-Hye Yoo[1]* ⓘ, Patrick Brown[2] and Youngseob Eum[1]

Abstract

Background: Air pollutants have been associated with various adverse health effects, including increased rates of hospital admissions and emergency room visits. Although numerous time-series studies and case-crossover studies have estimated associations between day-to-day variation in pollutant levels and mortality/morbidity records, studies on geographic variations in emergency department use and the spatial effects in their associations with air pollution exposure are rare.

Methods: We focused on the elderly who visited emergency room for cardiovascular related disease (CVD) in 2011. Using spatially and temporally resolved multi-pollutant exposures, we investigated the effect of short-term exposures to ambient air pollution on emergency department utilization. We developed two statistical models with and without spatial random effects within a hierarchical Bayesian framework to capture the spatial heterogeneity and spatial auto-correlation remaining in emergency department utilization.

Results: Although the cardiovascular effect of spatially homogeneous pollutants, such as PM2.5 and ozone, was unchanged, we found the cardiovascular effect of NO_2 was pronounced after accounting for the spatially correlated structure in emergency department utilization. We also identified areas with high ED utilization for CVD among the elderly and assessed the uncertainty associated with risk estimates.

Conclusions: We assessed the short-term effect of multi-pollutants on cardiovascular risk of the elderly and demonstrated the use of community multiscale air quality model-derived spatially and temporally resolved multi-pollutant exposures to an epidemiological study. Our results indicate that NO_2 was significantly associated with the elevated ED utilization for CVD among the elderly.

Keywords: Cardiovascular disease (CVD), Emergency department (ED) visits, Hierarchical Bayesian model, Community multiscale air quality (CMAQ), Ambient air quality, Spatial effects

Background

Adverse health effects of air pollutants have been documented in numerous past studies, investigating the associations between various health outcomes and exposures to ambient air pollution [1–4]. Some studies focused on the impact of long-term accumulated exposures on chronic health outcomes, whereas others focused on the acute effect of exposure by exploring the associations between short term changes in air pollution exposure and daily deaths or hospital admissions. A number of studies of emergency department (ED) utilization, which is a relatively sensitive health outcome for respiratory conditions and cardiovascular illnesses [5], have also demonstrated the effect of increased ambient particulate matter on acute health outcomes [4, 6, 7].

It is worth noting, however, that the majority of studies that have investigated associations between air pollution exposure and emergency department visits were conducted using case-crossover or time-series designs [7–12], whereas little to no attention was given

*Correspondence: eunhye@buffalo.edu
[1] Department of Geography, University at Buffalo, Buffalo, NY, USA
Full list of author information is available at the end of the article

to geographical variations in ED use. In our review of 167 studies on health effects of air pollution published between 1999 and 2017, a total of 55 studies (33%) used a case-crossover approach, 106 studies (64%) used a variant of time-series design, and 4 studies utilized both study designs [13–16]. Our search was conducted in Pub-Med and ScienceDirect databases up to November 2017 using a combination of the following keywords: emergency department/room and air pollution. Among these studies, spatially and temporally varying air pollution exposure were considered only in 14 studies and these following studies by Carlin et al. [17], Zhu et al. [18], Wannemuehler et al. [19], and Sarnat et al. [20] assessed the effect of air pollution on geographical variations of ED utilization.

Perhaps the popularity of these two modeling approaches compared to spatial models might be due to the well-established associations between ambient air pollution and respiratory outcomes [21], but also the limited availability of spatially and temporally resolved air quality data. The population-weighted spatial average of measurements from monitoring sites have been used in both time-series analysis and case-crossover studies to approximate city-wide or regional average ambient concentrations. This approach is relevant as long as the spatial homogeneity assumption is met, but can lead to increased uncertainty and potential bias in their estimates of health risk when the spatiotemporal heterogeneity of pollutants is pronounced [20]. Meanwhile, considerable improvements have been made in spatially and temporally dynamic air quality modeling efforts, which include community multiscale air quality (CMAQ) model [22] and optimal aerosol depth values retrieved from remote sensing [23]. CMAQ is one of the most widely used regional air quality modeling systems, which has been used to evaluate pollution control measures and to determine source contributions to air pollutants, but also to provides air pollution exposure estimation in epidemiological studies [24, 25]. Recently Environmental Protection Agency (EPA) released fine scale predictions of pollutant levels, which were obtained by fusing monitoring data with the CMAQ model outputs. Although these spatially and temporally resolved pollutant surface estimates are subject to calibration bias and uncertainties [26–28], there is the potential of improving the quality of individual and population exposure to ambient pollution. Meanwhile, the applications of CMAQ related air quality data to population-level epidemiological studies are still rare with a few exceptions [29, 30].

The other issue in epidemiological studies on cardiovascular and respiratory effect of air pollution is that health associations with exposure to air pollutants are affected by neighborhood effects. A recent study by O'lenick et al. [31] reported that neighborhood-level socioeconomic status (SES) is a key factor that contributes to short-term vulnerabilities to air pollution-related respiratory morbidity, such as asthma, among children (5–18 years old). Likewise, Winquist et al. [32] argued that this SES effect is generalizable based on their multi-city study. However, it is still questionable if their neighborhood-level SES effects hold for different study locations, study periods, or health outcomes other than respiratory disease. Given that the vulnerability of subgroups to CVD is more pronounced than other types of diseases [33–35], it is necessary to account for the effect of neighborhood-level SES to identify the vulnerabilities among the most susceptible individuals to air pollution related CVD.

From a statistical standpoint, a Poisson process model appears to be a natural choice to explore geographic variation in ED use with respect to neighborhood health effects. However classical Poisson regression models may be problematic for ED visit counts aggregated over spatial units, such as zip codes. First, there might be missing or confounding variables that were not captured at the scale of analysis, which consequently may yield overdispersion problems. Second, cardiovascular effects of air pollution are not likely to occur along the spatial boundaries of zip code units but rather smoothly change across boundaries of areal units. To reduce a bias in the model estimation and inference of cardiovascular effect of air pollution associated with a specific scale of analysis in the present study, we need a spatial model that explicitly address issues of spatially correlated structure in data.

In this paper, we aim to fill the gap in the literature by evaluating the short-term cardiovascular effect of ambient air pollution to the elderly, while increasing our understanding of the spatio-temporal patterns of CVD risks. We focused on the elderly in the present study because CVD related mortality is the most pronounced among this age group both in our preliminary data analysis and CVD related literature [4]. The associations between exposure to air pollution and CVD risks will be assessed after controlling for neighborhood characteristics that potentially impact patients' health. To achieve our goal, we linked ED visit records for CVD of individuals age 65 years and above to spatially and temporally resolved multi-pollutant exposures derived from CMAQ models in Western New York, US, in 2011. We used a Bayesian hierarchical model to assess the effect of patients' residential environments for physical activity and diet, as well as exposure to air pollutants on CVD risk, while accounting for spatial effects and uncertainty in the model inference.

Methods

Data and study area

The study area encompasses the Buffalo-Niagara region within Erie and Niagara counties of western New York, U.S. The records of Emergency Department (ED) visits for cardiovascular disease (CVD) were obtained from Statewide Planning and Research Cooperative System operated by New York State Department of Health. We focused on the records collected between January, 1, 2011, and December, 31, 2011. The original records contain information on admission date, discharge date, date of birth, 5 digit zip code of residence and demographic information (age, gender, ethnicity, and race) of individuals. We used residential 5 digit zip code and the day of visit as the finest spatial and temporal unit, respectively, for subsequent statistical analyses. The records also include the primary and secondary international classification of disease 9th (ICD-9) revision codes for diagnosis. Using the primary ICD-9 diagnosis code, we defined several cardiovascular disease groups. The diagnosis of CVD incorporates few sub-categories: hypertensive disease (401–405), ischemic heart disease (410–414), pulmonary heart disease (415–417), other forms of heart disease (420–429), cerebrovascular disease (430–438), and atherosclerosis (440). Our grouping and selection of records are largely based on published studies [3, 36].

Daily particulate matter with an aerodynamic diameter less than or equal to $2.5 \, \mu g/m^3$ (PM2.5) and ozone (O_3, in ppb) surfaces were obtained from the Downscaler (DS) model (https://www.epa.gov/air-research/downscaler-model-predicting-daily-air-pollution). The DS model fuses output from a gridded atmospheric model, the community multi-scale air quality model (CMAQ), with point air pollution measurements from fixed monitoring network, and predicts spatially and temporally resolved air quality, such as daily concentration at U.S. census tract centroid locations. To address the known issues of CMAQ estimates—CMAQ calibration bias and uncertainties [26–28], the DS model used a spatially-varying weighted model that regresses monitoring data on a derived regressor obtained by smoothing the entire CMAQ output with weights that vary both spatially and temporally. The DS model provides only PM2.5 and ozone, so we directly derived daily nitrogen dioxide (NO_2, in ppmv) levels from CMAQ model at $12 \times 12 \, km$ resolution. Our research team conducted an extensive accuracy assessment of CMAQ model across western New York for 2011 [37]. To resolve the differences between the spatial unit of analysis—5 digit zip code units (Zips) and those at which pollutant data are available, we processed daily average of these multi-pollutant concentrations using GIS polygon overlay, more specifically, using the maximum function, to estimate

daily air quality at Zips. Daily meteorological data were obtained from National Center for Environmental Information Climate Data Online system (http://www7.ncdc.noaa.gov/CDO/cdopoemain.cmd?datasetabbv=DS3505&countryabbv=&georegionabbv=&resolution=40) for two land-based monitoring stations within Erie/Niagara counties from January, 1, 2011 to December, 31, 2011. They include average temperature, dew point temperature, apparetus temperature, as well as relative humidity, wind speed and wind direction.

Socioeconomic data of the study region were obtained from 2010 Census and 2012 American Community Survey (ACS) at Zips. We summarized information on age- and gender-specific background population, and considered median household income, housing vacancies, education level less than high school graduate degree among adults over 18 years old, and health insurance coverage as proxy measures of poverty and economic status of each Zip. Health insurance coverage was quantified by calculating the percentage of population in each Zip who does not have health insurance coverage based on five year estimates between 2008 and 2012. Other SES variables were obtained from ACS five year estimates between 2007 and 2011. The one year gap between the health insurance coverage and other SES variables was due to the ACS data availability, as health coverage for the study area was published since 2012.

We also included the total number of healthcare facilities within Zips, which included hospitals, medical centers, federally qualified health centers, and home health services except nursing homes. The data from Department of Health and Human Services in 2012 were exploited to generate the locational information of healthcare facilities. The local food environment was characterized by the total number of grocery stores in each Zip. We obtained a list of businesses from 2016 InfoUSA (https://www.infousa.com) and identified grocery markets based on their business types, such as grocery-retail, grocery-wholesale, and food market. Using the information on their geographical coordinates, we counted the total number of grocery markets in each Zip. Similarly we assume that the spatial variation of local environment may promote a range of elderly populations' physical activities [33, 38] and quantified the availability of areas designated as state, county, or municipal parks per Zip. Specifically, we quantified the availability of physical activity resources based on the following two GIS data sources—boundary of state parks and the tax parcels data of Erie/Niagara counties. Both of them were obtained from New York State GIS clearinghouse (https://gis.ny.gov). We extracted parcels of county/municipal park based on the property types of parcels, including public parks, playgrounds, picnic grounds, and recreational facilities. For each Zip, the total areas of the parks was calculated and divided by the area of the Zip, then multiplied by a hundred to derive the percentage of park areas.

Ecological analysis: spatio-temporal models

Ecological time-series is a statistical approach established in environmental epidemiology to investigate the acute effect of air pollution [10]. Disease mapping has been used to elucidate the geographical distribution of underlying disease rates and to identify areas with low or high rates of incidences or mortality. However, the consideration of both spatial and temporal aspects of health outcomes with respect to the spatially and temporally varying air pollution is relatively rare. To fully explore the effect of air pollution while controlling spatially and temporally varying confounding factors, we developed a Bayesian hierarchical Poisson linear model for total counts of daily ED visits for CVD and used integrated nested Laplace approximations [INLA, see 39] for estimation.

Our goal was to assess potential cardiovascular effect of ambient air pollution exposure on the elderly and to identify areas with unusually high or low ED use. Total count of daily ED visits for CVDs among the elderly per Zip based on patients' home address was used as a response and denoted as Y_{it}, $i = 1, \ldots 84$, $t = 1, \ldots, 365$. Given that the fraction of the population suffering from serious cardiac emergency on a given day is quite small, we assume that the count of independent events of ED visit that are randomly occurring in time follows the Poisson distribution [40]. Specifically, the observed daily ED visit counts Y_{it} for CVD at a Zip was modeled using a Poisson likelihood as $Y_{it} \sim \text{Poisson}(E_i \lambda_{it})$, where E_i denotes the expected counts of daily ED utilization from unit i and λ_{it} is the corresponding relative risk on day t. An expected count for Zips can be derived either from known national rates for CVD or from a more local standard population [41], but we obtained E_i from age-specific standardized mortality ratio (SMR) using our ED records as $E_i = \sum_{j=1}^{J} n_{j,i} \hat{p}_j$ where $\hat{p}_j = \sum_i Y_{j,it} / \sum_i n_{j,i}$ denotes the observed overall visit rate for the age-group category $j = 1, \ldots, J$.

For the log-relative risk $\log(\lambda_{it})$, we identified potential risk factors of ED utilization for CVD via exploratory data analyses, which include a set of spatially and temporally resolved air pollution exposure variables X_k, $k = 1, \ldots, 3$. Our exploratory analysis indicated that there are considerable amounts of multicollinearity among weather conditions with a linear trend/a within-year cyclical pattern and among SES variables including housing vacancy/education achievements and median household income, and we omitted variables with weak

correlation with ED visits. The final model consisted of temporal variables T_l, $l = 1, \ldots, 12$ to capture temporal pattern of ED utilization among the elderly, and spatial variables Z_m, $m = 1, \ldots, 5$ to represent socioeconomic conditions of patients' residential location and their local environments for physical activity and diet, and is written as

$$\log(\lambda_{it}) = \beta_0 + \sum_{k=1}^{3} \beta_k X_{k,it} + \sum_{l=1}^{12} \alpha_l T_{l,t} + \sum_{m=1}^{5} \eta_m Z_{m,i} + U_i$$

$$(1)$$

Here, β_0 is an intercept term, and $\beta_1, \beta_2, \beta_3$ denotes the effect of daily NO_2, ozone, and PM2.5 exposure in Zip i during day t. Regarding the daily pattern of ED utilization among the elderly, we found that a within-year cyclical pattern is present, visits vary by day of the week, and there appears to be an overall declining trend. Specifically, the explanatory variables included in T_l are following:

- a within-year cyclical pattern, represented as two sine and two cosine functions with periods of 12 and 6 months evualted at time t;
- a day of the week effect with 8 levels (7 days plus one level for holidays) at time t;
- a linear trend;

Following Diez-Roux [34], we hypothesized that geographic variations of ED utilization are associated with socioeconomic status, the accessibility to healthcare facilities, and local environments for physical activities and diet. These Zip-specific covariates Z_m include

- Median household income and health insurance coverage at the Zip i
- Total number of healthcare facility, except nursing homes
- Percentage of park area
- Total number of grocery markets

The spatial random effects, denoted as U_i, are fully structured to accommodate spatial dependence through a Besag-York-Mollie [or BYM, see 42 model as $(U_1 \ldots U_N)' \sim \text{BYM}(\sigma_1^2, \sigma_2^2)$, where the Zip-specific random effects U_i are designed to capture extra-Poisson variability in the observed ED visit rates. These random effects U_i are modeled as a sum of a spatially structured component V_i (or more specifically, a first-order Markov random field) and a spatially independent term W_i. The independent term is modeled as $W_i \sim N(0, \sigma_2^2)$ thus modeling overall heterogeneity [18], while the spatial term is defined using a conditionally autoregressive (CAR) specification as

$$[V_i|V_j, j \neq i] \sim N\left(\frac{\sum_{j \sim i} V_j}{|j \sim i|}, \frac{c\sigma_1^2}{|j \sim i|}\right) \qquad (2)$$

where $j \sim i$ indicates that j-th Zip is a neighbour of region i with at least one boundary point in common. Following Simpson et al. [43], c is a scaling factor making σ_1^2 approximately equal to the marginal variance of V_i and penalized complexity prior distributions are assigned to combinations of the two variance parameters. The sum of the variances (square-rooted) has an exponential prior distribution with $pr\left(\sqrt{\sigma_1^2 + \sigma_2^2} > 0.5\right) = 0.1$, a fairly uninformative prior which on the upper end of 0.5 will give log relative risks as large as 1.0 and as small as -1.0 with corresponding relative risks close to 3 and $1/3$. The fraction of the variation due to the spatial process has a penalized compliexity prior with $pr\left(\sigma_1/\sqrt{\sigma_1^2 + \sigma_2^2} < 0.1\right) = 0.8$, favouring a spatially independent model (where this fraction is zero) but allowing for a large degree of spatial dependence (with the fraction close to one) should the data warrant it. The BYM model was fitted using the diseasemapping package (v 1.4.2) in R (v 3.4.0).

As a diagnostic tool, a zero-inflated Poisson distribution was substituted for the Poisson distribution for incidence counts. A large portion of the daily visit counts are zero, and the zero-inflated model introduces an additional parameter to induce more zeros than the Poisson distribution allows for. Were the Poisson model correct, and zeros are meerly the result of small expected counts for daily data at the Zip level, the estimate of the zero-inflation parameter would be expected to be small. This model was implemented as the `zeroinflated1` distribution in INLA, with the zero-inflation parameter having a Beta(1,9) distribution.

Results

Descriptive statistics of data

The characteristics of ED utilization in the study area during 2011 are summarized in Table 1. The gender differences in the ED visit for CVD are not substantial unlike the differences by age group. Individuals age over 65 take the majority of the 2011 ED utilization (46.0 %) compared to their demographic composition (15.8%) in this region. The seasonal differences of ED utilization are not substantial. Although the proportion of ED utilization in summer and winter (33.0 and 33.2%) are about twice large as those of spring and fall (16.7 and

Table 1 ED utilization by age group, sex, season, and day of week

	Patients (%)	Population (%)
All ages	5798	1,135,474
Sex		
Female	2997 (51.7%)	587,469 (51.7%)
Male	2801 (48.3%)	548,005 (48.3%)
Age		
0–64	3136 (54.1%)	955,556 (84.2%)
65–74	983 (17.0%)	87,569 (7.7%)
75+	1679 (29.0%)	92,349 (8.1%)
Aged over 65	2662	179,918
Sex		
Female	1549 (58.2%)	106,292 (59.1%)
Male	1113 (41.8%)	73,626 (40.9%)
Season		
Winter	879 (33.0%)	
Spring	445 (16.7%)	
Summer	885 (33.2%)	
Fall	453 (17.0%)	
Day of week		
Sunday	431 (16.2%)	
Monday	404 (15.2%)	
Tuesday	339 (12.7%)	
Wednesday	313 (11.8%)	
Thursday	393 (14.8%)	
Friday	409 (15.4%)	
Saturday	373 (14.0%)	

17.0%), the summer and winter months are defined as four months, whereas the spring and fall are defined as two months based on the seasonal variability in the study region. The effect of the day of week is more noticeable such that Tuesday and Wednesday are the lowest (12.3 and 11.6%) and Sunday and Monday are highest (16.2 and 15.2 %).

The spatial distribution of the ED utilization in 2011 was examined under the consideration of the underlying population at risk, the spatial distribution of the elderly age over 65 at each Zip. The size of the elderly per Zip varies from 17 to 12,680 people with the mean of 2192 and the standard deviation 2370. The spatial distribution of the elderly in Fig. 1 shows that the elderly resides in suburbs around the city of Buffalo forming a ring pattern centered at the city center. The Zips with more than 2829 elderly residents (75th percentile) have the median household income between $31,383 and $80,302, which correspond to 0.25 quantile and 0.75 quantile of the regional median household income levels. The raw counts of daily ED visit per Zip vary from zero to three with an average 0.09 with a standard deviation of 0.31

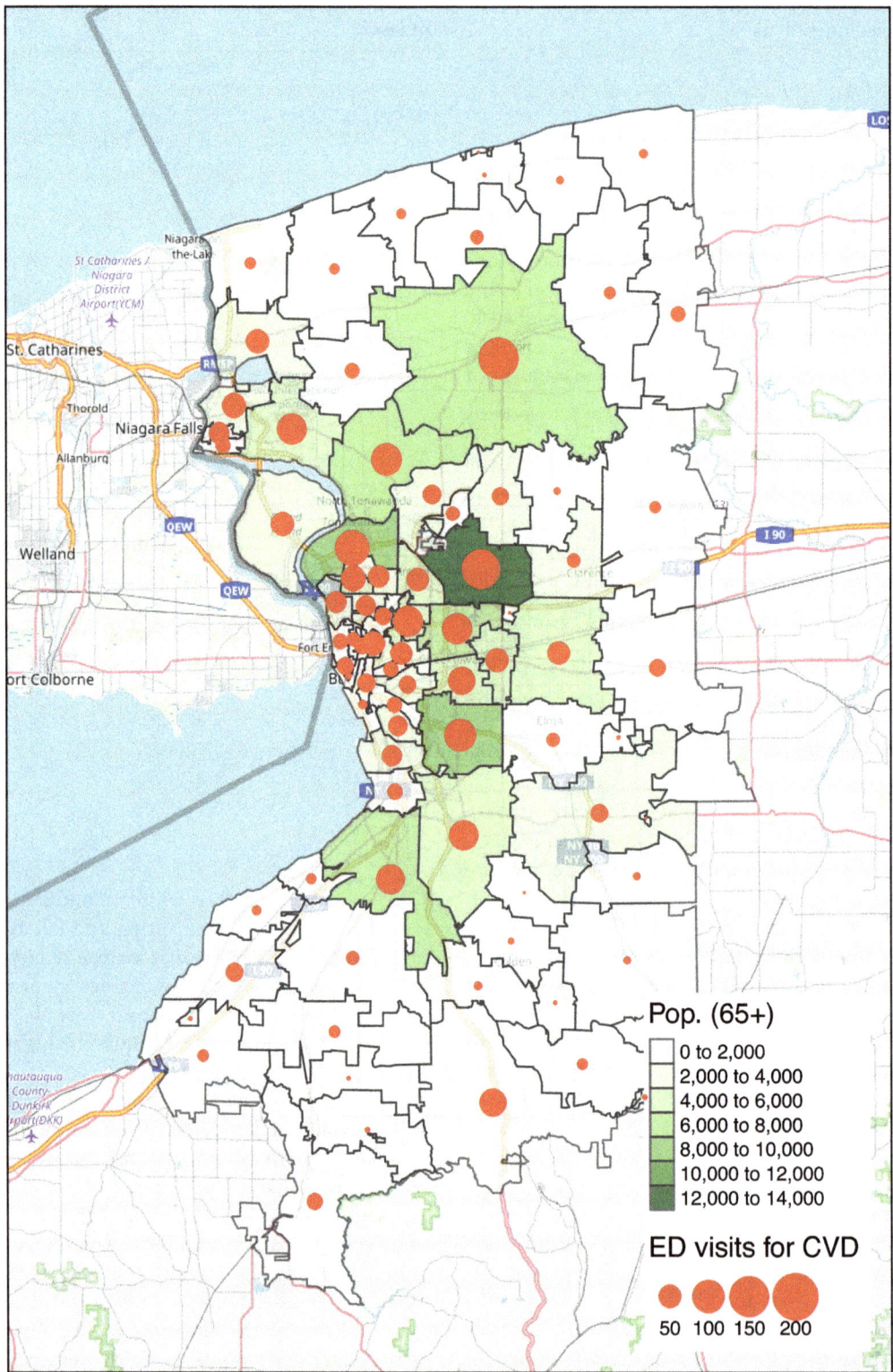

Fig. 1 Spatial distribution of population age over 65 and ED visits for CVD

Table 2 Spatio-temporal distribution of cardiovascular ED visits and air pollutants

	Mean ± SD	Min.	1st Q.	Median	3rd Q.	Max.
ED visits						
Daily counts per zip	0.09 ± 0.31	0.00	0.00	0.00	0.00	3.00
Total counts per zip	31.69 ± 32.39	0.00	7.75	22.50	45.75	153.00
Total counts per day	7.29 ± 2.75	0.00	5.00	7.00	9.00	16.00
Air pollutants						
NO_2 (ppmv)	6.26 ± 4.31	0.38	2.87	5.15	8.59	24.29
PM2.5 ($\mu g/m^3$)	9.48 ± 4.76	1.13	5.88	8.60	12.00	29.22
Ozone (ppb)	39.63 ± 10.81	13.77	31.87	38.65	45.44	87.21

(see Table 2). The spatial distribution of ED utilization was quantified by aggregating counts of ED visits per Zip over the year 2011 and visualized in bubble plot of Fig. 1. The size of bubbles is proportional to the total counts of cadiovascular ED visit in 2011. As expected, this pattern is strongly correlated ($r = 0.92$) with the spatial distribution of the elderly. A few exceptions were found in the south and south west areas of the Erie county, where relatively high ED visits were observed despite their small population. The temporal distribution of ED utilization is characterized by a mean of 7.29 cases per day with the standard deviation 2.75. The day with the highest utilization in 2011 had a total of 16 cases across the study region.

The distribution of the three air pollutants are summarized in Table 2 and mapped in Fig. 2. Zip level daily NO_2 ranged from 0.38 to 24.29 ppmv with a mean of 6.26 ppmv and the standard deviation of 4.31. Similarly, daily PM2.5 concentrations at Zip ranged from 1.13 to 29.22 $\mu g/m^3$ with a mean of 9.48 $\mu g/m^3$ and standard deviation of 4.76. Both PM2.5 and NO_2 have relatively small variability year-round as shown in monthly time scale of box plots (see Fig. 2), although their spatial patterns are quite different from each other. High concentrations of NO_2 are centered at the city of Buffalo where high traffic volume exists, while PM2.5 is high at the north west of the study area including Tonawanda in which a violation of the Clear Air Act by Tonawanda Coke Corporation was reported [44, 45]. Daily ozone concentration shows a cyclical pattern—high in summer months with a peak in July and low in cold months with the mean and standard deviation 39.63 ppm and 10.81, respectively, and a wider range of lowest value 13.77 and maximum 87.21 ppb. This seasonal variability is observed in both PM2.5 and ozone, but is slightly different as ozone is lower in both spring and winter whereas the PM2.5 is lowest in spring and fall. The spatial pattern of ozone is quite different from PM2.5 and NO_2, as the high concentration of ozone is found in east side of the study area and lowest at the city of Buffalo (see Fig. 2).

Spatio-temporal ecological models

To allow a proper assessment of the spatio-temporal ecological model, we began fitting a Poisson generalized linear model (GLM) with the full set of covariates used for the spatio-temporal random effect model in Eq. (1). The model fits are summarized in Table 3.

Compared to the ED utilization on Mondays, a low utilization of emergency department visits for CVD was observed on both weekend and holidays with statistical significance. A cyclical term for sine 12 was also significant. Figure 3 shows the estimated seasonal effect for both the Poisson GLM and the spatial random effects model. The estimated coefficients for the sine and cosine functions in Table 3 determine these seasonal effect. Both models agree that the period of peak ED use is from September to November, with February to June being the time of year with the fewest ED visits.

Among the spatial covariates associated with socioeconomic status, both the median household income and the total number of healthcare facilities located in each Zip have statistically significant associations with ED utilization. Strong and negative association with median household income corroborates the previous finding that high ED utilization pattern is an indicator of poor economic status at community level [46], meanwhile a small but positive association with healthcare facilities might be associated with the fact that our study is purely based on the elderly who prefer to reside near healthcare facilities. In terms of neighborhood environments for physical activities, we did not find the percentage of green space in each Zip being significant at 95% credible intervals. The number of grocery stores in each Zip was negatively associated with the high ED use as one would expect. In the Poisson GLM, none of the three air pollutants were significant. For a purpose of model validation, we examined the residuals of the Poisson GLM for the possible presence of autocorrelation in space and time. First we computed the temporal autocorrelation function of daily residuals aggregated over the entire study area and found no significant temporal auto-correlation remaining in the

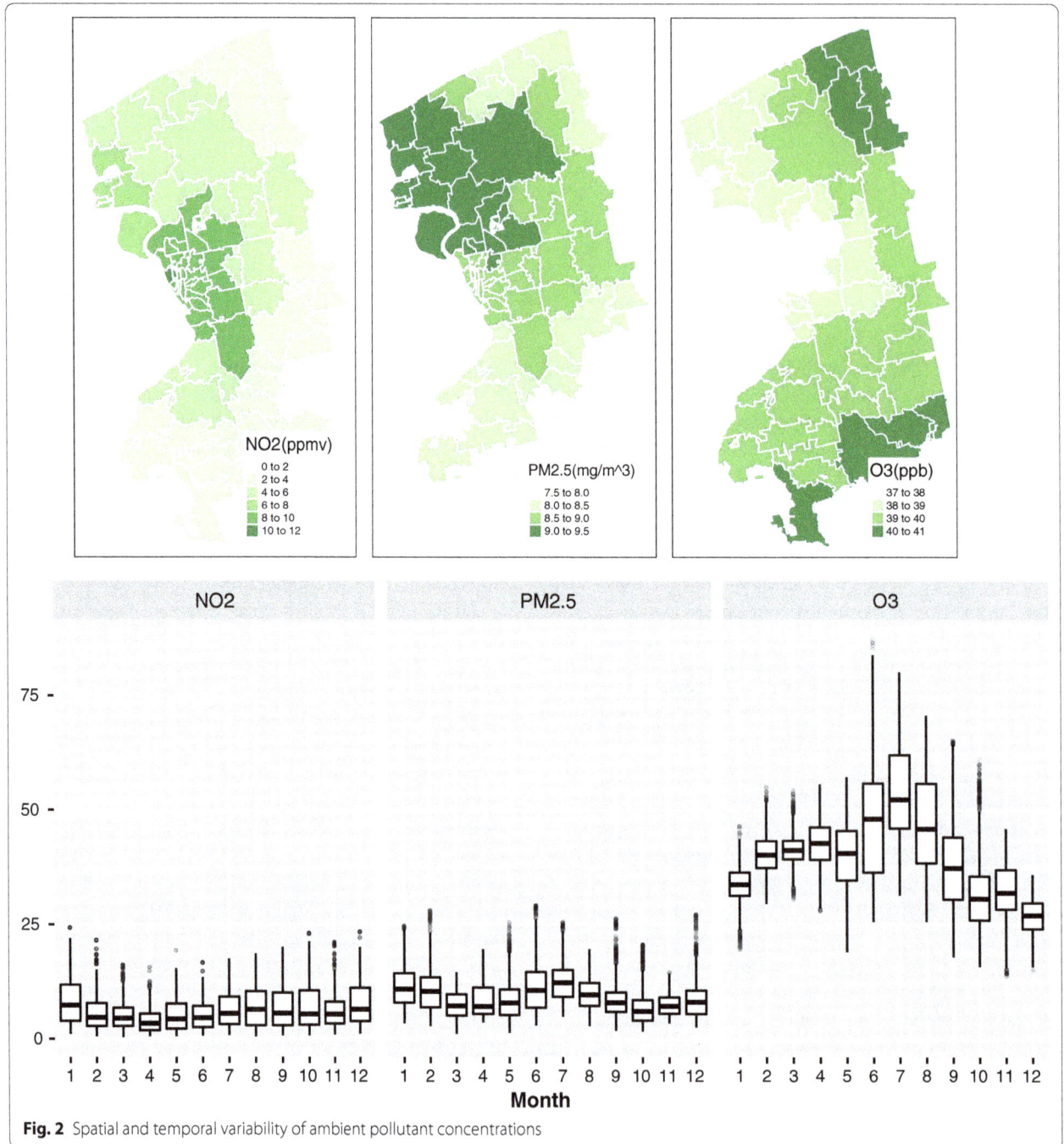

Fig. 2 Spatial and temporal variability of ambient pollutant concentrations

Poisson GLM. On the other hand, Moran's I index [47], a summary statistic widely used to evaluate the presence of spatial autocorrelation, was 0.381 with the p-value of 0.0001. This result suggested that there is considerable spatial autocorrelation in the residuals and an inclusion of a spatial correlation structure in the model will be appropriate.

For the spatial random effect model in Eq. (1), the model coefficient estimates are similar to the Poisson GLM for the temporal covariates but not for neighborhood health effects, including daily exposure to air pollutants. The positive associations observed in Poisson GLM between the neighborhood level accessibility to healthcare facilities/the percentage of residents without

Table 3 Fitted relative risk for the parameters of interests via Poisson regression and spatial random effect model

	Poisson regression model				Spatial random effect model			
	Mean	0.025Q	0.975Q	SD	Mean	0.025Q	0.975Q	SD
(Intercept)	*1.16*	1.04	1.29	1.06	*1.19*	1.06	1.35	1.06
sin12	*0.89*	0.80	0.99	1.05	0.92	0.83	1.02	1.06
cos12	1.02	0.95	1.09	1.04	1.00	0.93	1.07	1.04
sin6	0.99	0.92	1.07	1.04	0.99	0.92	1.06	1.04
cos6	0.98	0.92	1.03	1.03	0.97	0.91	1.02	1.03
Tuesday	1.00	0.86	1.15	1.07	0.99	0.86	1.14	1.07
Wednesday	0.90	0.78	1.04	1.08	0.91	0.79	1.05	1.08
Thursday	0.97	0.84	1.12	1.08	0.97	0.84	1.12	1.08
Friday	1.05	0.91	1.21	1.07	1.06	0.92	1.21	1.07
Saturday	*0.80*	0.69	0.93	1.08	*0.82*	0.71	0.96	1.08
Sunday	*0.76*	0.65	0.88	1.08	*0.79*	0.68	0.92	1.08
Holidays	*0.68*	0.49	0.93	1.18	*0.71*	0.51	0.98	1.18
Day	0.77	0.58	1.01	1.15	0.78	0.59	1.04	1.15
Median Income	*0.88*	0.81	0.95	1.04	*0.80*	0.70	0.92	1.07
% No-insurance	*1.13*	1.03	1.24	1.05	1.00	0.86	1.16	1.08
No. Health Fac.	*1.04*	1.01	1.07	1.01	1.05	0.98	1.12	1.03
% Green space	0.99	0.94	1.04	1.03	1.01	0.92	1.12	1.05
Grocery stores	*0.94*	0.90	0.99	1.02	0.97	0.88	1.06	1.05
NO_2	0.93	0.83	1.04	1.06	*1.15*	1.01	1.30	1.06
PM2.5	1.00	0.95	1.05	1.03	1.00	0.95	1.06	1.03
O_3	0.97	0.87	1.07	1.05	0.92	0.83	1.02	1.06
Non-spatial $\sqrt{\sigma_1^2 + \sigma_2^2}$					1.40	1.29	1.55	
Spatial $\sigma_1/\sqrt{\sigma_1^2 + \sigma_2^2}$					2.14	1.40	2.66	1.19
DIC	16427.89				16264.55			

The significance of italics was determined based on the 95% credible intervals for the fixed effects (known risk factors)

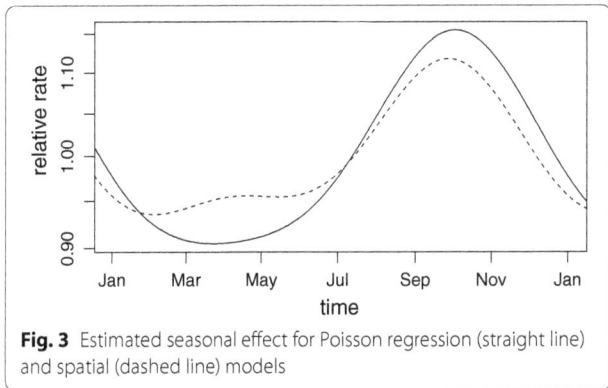

Fig. 3 Estimated seasonal effect for Poisson regression (straight line) and spatial (dashed line) models

health insurance coverage and high ED use are no longer significant, but the positive effect of NO_2 exposure became significant after accounting for the spatial correlation in ED utilization at Zips. An increase of 10 unit of

NO_2 exposure is associated with an increase of 15.00 % in the relative risk of ED utilizations for CVD among the elderly according to the Bayesian hierarchical model.

The estimate of the spatially-structured contribution to the Zip-level variation in ED use, shown as $\hat{\sigma}_1/\sqrt{\hat{\sigma}_1^2 + \hat{\sigma}_2^2}$

in Table 3, suggests that non-trivial spatial patterns exist in ED utilizations. The moderately large estimate of 0.76 and the very large upper 97.5% quantile of 0.98 indicate the spatial model should be trusted over the Poisson GLM. The latter ignores all this spatially structured random error, which is likely to result in incorrect (narrower) estimates of uncertainty intervals of parameters that we are interested in, such as NO_2.

The zero-inflated model produced estimates nearly identical to those of the Poisson model (results appear in the Appendix), with the zero-inflation parameter having a posterior mean of 0.04. This suggests the Poisson assumption is appropriate and there are no 'structural' effect inducing excess zeros.

Mapping relative risk of cardiovascular disease

In a Bayesian hierarchical model the relative risk of a disease is estimated as a posterior distribution instead of a single value. However, Bayesian disease mapping analysis results are typically presented as a map of a point estimate (usually the mean or median of the posterior distribution) of the relative risk for each area. To interpret such maps, one needs to understand the extent to which the statistical model is able to smooth the risk estimates to eliminate random noise while at the same time

avoiding over-smoothing that might flatten any true variations in risk [48]. Figure 4a presents the posterior mean for the Zip-level random effect of relative risk estimates of cardiovascular disease of elderly in Erie/Niagara counties. The total number of Zips with relative risk above the overall average (Relative Risk > 1) was a total of 37, which corresponds to 44.04 %. The majority areas in the north and south of the study area have the high relative risks including one Zip in the south whose risk is above more than double of the region-wide overall risk. It is also noticeable that areas around the city of Buffalo have a relatively lower risk of CVD despite the considerable

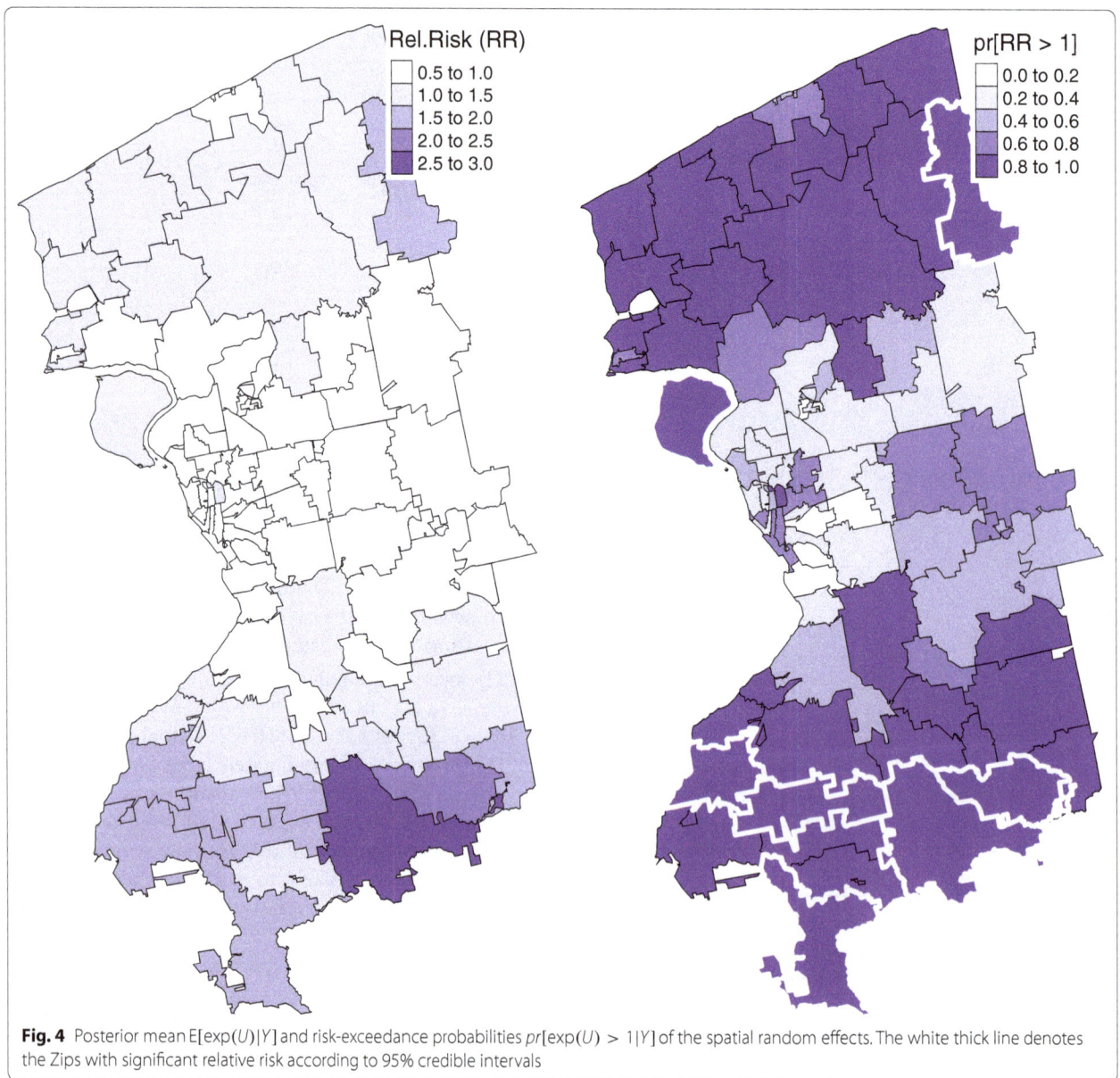

Fig. 4 Posterior mean E[exp(U)|Y] and risk-exceedance probabilities pr[exp(U) > 1|Y] of the spatial random effects. The white thick line denotes the Zips with significant relative risk according to 95% credible intervals

number of elderly residents as shown in the background map of Fig. 1.

To assess the uncertainty associated with the point estimate (posterior mean) of relative risk, we followed Richardson et al. [48] and Blangiardo and Cameletti [49] and mapped the likelihood of excessive risk based on the posterior probability (termed as "risk-exceedence probabilities"). That is, the probability that the relative risks (or spatial random effects) are greater than the region-wide risk, i.e., $p\{\exp(U_i) > 1|(y_1, \ldots, y_N)\}$, is visualized in Fig. 4b. The risk-exceedence probabilities associated with the 37 areas whose Relative Risk > 1 ranged between 0.82 and 1.00 with mean and standard deviation of 0.97 and 0.05, respectively. These high risk-exceedence probabilities imply that the uncertainty associated with the relative risk estimates of these Zips are quite small. We also identified Zips with significant relative risks based on the 95 % credible intervals of relative risk estimates. The results are shown in Fig. 4b using extra thick border lines. The results indicated that a total of 9 Zips with statistical significance relative risk all also had high risk-exceedence probabilities.

Discussion

We explored the spatio-temporal variability of ED utilizations for CVD in relation to the spatial variation of daily exposure to air pollutants, such as NO2, PM2.5 and ozone, at Zips. Our study advanced previous findings in western New York [50–52] in that we assessed the association between air pollution and ED utilization using spatially and temporally resolved air pollution exposure derived from the state-of-art atmospheric models (CMAQ). In a closely related study Castner et al. [52] assessed the short-term health effect of daily concentrations of multi-pollutants, including Carbon monoxide (CO), NO2, PM2.5, and ozone, using a region-wide ambient air quality based on measurements obtained from a small number of monitors (two to five depending on the pollutant types). We argue that such approach may be appropriate for pollutants with limited spatial and temporal heterogeneity, but is problematic for certain pollutants, such as NO2 or CO, which exhibit significant spatial heterogeneity [53]. Castner et al. [52] found no significant associations between ED asthma utilization and air pollution, but a positive and significant effect of NO2 on ED utilization among the elderly for CVD was found in the present study. This difference might be due to that we have examined only one year (2011) instead of multi-year data (2007–2012), or the focus on different health outcomes, specifically, CVD rather than asthma. However, it is also possible that the explicit consideration of geographic variations of ED utilization and the spatially heterogeneity of air pollutant concentrations played a

crucial role in revealing the CVD effects of NO2 among the elderly.

To properly assess the cardiovascular effect of pollutants, we fitted two models with and without spatial random effects. Both models indicated that community level socioeconomic status is a determinant of ED utilization for CVD. The Poisson GLM also suggested that the associations with known spatial risk factors, such as the accessibility to healthcare facilities and the reduced access to healthy food options in Zips, were significant in addition to the temporal trend. Our findings on these significant temporal covariates concur with the existing literature [54–56] including the recent work by Castner et al. [51] that the day of week is the most influential predictor of ED utilization. As argued by Wargon et al. [56], the Monday effect appears to be a common driver that increases adult ED utilization across different study areas and study periods. This effect might be attributed to the return of patients from a weekend absence or return of primary care practitioners to their office and sending their patients to ED.

We found the spatial random effect model was more effective to investigate the spatial pattern of ED utilizations of the elderly in the study area than a Poisson GLM from the following reasons. Both the Moran's I index of Poisson GLM and the conditional autoregressive specification parameter estimate from the BYM model suggested that there was a statistically significant autocorrelation in the residuals of Poisson GLM. We suspect that the presence of spatial autocorrelation is a natural outcome of using aggregated data—both for ED utilization and neighborhood-level covariates. However, the presence of spatial heterogeneity and autocorrelation might be associated with the measures of residential environments for physical activity, diet, and air quality in our study. We used Zip as a unit of analysis and summarized other covariates, including exposure to air quality and residential environments for green space and healthy food access, within the unit, but other spatial scales might have been more relevant to properly capture geographic variations of covariates. The literature on spatial statistics [41, Chap. 4 and 5] warns that the spatial scale or unit of analysis may induce the spatial heterogeneity and/or autocorrelation, as unmeasured covariates do. After accounting for the spatially correlated structure, we found that the neighborhood level exposure to NO2 was positively associated with the risk of CVD, but several spatial risk factors, such as the percentage of people without health insurance, the number of healthcare facilities, and the number of grocery stores, were no longer significant in the spatial random effect model. One may suspect these changes are due to correlations between NO2 concentration and spatial risk factors or the population

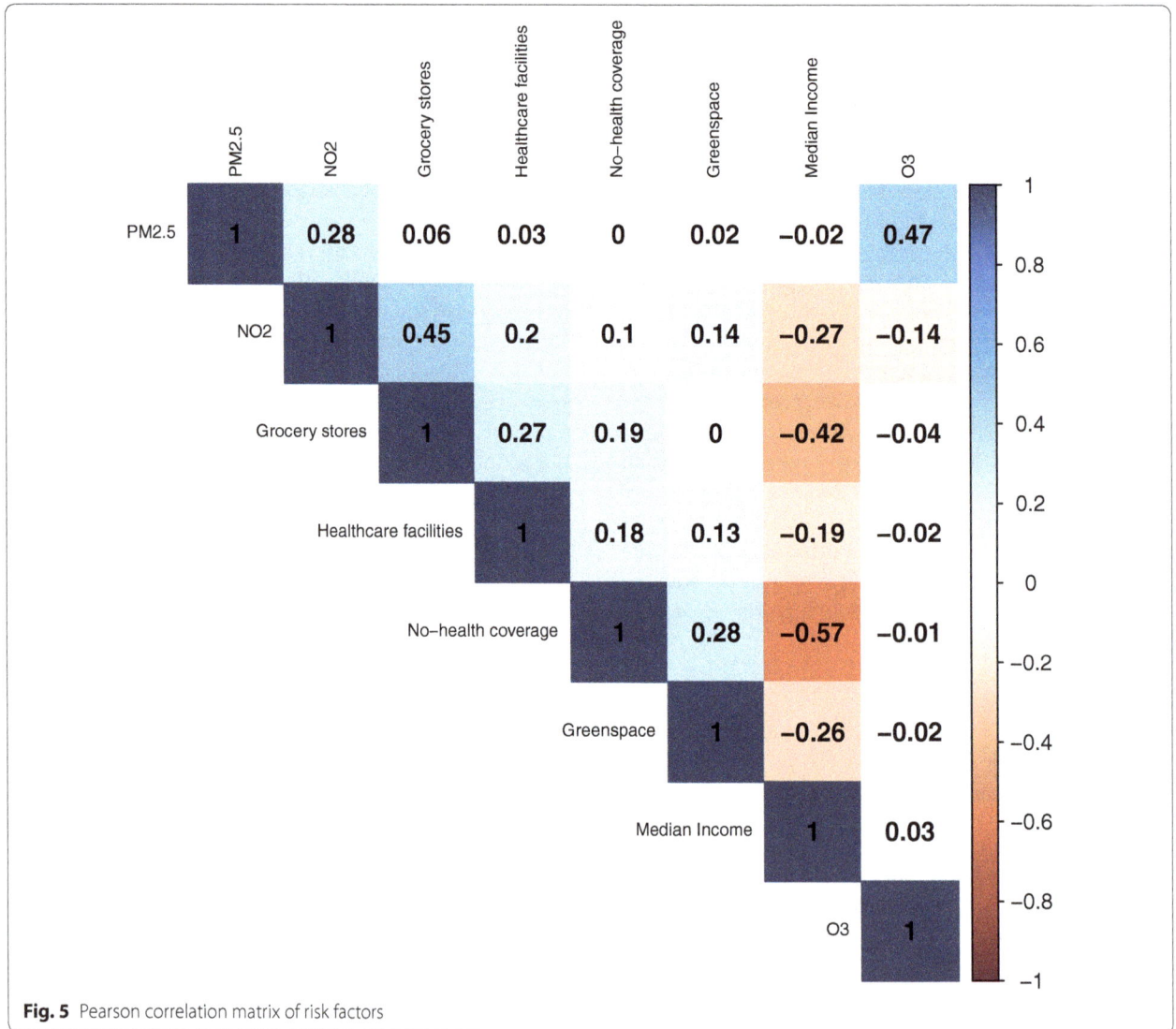

Fig. 5 Pearson correlation matrix of risk factors

at risk considered in our study. However, Fig. 5 indicated that the correlation between NO$_2$ and spatial risk factors, including the number of healthcare facilities at Zips, was low in the range of -0.27 and 0.14 except the accessibility to grocery stores (0.45). Meanwhile, the strong negative correlation between median income and risk factors (up to -0.57 with no health insurance coverage) and the noticeable changes in the effect median income from -0.13 in Poisson GLM to -0.22 in the spatial random effect model might affect the results. In addition, the target population considered in this study was elderly whose health insurance is covered by Medicare.

Mapping the area-specific random effects for CVD of the elderly suggests that the CVD risk is spatially heterogeneous even after we accounted for the geographic variation of the spatial and temporal risk factors. Interestingly the areas with high CVD risk above the region-wide risk (Relative Risk > 1) are concentrated in north and south of the study region with one Zip of the highest risk 2.92 (almost three times higher than the overall ED utilization for CVD) in the south border. This result is rather surprising because the raw ED visit counts in Fig. 1 show high ED utilization around the first ring around the city of Buffalo and small ED visits at the outer edges where the elderly is sparse. After taking into account demographic characteristics and risk factors together, the north and south side of the study regions were identified as having high ED utilization for

CVD among the elderly. To fully understand the outputs from the Bayesian hierarchical model, we also visualized the uncertainty associated with relative risk estimates as shown in Fig. 4b. Based on this uncertainty assessment, we concluded that our identification of Zips with high cariodvascular risk are almost certain. Our study is not free of limitations and a number of issues still remain unresolved. First, potential errors in CMAQ-based air pollution exposure estimates have not been explicitly discussed in our study. Our decision is based on the fact that many studies including those sponsored by EPA (https://www.epa.gov/hesc/rsig-related-downloadable-data-files) and the Centers for Disease Control and Prevention (https://ephtracking.cdc.gov/DataExplorer/#/) have used spatially fused air quality surface in their regulation and decision making processes, but also our team's recent study was directly related with the sensitivity assessment of CMAQ outputs and calibration [37]. We are confident that the quality of our CMAQ modeling outputs is sufficient to be used in epidemiological studies. Second, the present study related residential environments to observed cardiovascular risk, in which individual-level characteristics, such as existing chronic conditions, smoking and leisure time physical activities, were not statistically controlled. This problem, referred to as residual confounding, is common to ecological studies, and requires caution in interpreting results [34]. Third, we found that residential environments for diet and physical activities were not significant despite the growing literature supporting their associations. We suspect that the lack of associations might be related with measurements of such environments and the spatial scale at which those characteristics were captured. For example, aesthetically pleasing environment might be more encouraging physical activity participation for the elderly rather than a mere measure of accessibility to or availability of green space [57]. Similarly, the spatial scale of analysis at which both health outcome and spatial risk factors are characterized might have played an important role to determine their associations. The other critical issues lie in the potential multicollinearity among covariates. For example, Zip level ozone and PM2.5 are strongly correlated as median household income is negatively associated with health insurance coverage and the percentage of green space. These correlated variables may induce bias in the estimated model coefficients. The correlation among multi-pollutants is of particular concern. Our exploratory analysis indicates that the strong positive correlation (0.47) exists between O_3 and PM2.5 (see Fig. 5), but the correlations between NO_2 and the other two pollutants are relatively weak as -0.14 for O_3 and 0.28 for PM2.5, respectively. This suggests that our finding on the effect of NO_2 on the ED utilization for CVD is less likely to be affected by the collinearity problem. We also evaluated the collinearity problem by running three single-pollutant models and compared these results with those from the proposed multi-pollutant models. We found that only NO_2 was significant at 90 % credible intervals, and none of the individual pollutants was significant at 95% credible intervals. We concluded that the collinearity was present among the three pollutants, but it was not influential in the present study. Liverani et al. [58] have developed profile regression specifically to address this problem of severe correlation among covariates, and we are taking this approach in future work to investigate how multicollinearity among covariates affects or modifies the cardiovascular effect of air pollution. We will be able to better understand the role of neighborhood health effects using profile regression. Lastly we will extend our study to multi-year ED utilization data in future work along with corresponding CMAQ driven multi-pollutant profile to evaluate our hypothesis on the cyclical patterns of ED visits.

Our findings have multiple public health implications. We identified neighborhoods with unusually high ED utilization for CVD among the elderly in the present study. The investigation of the factors responsible for health disparities in the study region and taking measures to improve health and healthcare delivery, increase access to care should be a topic for further investigation. One of our long-term goals is to translate our findings to local practice, that is, to improve population health. Our study parallels with on-going community efforts, such as Keys to Health (http://www.pophealthwny.org/), to develop preventive strategies, such as health education or chronic care managements, for residents in Western New York whose socioeconomic status and quality of health vary geographically. Our findings can be further used to effectively reallocate local healthcare resources to address population at greater risk, such as the elderly and the individuals with chronic diseases. We expect that dissemination of information on alternative healthcare facilities other than ED and the improvement on the accessibility of the elderly to non-ED health facilities may alleviate the ED burden. Lastly, our result suggests that NO_2 has significant associations with cardiovascular ED utilization among the elderly in the study region, and more stringent control for emission sources for NO_2 below normal health guidelines is needed to protect them.

Conclusions

We assessed the short-term effect of exposure to NO_2 on the risk of ED visits for cadiovascular related disease among the elderly using a Bayesian hierarchical model. The model fit indicated there is a statistically significant association between daily exposure to NO_2 and the elevated ED utilizations for CVD when the spatial autocorrelation in the observed ED visit counts is accounted for. The results also indicated that there are areas with unusually high ED utilization for CVD compared to region-wide overall use of ED with little uncertainty. While our findings have the potential to be useful to improve our understanding of both the CVD risk among the elderly in the western New York and spatial disparity in ED utilization for CVD, further investigation is warranted to explore the multidimensional aspect of associations between air pollution exposure and ED visits.

Author's contributions

EHY developed the study design. EHY and PB conducted the data analysis. EHY and YSE provided input on spatial analysis. EHY and PB wrote the manuscript. All authors read and approved the final manuscript.

Author details

[1] Department of Geography, University at Buffalo, Buffalo, NY, USA. [2] Department of Statistical Sciences, University of Toronto, Toronto, Canada.

Acknowledgements

We would like to thank to IT supports from the college of Arts and the Center for Computational Science atthe University at Buffalo. We also appreciate the support provided by the Center for Computational Research and the Research and Education in Energy, Environment and Water (RENEW) seed projectfunding at the University at Buffalo and the University of Toronto. We are grateful for helpful comments from Dr. Castner and Dr. Roberts, and Xiangyu Jiang's assistance in producing and sharing the CMAQ model outputs on the manuscript. The opinions expressed herein are those of the authors and do not necessarily reflect the views of the University at Buffalo.

Competing interests

The authors declare that they have no competing interests.

Appendix

The ED utilization data have more zeros than expected, based on the Poisson distribution. To account for the extra zero in daily ED uses we developed a zero-inflated Poisson regression model and the results are summarized in Table 4. The model fit is nearly identical to the spatio-temporal model in Table 3, which indicated that the spatio-temporal Poisson model is appropriate for the data.

Table 4 Fitted relative risk for the parameters via zero-inflated Poisson regression model

	Mean	0.025Q	0.975Q	SD
(Intercept)	*1.25*	1.10	1.44	1.07
sin12	0.92	0.83	1.02	1.06
cos12	1.00	0.93	1.07	1.04
sin6	0.99	0.92	1.06	1.04
cos6	0.97	0.91	1.02	1.03
Tuesday	0.99	0.86	1.14	1.07
Wednesday	0.91	0.79	1.05	1.08
Thursday	0.97	0.84	1.12	1.08
Friday	1.05	0.92	1.21	1.07
Saturday	*0.82*	0.71	0.96	1.08
Sunday	*0.79*	0.68	0.92	1.08
Holidays	*0.71*	0.51	0.98	1.18
Day	0.78	0.59	1.03	1.15
Median income	*0.80*	0.70	0.92	1.07
% No-insurance	1.00	0.87	1.16	1.08
No.Health Fac.	1.05	0.99	1.12	1.03
% Green space	1.01	0.92	1.12	1.05
Grocery stores	0.97	0.88	1.06	1.05
NO_2	*1.14*	1.01	1.30	1.06
PM2.5	1.00	0.95	1.06	1.03
O_3	0.92	0.83	1.02	1.06
Non-spatial	1.40	1.29	1.56	
Spatial	2.15	1.42	2.66	1.19
DIC	16266.54			

The significance of italics was determined based on the 95% credible intervals for the fixed effects (known risk factors)

References

1. Pope CA III, Schwartz J, Ransom MR. Daily mortality and $PM_{1}0$ pollution in utah valley. Arch Environ Health Int J. 1992;47(3):211–7.
2. Dockery DW, Pope CA, Xu X, Spengler JD, Ware JH, Fay ME, Ferris BG Jr, Speizer FE. An association between air pollution and mortality in six US cities. N Engl J Med. 1993;329(24):1753–9.
3. Laden F, Schwartz J, Speizer FE, Dockery DW. Reduction in fine particulate air pollution and mortality: extended follow-up of the harvard six cities study. Am J Respir Crit Care Med. 2006;173(6):667–72.
4. Brook RD, Rajagopalan S, Pope CA, Brook JR, Bhatnagar A, Diez-Roux AV, Holguin F, Hong Y, Luepker RV, Mittleman MA, et al. Particulate matter air pollution and cardiovascular disease. Circulation. 2010;121(21):2331–78.
5. Peel JL, Tolbert PE, Klein M, Metzger KB, Flanders WD, Todd K, Mulholland JA, Ryan PB, Frumkin H. Ambient air pollution and respiratory emergency department visits. Epidemiology. 2005;16(2):164–74.
6. Zanobetti A, Schwartz J. The effect of particulate air pollution on emergency admissions for myocardial infarction: a multicity case-crossover analysis. Environ Health Perspect. 2005;113(8):978.
7. Rückerl R, Schneider A, Breitner S, Cyrys J, Peters A. Health effects of particulate air pollution: a review of epidemiological evidence. Inhal Toxicol. 2011;23(10):555–92.
8. Poloniecki JD, Atkinson RW, de Leon AP, Anderson HR. Daily time series for cardiovascular hospital admissions and previous day's air pollution in London, UK. Occup Environ Med. 1997;54(8):535–40.

9.   Jalaludin B, Morgan G, Lincoln D, Sheppeard V, Simpson R, Corbett S. Associations between ambient air pollution and daily emergency department attendances for cardiovascular disease in the elderly (65+ years), Sydney, Australia. J Exposure Sci Environ Epidemiol. 2006;16(3):225–37.

10. Peng RD, Dominici F (2008) Statistical methods for environmental epidemiology with R. Springer, New York. https://doi.org/10.1007/978-0-387-78167-9

11. Sarnat SE, Winquist A, Schauer JJ, Turner JR, Sarnat JA. Fine particulate matter components and emergency department visits for cardiovascular and respiratory diseases in the St. Louis, Missouri–Illinois, metropolitan area. Environ Health Perspect. 2015;123(5):437.

12. Xu Q, Wang S, Guo Y, Wang C, Huang F, Li X, Gao Q, Wu L, Tao L, Guo J, et al. Acute exposure to fine particulate matter and cardiovascular hospital emergency room visits in Beijing, China. Environ Pollut. 2017;220:317–27.

13. Li S, Batterman S, Wasilevich E, Wahl R, Wirth J, Su F-C, Mukherjee B. Association of daily asthma emergency department visits and hospital admissions with ambient air pollutants among the pediatric medicaid population in detroit: time-series and time-stratified case-crossover analyses with threshold effects. Environ Res. 2011;111(8):1137–47.

14. Rappold AG, Diaz-Sanchez D, Neas LM, Devlin RB, Stone SL, Kilaru VJ, Cascio WE. Cardio-respiratory outcomes associated with exposure to wildfire smoke are modified by measures of community health. Environ Health. 2012;11(1):71.

15. Neuberger M, Moshammer H, Rabczenko D. Acute and subacute effects of urban air pollution on cardiopulmonary emergencies and mortality: time series studies in austrian cities. Int J Environ Res Public Health. 2013;10(10):4728–51.

16. Gleason JA, Fagliano JA. Associations of daily pediatric asthma emergency department visits with air pollution in Newark, NJ: utilizing time-series and case-crossover study designs. J Asthma. 2015;52(8):815–22.

17. Carlin BP, Xia H, Devine O, Tolbert P, Mulholland J. Spatio-temporal hierarchical models for analyzing Atlanta pediatric asthma ER visit rates. In: Case studies in Bayesian statistics. Springer; 1999. pp. 303–320.

18. Zhu L, Carlin BP, Gelfand AE. Hierarchical regression with misaligned spatial data: relating ambient ozone and pediatric asthma ER visits in Atlanta. Environmetrics. 2003;14(5):537–57.

19. Wannemuehler KA, Lyles RH, Waller LA, Hoekstra RM, Klein M, Tolbert P. A conditional expectation approach for associating ambient air pollutant exposures with health outcomes. Environmetrics. 2009;20(7):877–94.

20. Sarnat SE, Sarnat JA, Mulholland J, Isakov V, Özkaynak H, Chang HH, Klein M, Tolbert PE. Application of alternative spatiotemporal metrics of ambient air pollution exposure in a time-series epidemiological study in Atlanta. J Exposure Sci Environ Epidemiol. 2013;23(6):593–605.

21. Strickland MJ, Darrow LA, Klein M, Flanders WD, Sarnat JA, Waller LA, Sarnat SE, Mulholland JA, Tolbert PE. Short-term associations between ambient air pollutants and pediatric asthma emergency department visits. Am J Respir Crit Care Med. 2010;182(3):307–16.

22. Byun D, Schere KL. Review of the governing equations, computational algorithms, and other components of the models-3 community multiscale air quality (cmaq) modeling system. Appl Mech Rev. 2006;59(2):51–77.

23. Liu Y, Franklin M, Kahn R, Koutrakis P. Using aerosol optical thickness to predict ground-level PM2.5 concentrations in the St. Louis area: a comparison between MISR and MODIS. Remote Sens Environ. 2007;107(1–2):33–44.

24. Chang HH, Reich BJ, Miranda ML. Time-to-event analysis of fine particle air pollution and preterm birth: results from north carolina, 2001–2005. Am J Epidemiol. 2012;175(2):91–8. https://doi.org/10.1093/aje/kwr403.

25. Zhang H, Chen G, Hu J, Chen S-H, Wiedinmyer C, Kleeman M, Ying Q. Evaluation of a seven-year air quality simulation using the weather research and forecasting (wrf)/community multiscale air quality (cmaq) models in the eastern United States. Sci Total Environ. 2014;473:275–85.

26. Tesche T, Morris R, Tonnesen G, McNally D, Boylan J, Brewer P. Cmaq/camx annual 2002 performance evaluation over the eastern US. Atmos Environ. 2006;40(26):4906–19.

27. Kang D, et al. Bias adjustment techniques for improving ozone air quality forecasts. J Geophys Res Atmos. 2008. https://doi.org/10.1029/2008J D010151.

28. Lee P, Kang D, McQueen J, Tsidulko M, Hart M, DiMego G, Seaman N, Davidson P. Impact of domain size on modeled ozone forecast for the northeastern United States. J Appl Meteorol Climatol. 2008;47(2):443–61.

29. Hao Y, Flowers H, Monti MM, Qualters JR. Us census unit population exposures to ambient air pollutants. Int J Health Geogr. 2012;11(1):3.

30. Weber SA, Insaf TZ, Hall ES, Talbot TO, Huff AK. Assessing the impact of fine particulate matter (pm 2.5) o respiratory-cardiovascular chronic diseases in the New York City metropolitan area using hierarchical bayesian model estimates. Environ Res. 2016;151:399–409.

31. O'lenick CR, Winquist A, Mulholland JA, Friberg MD, Chang HH, Kramer MR, Darrow LA, Sarnat SE. Assessment of neighbourhood-level socioeconomic status as a modifier of air pollution–asthma associations among children in Atlanta. J Epidemiol Community Health. 2017;71(2):129–36.

32. Winquist A, O'Lenick CR, Chang HH, Mulholland JA, Friberg MD, Kramer MR, Sarnat SE. Ozone and childhood respiratory disease in three US cities: evaluation of effect measure modification by neighborhood socioeconomic status using a bayesian hierarchical approach. Environ Health. 2017;16(1):36.

33. Diez-Roux AV. Investigating neighborhood and area effects on health. Am J Public Health. 2001;91(11):1783–9.

34. Diez-Roux AV. Residential environments and cardiovascular risk. J Urban Health. 2003;80(4):569–89.

35. Sundquist K, Winkleby M, Ahlén H, Johansson S-E. Neighborhood socioeconomic environment and incidence of coronary heart disease: a follow-up study of 25,319 women and men in Sweden. Am J Epidemiol. 2004;159(7):655–62.

36. Lepeule J, Laden F, Dockery D, Schwartz J. Chronic exposure to fine particles and mortality: an extended follow-up of the Harvard Six Cities study from 1974 to 2009. Environ Health Perspect. 2012;120(7):965.

37. Jiang X, Yoo E-H. The importance of spatial resolutions of community multiscale air quality (CMAQ) models on health impact assessment. Sci Total Environ. 2018;627(15):1528–43.

38. Diez-Roux AV, Evenson KR, McGinn AP, Brown DG, Moore L, Brines S, Jacobs DR Jr. Availability of recreational resources and physical activity in adults. Am J Public Health. 2007;97(3):493–9.

39. Rue H, Martino S, Chopin N. Approximate Bayesian inference for latent Gaussian models by using integrated nested Laplace approximations. J R Stat Soc Ser B (Statistical Methodology). 2009;71(2):319–92.

40. Schwartz J, Slater D, Larson TV, Pierson WE, Koenig JQ. Particulate air pollution and hospital emergency room visits for asthma in seattle. Am Rev Respir Dis. 1993;147(4):826–31.

41. Lawson AB. Statistical methods in spatial epidemiology., Wiley series in probability and statisticsNew York: Wiley; 2013.

42. Besag J, York J, Mollié A. Bayesian image restoration, with two applications in spatial statistics. Ann Inst Stat Math. 1991;43(1):1–20.

43. Simpson D, Rue H, Riebler A, Martins TG, Sorbye SH. Penalising model component complexity: a principled, practical approach to constructing priors. Stat Sci. 2017;32(1):1–28. https://doi.org/10.1214/16-STS576.

44. Tonawanda Coke Corporation: United States versus Tonawanda Coke Corporation & Mark L. Kamholz 10- CR-219-S (2013). https://www.justi ce.gov/sites/default/files/usao-wdny/legacy/2014/03/04/Victim_Quest ionaire.pdf.

45. Baldwin HL. Clearing the air: how an effective transparency policy can help the us meet its paris agreement promise. JL & Com. 2016;35:79.

46. Cunningham PJ. What accounts for differences in the use of hospital emergency departments across us communities? Health Aff. 2006;25(5):324–36.

47. Cliff AD, Ord JK. Spatial autocorrelation. London: Pion; 1973.

48. Richardson S, Thomson A, Best N, Elliott P. Interpreting posterior relative risk estimates in disease-mapping studies. Environ Health Perspect. 2004;112(9):1016.

49. Blangiardo M, Cameletti M. Spatial and spatio-temporal bayesian models with R-INLA. New York: Wiley; 2015.

50. Castner J, Wu Y-WB, Mehrok N, Gadre A, Hewner S. Frequent emergency department utilization and behavioral health diagnoses. Nurs Res. 2015;64(1):3–12.

51. Castner J, et al. Medical mondays: Ed utilization for medicaid recipients depends on the day of the week, season, and holidays. J Emerg Nurs. 2016;42(4):317–24.

52. Castner J, Guo L, Yin Y. Ambient air pollution and emergency department visits for asthma in Erie county, New York 2007–2012. Int Arch Occup Environ Health. 2018;91(2):205–14.

53. Ozkaynak H, Baxter LK, Burke J. Evaluation and application of alternative air pollution exposure metrics in air pollution epidemiology studies. J Eposure Sci Environ Epidemiol. 2013;23(6):565.

54. Holleman DR, Bowling RL, Gathy C. Predicting daily visits to a waik-in clinic and emergency department using calendar and weather data. J Gen Intern Med. 1996;11(4):237–9.

55. Batal H, Tench J, McMillan S, Adams J, Mehler PS. Predicting patient visits to an urgent care clinic using calendar variables. Acad Emerg Med. 2001;8(1):48–53.

56. Wargon M, Guidet B, Hoang T, Hejblum G. A systematic review of models for forecasting the number of emergency department visits. Emerg Med J. 2009;26(6):395–9.

57. Booth ML, Owen N, Bauman A, Clavisi O, Leslie E. Social-cognitive and perceived environment influences associated with physical activity in older Australians. Prev Med. 2000;31(1):15–22.

58. Liverani S, Hastie DI, Azizi L, Papathomas M, Richardson S. Premium: an r package for profile regression mixture models using dirichlet processes. J Stat Softw. 2015;64(7):1.

10

Spatial variability of excess mortality during prolonged dust events in a high-density city: a time-stratified spatial regression approach

Man Sing Wong[1], Hung Chak Ho[1*] ⓘ, Lin Yang[2], Wenzhong Shi[1], Jinxin Yang[1] and Ta-Chien Chan[3]

Abstract

Background: Dust events have long been recognized to be associated with a higher mortality risk. However, no study has investigated how prolonged dust events affect the spatial variability of mortality across districts in a downwind city.

Methods: In this study, we applied a spatial regression approach to estimate the district-level mortality during two extreme dust events in Hong Kong. We compared spatial and non-spatial models to evaluate the ability of each regression to estimate mortality. We also compared prolonged dust events with non-dust events to determine the influences of community factors on mortality across the city.

Results: The density of a built environment (estimated by the sky view factor) had positive association with excess mortality in each district, while socioeconomic deprivation contributed by lower income and lower education induced higher mortality impact in each territory planning unit during a prolonged dust event. Based on the model comparison, spatial error modelling with the 1st order of queen contiguity consistently outperformed other models. The high-risk areas with higher increase in mortality were located in an urban high-density environment with higher socioeconomic deprivation.

Conclusion: Our model design shows the ability to predict spatial variability of mortality risk during an extreme weather event that is not able to be estimated based on traditional time-series analysis or ecological studies. Our spatial protocol can be used for public health surveillance, sustainable planning and disaster preparation when relevant data are available.

Keywords: Spatial analytics, Extreme weather event, Dust mortality, Spatial variability, Community vulnerability, Geospatial modelling

Background

Dust events are extreme pollution events that can induce adverse health effects in global cities, as studies have found for major cities in the United States, Australia, Asia and Europe [6, 12, 16, 31, 34, 40, 49]. Previous studies extensively applied temporally stratified models to quantify mortality risk during dust events, with promising results [31, 40, 49]; for example, one study showed that extreme events can lead to a 16% increase in dust mortality in a downwind city [31]. However, there has been no study to investigate the spatial variability of mortality risk during a prolonged dust event. In contrast to a lack of research on this issue, extensive environmental health studies on extreme weather and pollution have pointed out the necessity of predicting spatial variability of mortality and morbidity [2, 20, 23, 27, 29], for the purpose of measuring community vulnerability and public health planning. Estimating community vulnerability is particularly important to a high-density city, as the urban morphology of a

*Correspondence: derrick.hc.ho@polyu.edu.hk
[1] Department of Land Surveying and Geo-informatics, Hong Kong Polytechnic University, Kowloon, Hong Kong
Full list of author information is available at the end of the article

high-density city influences air pollutant dispersion [58], resulting in extreme conditions with severe health risk, in particular at the district level. The prolonged effect of dust combined with urban morphology is expected to induce an additional effect on mortality in a downwind city.

In order to measure community vulnerability, both governmental health guidelines and previous studies have suggested investigating the environmental and socioeconomic factors that can additionally elevate the health risk [11, 17, 19, 24, 38, 41, 42]. Some studies have also proposed combining significant environmental and socioeconomic factors to pinpoint the hotspots of health risk [26, 44, 47, 50]. In order to enhance health planning to minimize adverse health effects of prolonged dust events, this study develops a set of protocols for (1) evaluating potential environmental and socioeconomic factors that can elevate mortality risk during a prolonged dust event, (2) including spatial influences of neighboring communities to adjust for environmental and socioeconomic effects on mortality risk, and (3) locating communities with higher mortality risk for disaster risk management during future dust episodes. The approach developed from this study could be applied to other regions where data on city-specific environmental and socioeconomic factors are available.

Urban and climate settings of Hong Kong

Hong Kong is a typical high-density city located in a subtropical region. There have been ten reported days with dust events in the past decade in Hong Kong, including 2 days in 2006 (Apr 16–17, 2006), 4 days in 2009 (Apr 27–30, 2009), and 4 days in 2010 (Mar 23–26, 2010) [53, 54]. Two of these three dust events (8 of 10 days) were prolonged dust events with ≥ 3 consecutive dusty days. Significant mortality risk was observed on those days, with 7% increase in all-cause mortality and 7% increase in cardiorespiratory mortality during a dusty day. There was also significant air pollution during those dusty days, with average $PM_{10-2.5}$ concentrations 147.6% higher than the days without dust. There is also an extreme population pattern in Hong Kong. The population density of Hong Kong is approximately 6500 persons per km^2. The significant clustering of the urban population in Hong Kong potentially introduces significant intra-urban differences in mortality risk, due to the built environment and demographic structure [13, 33, 52].

Methods
Evaluation of community and environmental characteristics related to mortality risk

Mortality for dusty days and non-dusty days was calculated for each of 287 tertiary planning units (TPU), which is the smallest spatial unit in Hong Kong with mortality and census data available, in order to measure region-specific mortality risks across the entire territory of Hong Kong. The all-cause mortality dataset for dusty days was retrieved from mortality data of the Hong Kong Census and Statistics Department, based on 8 dust days (Apr 27–30, 2009 and Mar 23–26, 2010) associated with prolonged dust events (≥ 3 consecutive dust days), and by excluding all traffic-related deaths (ICD-10 codes V01–V99) during these prolonged dust episodes. Mortality on non-dusty days for each TPU was used to represent the baseline mortality. Deaths of the same weekday of four control weeks before and four control weeks after each dusty day were used to represent the mortality on non-dusty days, in order to minimize bias of seasonality and weekday/weekend effect; and this was divided by the numbers of control weeks for the purpose of comparison with the total mortality on all dusty days in Hong Kong.

To evaluate the potential community and environmental factors that influence mortality risk during a dust storm in Hong Kong, multivariate linear regression was firstly applied to estimate total mortality during the prolonged dust events. Six variables were included as independent variables to evaluate the environmental and socioeconomic effects on mortality in each TPU: (1) sky view factor (SVF), (2) percentage of vegetation, (3) land surface temperature (LST), (4) percentage of low education, (5) percentage of low income, and (6) percentage of elderly:

$$\begin{aligned} Total\ mortality = \ & SVF + \%\ vegetation + average\ LST \\ & + \%\ low\ education + \%\ low\ income \\ & + \%\ elderly \end{aligned}$$

where *total mortality* is the total mortality within 8 days of each TPU, *average SVF* is the average SVF of each TPU, *% vegetation* is the percentage of vegetation of each TPU, *average LST* is the average LST of each TPU, *% low education* is the percentage of low education population of each TPU, *% low income* is the percentage of low income population of each TPU and *% elderly* is the percentage of elderly of each TPU.

Urban geometric characteristics can be depicted by different parameterization indices such as building height, building density, frontal area index (FAI), planar area index (PAI), height/width ratio (H/W), and SVF. The SVF is an indicator representing combinations of building height, building density and topography [22]. The SVF is a ratio to measure the openness of a particular area within an urban setting and in general a terrestrial landscape, which has significant implications for the incoming and outgoing radiation [9]. SVF has been widely used in urban climate research [15, 21, 25, 28, 35, 45, 56], especially to improve spatial models of air pollution prediction [18, 39]. In this study, the SVF was used to locate high-density environments that can potentially trap air pollutants and prohibit air ventilation during prolonged dust events. Average SVF of each TPU was calculated based a raster-based SVF image of Yang et al. [56] derived from airborne Lidar data (Fig. 1). The SVFs at both rooftop and ground levels of this raster-based image were estimated and the spatial resolution of the airborne LIDAR data is 1 m. The building GIS data of Hong Kong were used to calculate the SVF for vertical facets using the planar area index (PAI) and the frontal area index (FAI).

Vegetation coverage (measured in percentage) can potentially influence or absorb ground-level air pollution in each TPU. In this study, the territory-wide vegetation coverage was estimated using the land use and land cover map derived from the Planning Department of Hong Kong (Fig. 2).

Land surface temperature (LST) images are commonly used to represent spatial variations of surface temperature that can affect health risk [29, 36, 55]. Landsat Thematic Mapper TM 5 on March 25, 2010 was used to estimate LST to demonstrate typical temperature variations during prolonged dust events in Hong Kong.

Average LST (Fig. 3) was estimated using an improved urban emissivity model based on the SVF [57].

Lower education is associated with higher social vulnerability during air pollution events [32, 52], and lower income is related to low socioeconomic status, which may induce adverse health effects on a day with heavy pollution [52]. The elderly are identified as one of the major age groups that are highly vulnerable during days with heavy air pollution [8, 32]. Therefore, the percentages of low education, low income and elderly were extracted from the 2006 census data of Hong Kong, and were used to represent the socioeconomic influence of each TPU. The percentage of low education was calculated based on the percentage of persons who had a primary school education or less (Fig. 4). The percentage of low income was the percentage of persons who were unpaid or had monthly income lower than HKD$10,000 (Fig. 5). The percentage of elderly was the percentage of persons aged ≥65 in each TPU (Fig. 6). Two TPUs with missing data of low education, low income and elderly were excluded from this study.

Finally, the predicted total mortality and the 95% confidence interval (CI) were estimated to represent the

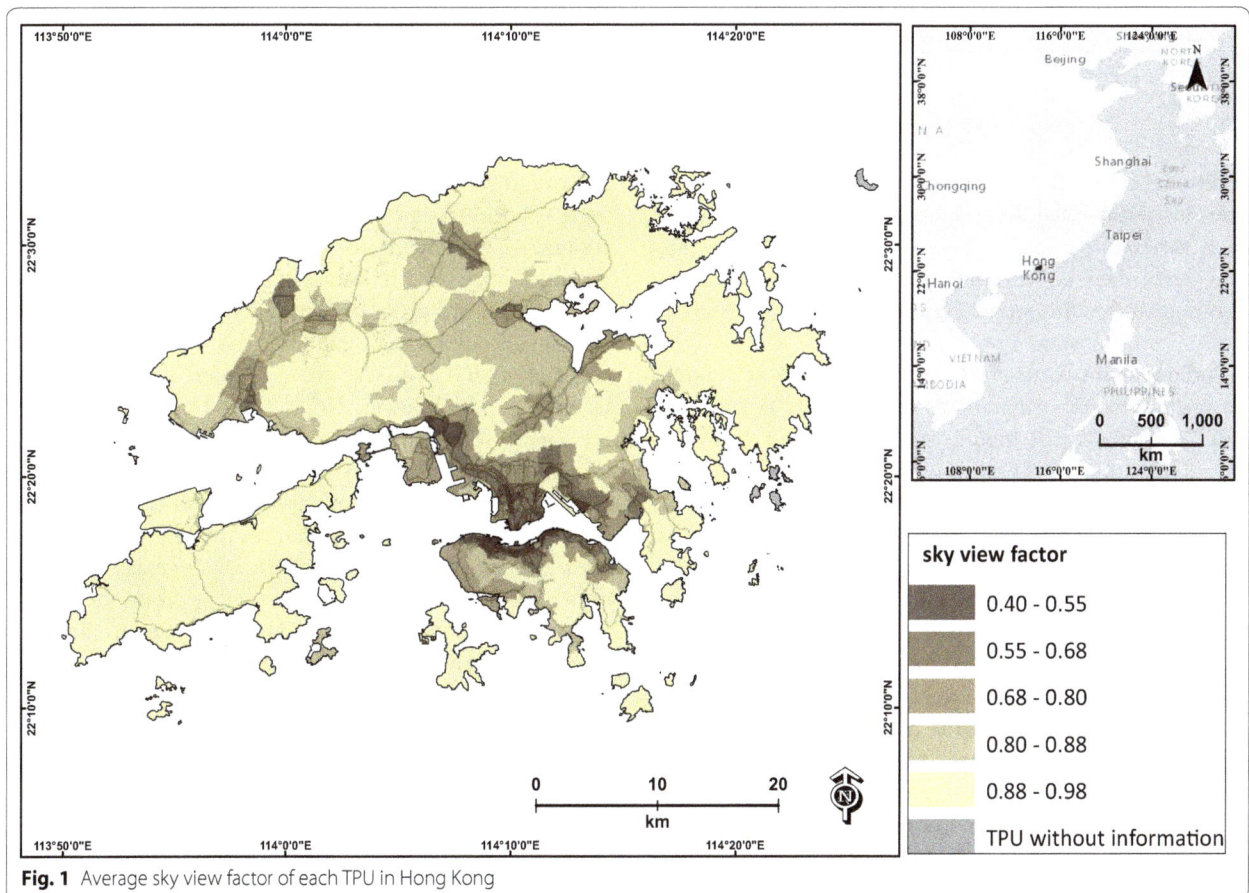

Fig. 1 Average sky view factor of each TPU in Hong Kong

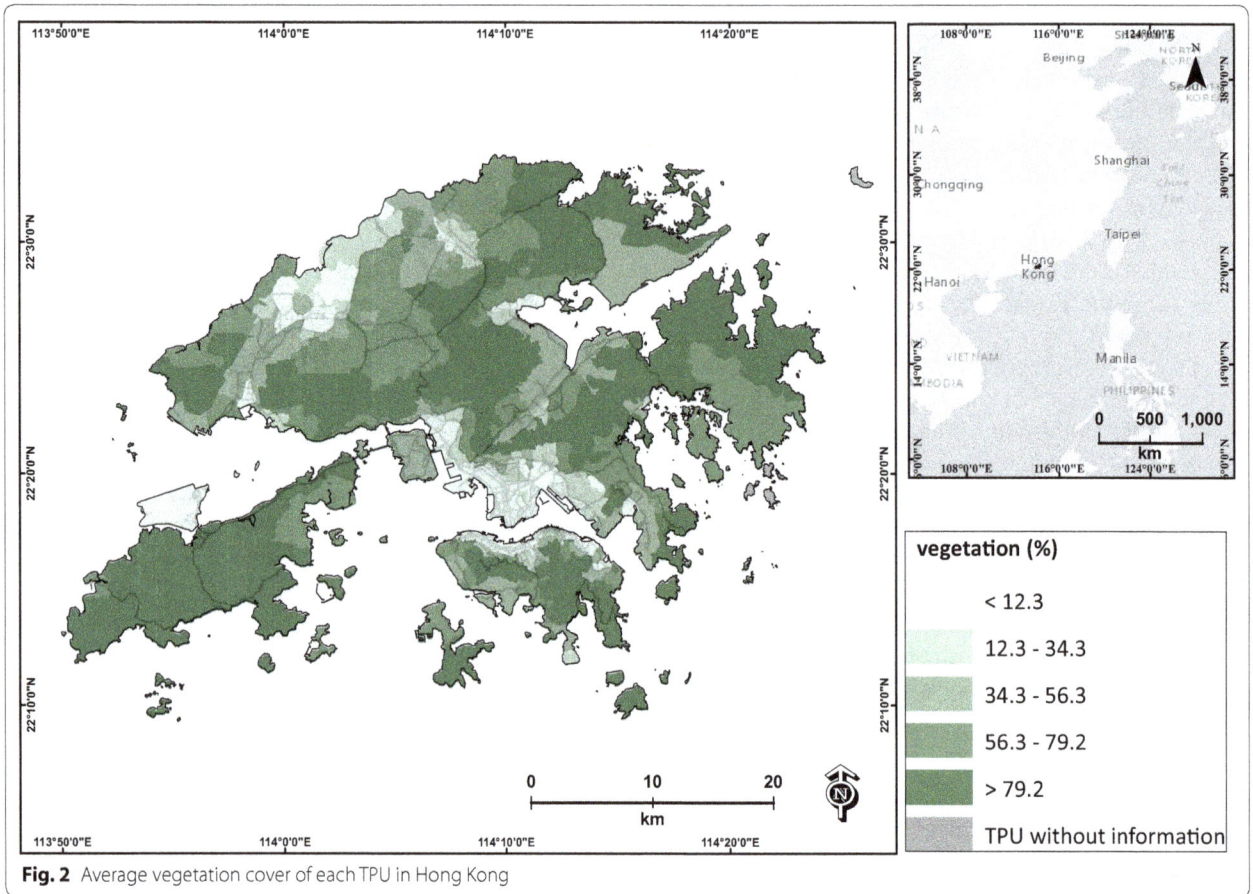

Fig. 2 Average vegetation cover of each TPU in Hong Kong

additional effect of mortality risk on both dusty days and non-dusty days (baseline) from the spatial variability of each variable. Excess mortality between dusty days and non-dusty days contributed by each spatial factor was also reported in this study (Fig. 7).

Including neighboring effects for mortality risk estimation

To include neighboring effects on mortality risk of each TPU, a spatial error model was applied and was compared with the results of multivariate linear regression. The spatial error model incorporated spatial autocorrelation in a regression error term (Lambda) to adjust spatial dependence in a multivariate linear regression model [3]. In our study, the spatial error model weights the neighboring TPUs to spatially adjust socioeconomic and environmental influences on total mortality. To spatially weight the TPUs, we applied the queen contiguity method. This method weights all spatial neighbors with shared borders and corners [4], based on a spatial distance with the order of contiguity. This study applied the queen contiguity method to adjust the mortality risk of each TPU based on all surrounding TPUs. To evaluate the appropriate spatial distance for adjustment, the 1st to

3rd orders of contiguity (lag 1–lag 3) were used to estimate total mortality and for comparison with the linear results. All significant environmental and socioeconomic variables were used to construct the spatial error models with the 1st–3rd order of contiguity, and the multivariate linear regression for comparison. The Akaike information criterion (AIC) [10] was then adopted to compare the models, in which lower AIC indicated better model performance. Total mortality and CIs representing the additional effects of mortality risk from the spatial variability of each variable were also reported, and the differences between models were further evaluated. Finally, predicted mortality change (increase or decrease) in numbers of deaths of each TPU from the appropriate models for both dusty and non-dusty days were used to illustrate the spatial variability of relative mortality across Hong Kong during prolonged dust events.

Results

Contributions of socioeconomic and environmental influences to mortality risk

There were in total of 802 decedents reported on all case days, and 6331 decedents reported on all control days.

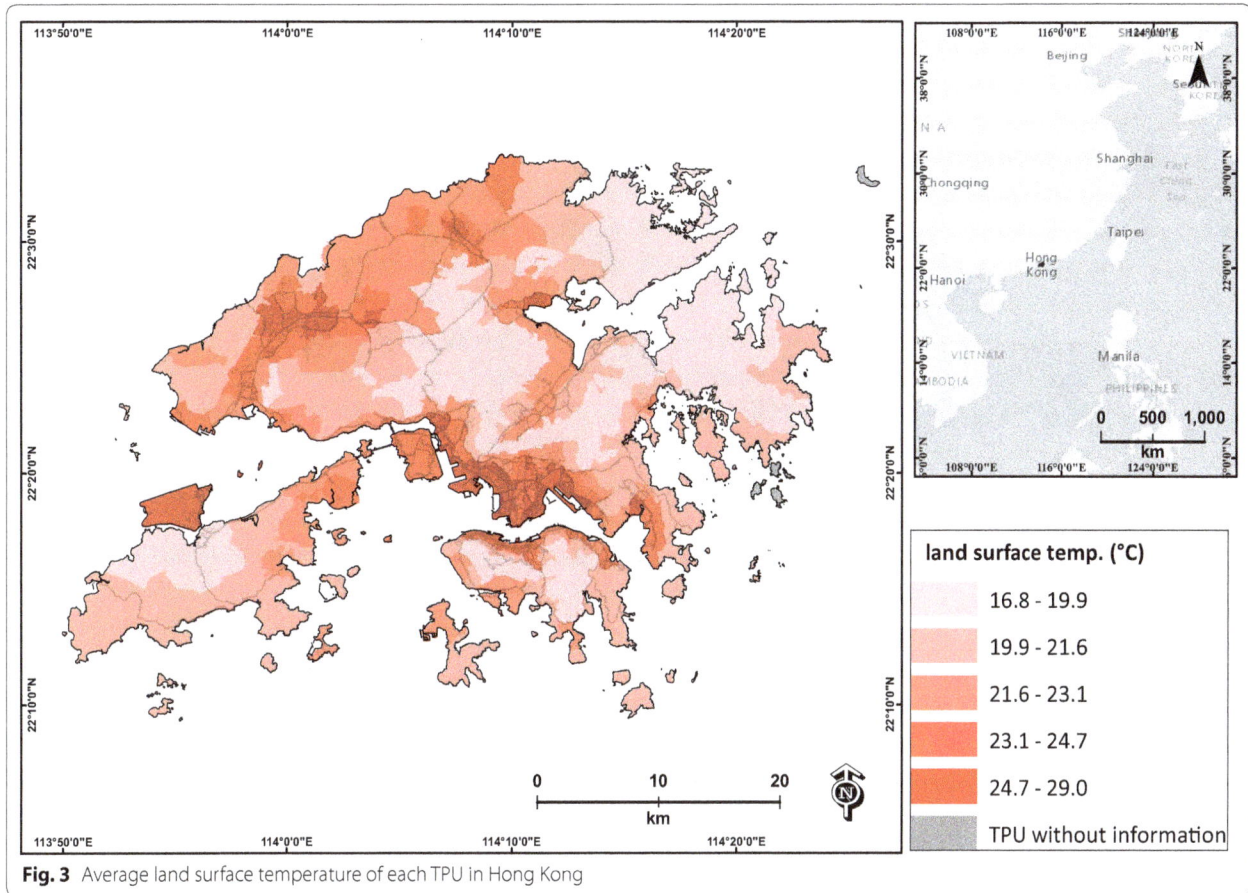

Fig. 3 Average land surface temperature of each TPU in Hong Kong

Based on the multivariate linear models, the SVF, percentage of low education, percentage of low income, and percentage of elderly show varied contributions to local mortality risk of each TPU during prolonged dust events (Table 1). Among all, percentage of low income is the highest risk factor of a community during prolonged dust events. A TPU with 10% more low-income population is found to have 12.5% higher mortality during a dusty day than a non-dusty day. At a TPU with 10% more population who education level was primary school or below, there is also 6.3% higher mortality during prolonged dust events than days without dust. In contrast, SVF has a negative association with mortality risk. A TPU with 10% higher SVF has 5.3% less mortality during a day with a dust storm. This indicates that a TPU with a high-density built environment generally has higher risk during prolonged dust events, while lower-density environments with higher SVF have less mortality risk.

In addition, there is no observation of an increase of total mortality in the TPUs with a higher percentage of elderly. Similar results have been found in other Hong Kong studies; for example, Chan et al. [13] estimated community vulnerability with census data and found that those aged ≥75 had significantly lower mortality risk than those aged <75, especially for the male population. Spatial differences in temperature and vegetation did not have significant contributions to mortality risk during prolonged dust events.

Including spatial influences for mortality risk estimation

Compared to the non-spatial model for dusty days using all variables with an AIC of 1692.3, the non-spatial model using only significant environmental and socioeconomic variables (SVF, % lower education, % lower income and % elderly) has a lower AIC of 1689.6, indicating a better model for prediction. By using all significant environmental and socioeconomic variables, it is observed that inclusion of neighboring effects as spatial influential factors has enhanced mortality risk estimation. By comparing all models for predicting mortality during dusty days with and without incorporating spatial autocorrelation (Table 2), the model considering the 1st order of queen contiguity (lag 1) has the best performance. The AIC of this lag-1 model is 1679.97, and it is the lowest among the others. There is a positive value of the regression error term of the lag-1 model (Lambda: 0.3), indicating

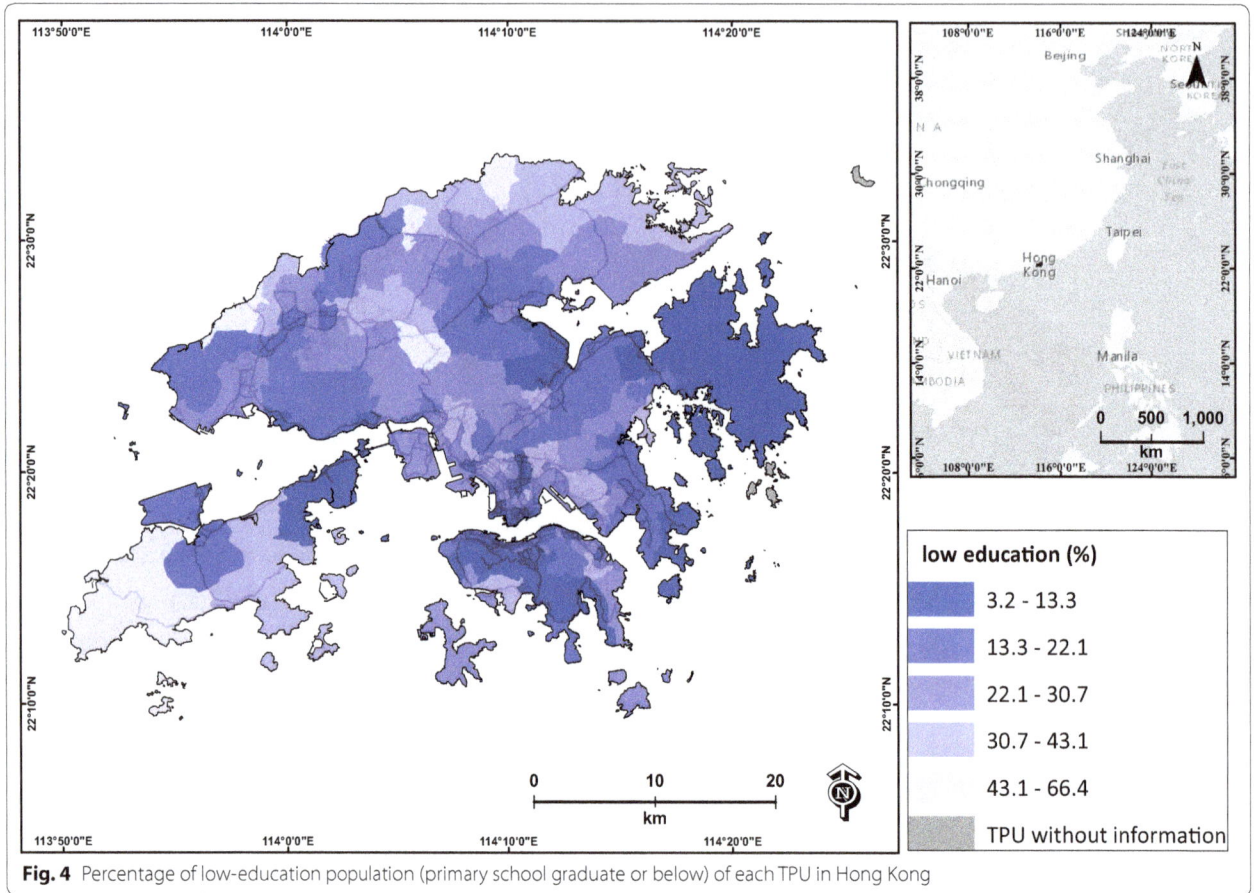

Fig. 4 Percentage of low-education population (primary school graduate or below) of each TPU in Hong Kong

that including neighboring effects of surrounding TPUs results in less spatial error for mortality risk prediction. It is also important to note that only including the 1st- or 2nd-order queen contiguity in modelling can enhance mortality risk estimation for prolonged dust events in Hong Kong. The 3rd-order queen contiguity does not improve the modelling, based on Lambda reported with the spatial error model. We also repeated the analyses for mortality predictions of non-dusty days (Table 3). We found similar results for model comparison, with the lag-1 model the best for predicting mortality during days without prolonged dust events (AIC: 1582.04).

By using the lag-1 model to include the neighboring effects (Table 4), areas with 10% higher SVF will have 5.3% less mortality risk than TPUs during a prolonged dust event, while a TPU with 10% more low-education population will have 6.7% higher mortality during prolonged dust events compared to non-dusty days, with all these reaching statistical significance.

Based on the comparison of spatial and non-spatial models, we applied a spatial error model incorporating the 1st order of queen contiguity to predict total mortality on dusty days and non-dusty days, and a predicted

change of total mortality as relative risk of each TPU is reported in this study (Fig. 8). The mortality risk map indicates that rural areas with low-density environments have a potential decrease in mortality during prolonged dust events compared to non-dusty days. In contrast, the TPUs with high-density environments and high socio-economic deprivation, such as TPUs in Tuen Mun, Sham Shui Po, Wong Tai Sin and Kwun Tong, generally have a higher increase in mortality during prolonged dust events compared to non-dusty days. These TPUs are predicted to have 0.1–0.5 more deaths in a period of 8 dust days than the control periods, controlling for SVF, percentage of low education, percentage of low income, percentage of elderly, and spatial autocorrelation.

Discussion

This study applied a spatial regression approach to estimate spatial variability of mortality risk across a high-density city during prolonged dust events. Based on this approach, the influence of the built environment is highlighted by the negative association between SVF and mortality increase. This result indicates that high-density urban areas may trap air pollutants during days with

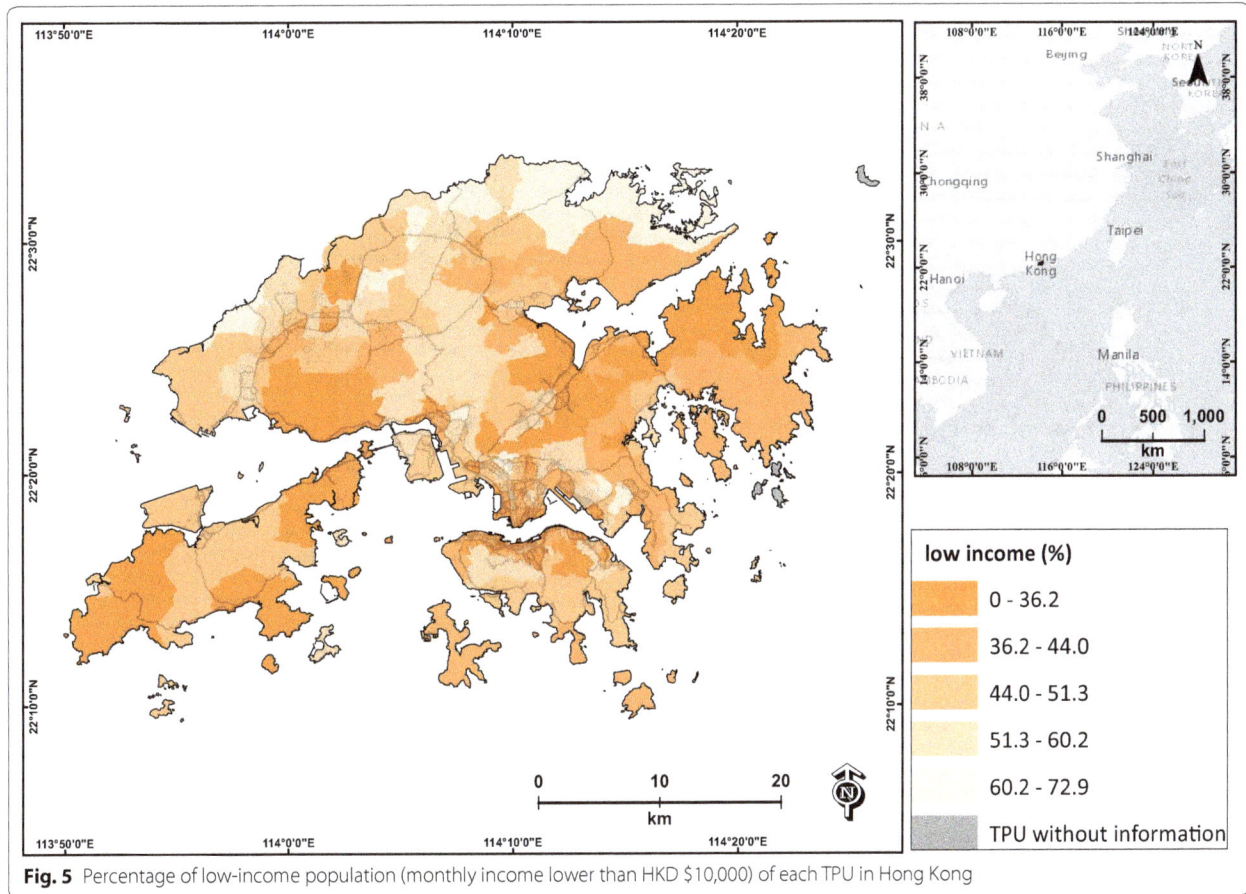

Fig. 5 Percentage of low-income population (monthly income lower than HKD $10,000) of each TPU in Hong Kong

dust storms, resulting in poorer air quality and severely increasing health risk; while areas with more openness allow better air ventilation and dispersion, therefore less health risk attributable to air pollution can be found in these areas during dusty days. Influence from socioeconomic deprivation is also determined by the positive association between total mortality, percentage of low education, and percentage of low income. In contrast, percentage of elderly of a TPU does not have a positive association with mortality risk. This might be due to the presence of more health facilities in communities with higher percentages of elderly, which reduces the mortality risk of such neighborhoods, while elderly in TPUs with lower percentages of older population may not benefit from such facilities, therefore increasing their risk. In conclusion, these findings are innovative, because previous studies only temporally stratified the dust mortality [12, 14, 31, 40, 49], without understanding the intra-urban difference in mortality risk during dust events.

In the context of spatial health planning, health risk mapping can characterize vulnerability of specific populations in a specific region [24], for the purpose of supporting health authorities, policymakers, and city officials to determine future health protocols in different communities [1]. This mapping technique has been widely used along with governmental actions to develop public health surveillance. For example, the City of Toronto in Canada initiated a heat vulnerability mapping project for minimizing summer risks [44], and Vancouver Coastal and Fraser Health Authorities gave impetus to the development of the Vancouver Area Neighborhood Deprivation Index (VANDIX) for general health risk estimation [7]. Mapping mortality risk adjusted for environmental and socioeconomic factors can help target a single disaster episode for comprehensive health planning. This is necessary because the general health vulnerability index can be somewhat useful, but may not be able to fully describe the spatial variability of a particular health risk [43]. One example is that VANDIX is related to heat mortality in the Vancouver area, but it is necessary to adjust it to pinpoint heat risks with accuracy [27]. Therefore, previous health studies indicate the need to calibrate spatial vulnerability assessments with health outcome data [5, 11, 26, 47, 50], while mortality data will be the most appropriate dataset for demonstrating

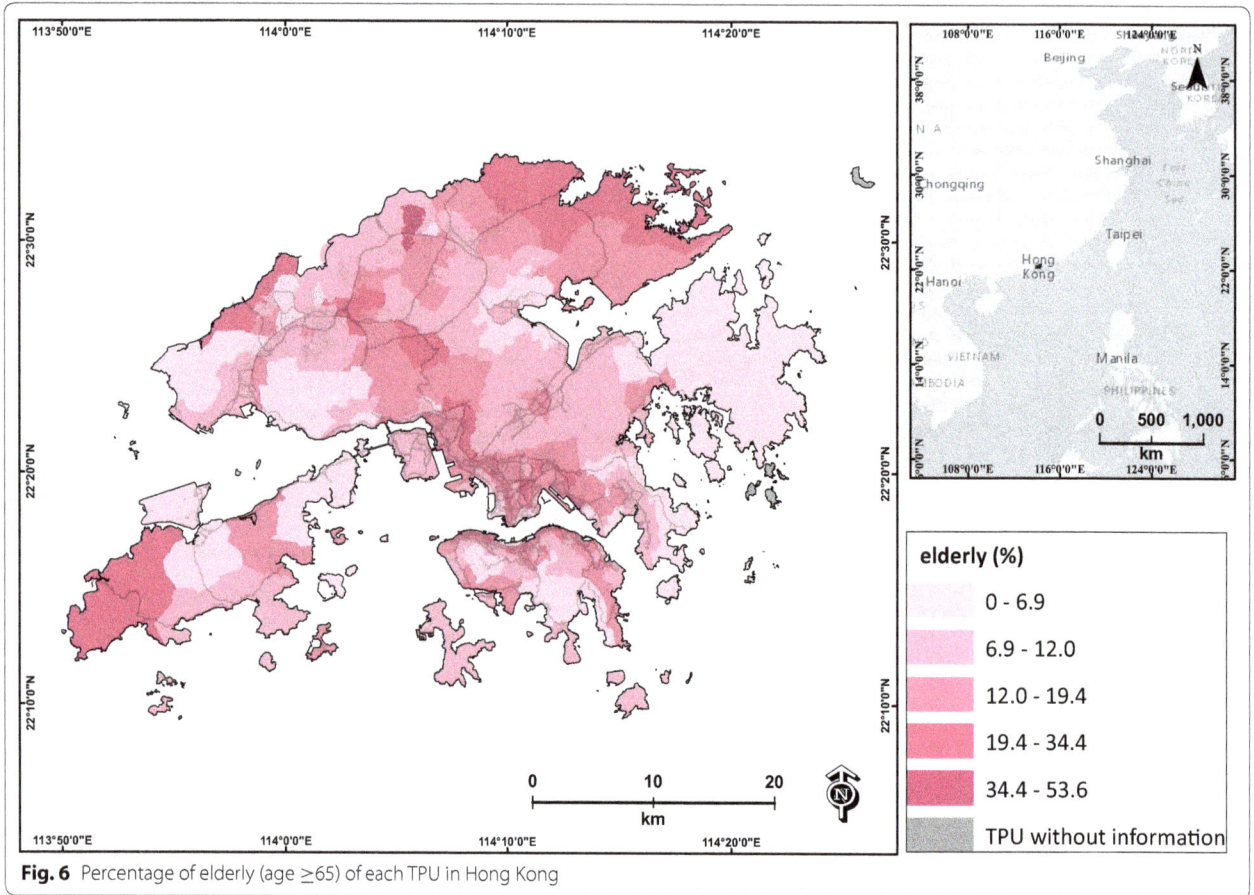

Fig. 6 Percentage of elderly (age ≥65) of each TPU in Hong Kong

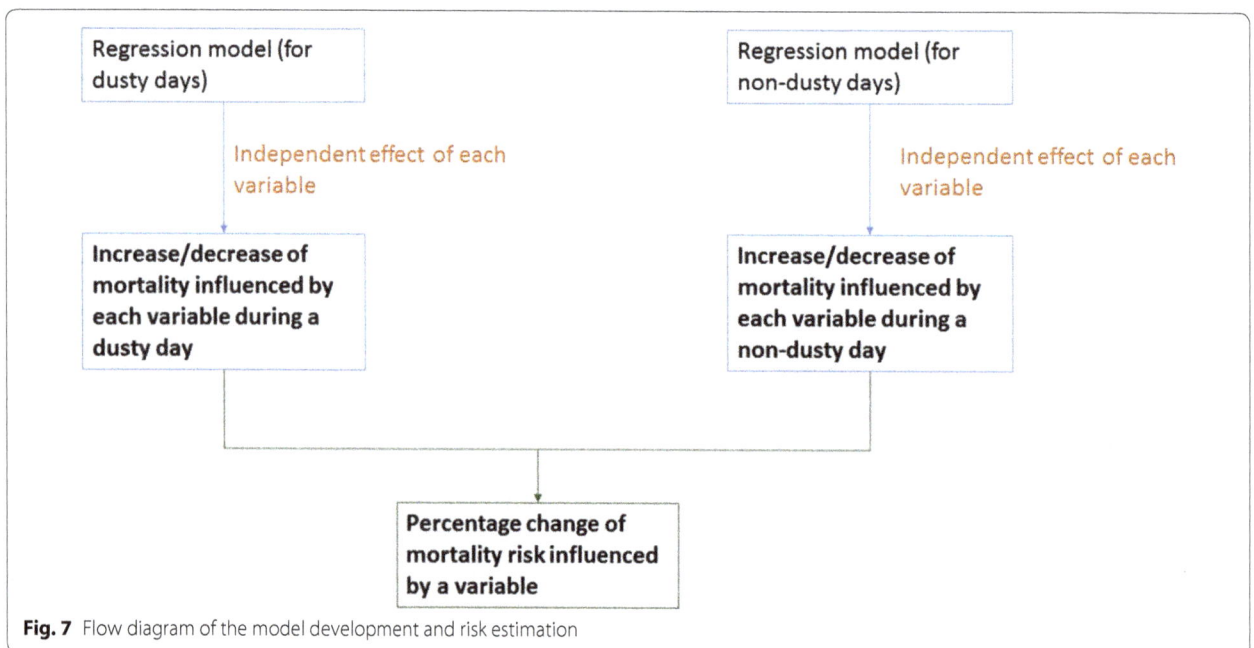

Fig. 7 Flow diagram of the model development and risk estimation

Table 1 Influences of community factors on excess mortality

Variables	Predicted total mortality		Excess mortality (%)
	Change in number of deaths on days with prolonged dust events (95% confidence intervals)	Baseline: number of deaths on days without prolonged dust events (95% confidence intervals)	
SVF (in 10%)	−2.0 [−2.6, −1.3]*	−1.9 [−2.5, −1.3]*	−5.3
% vegetation (in 10%)	0.0 [−0.4, 0.4]	0.0 [−0.3, 0.4]	0
LST (in 1 °C)	−0.1 [−0.6, 0.4]	−0.1 [−0.5, 0.3]	0
% low education (in 10%)	1.7 [0.8, 2.5]*	1.6 [0.9, 2.3]*	6.3
% low income (in 10%)	0.9 [0.2, 1.6]*	0.8 [0.2, 1.4]*	12.5
% elderly (in 10%)	−2.4 [−3.6, −1.1]*	−2.2 [−3.2, −1.1]*	−9.1

* Are the results with significant p values (<0.05)

disaster episodes. Therefore, mapping mortality risk during prolonged dust events is essential, since such spatial assessment can be used for local government action, as well as serving as a regional protocol for developing similar health indices in other cities.

Furthermore, previous research mostly developed health indices based on a simple spatial overlay technique [50]; there were issues related to spatial autocorrelation that these studies did not consider, and that might create potential biases in results. Our study adopting spatial error modelling is test-proven, with promising results showing that spatial autocorrelation can significantly improve the accuracy of predicting mortality during dust episodes. Its findings are similar to those of other spatial epidemiologic literature showing that analysis with spatial autocorrelation can help predict spatial variability of health risks [37, 51].

One limitation of this study is that the prolonged dust events were isolated episodes in Hong Kong. Based on only two dust events in Hong Kong, it was not able to employ time-series analysis for a more comprehensive spatio-temporal assessment. Application of an alternative method such as a time-stratified approach for estimating the standard mortality ratio of each small neighborhood is also problematic, since comparing rare death cases on non-dusty days in each neighborhood may create extreme estimation, resulting in statistical bias. To avoid the statistical bias, previous health studies generally applied spatial delineation techniques to stratify socioeconomic or environmental data by groups [27, 48, 52]. This method can capture spatial differences between groups, but is still insufficient to estimate the individual risk of each district. Our approach is applicable for the present case study, because we applied spatial regression to predict mortality on both dusty and non-dusty days for comparison. With the support of spatial regressions to compare total mortality between dusty and non-dusty days, the results of this study can be used to demonstrate

the additional mortality effect in each district due to spatial variability of environmental and socioeconomic factors during the isolated but fatal dust events.

For future study, inclusion of spatial data on air pollution exposure may enhance mortality risk mapping. However, existing pollution mapping methods such as land use regression are limited by the spatiotemporal coverage of the data, which may not be able to demonstrate extreme cases such as a prolonged dust event. In addition, there is an accuracy issue in using such mapping methods in a high-density city, because a complex urban built environment influences air ventilation, and as a result produces bias in pollution mapping [46]. Misuse of air pollution maps for a spatial study can induce a significant ecological fallacy, especially since community vulnerability is already influenced by the adverse effect due to aggregate-level data, instead of the association with individual-level response [13]. In order to tackle this issue, some studies have started to use moderate-resolution satellite images for mapping Aerosol Optical Depth (AOD) or Aerosol Optical Thickness (AOT) in order to demonstrate spatiotemporal variation in air pollution. However, there are varied associations between AOD/AOT and particulate matters (the main components of dust), depending on the size of particulate matters and spatial locations. While fine particulate matter is a common pollutant contributing to health risk in typical non-dust scenarios [30], there are also studies finding that PM_{10} or $PM_{10-2.5}$ concentration may severely increase the mortality risk during a dusty day [16, 31, 40]. Therefore, further investigation is needed on how to use AOD/AOT to map spatiotemporal variations of both fine and coarse particulate matters for determining how air pollution exposures actually influence mortality risk during a dusty day. A future study should, therefore, combine an existing city-based mapping method with satellite images to improve the spatio-temporal modelling of air pollution exposure, at the same time increasing the spatial

Table 2 Comparison of spatial and non-spatial models for predicting total mortality during days with prolonged dust events

Variables	Multivariate linear: predicted mortality on dusty days (95% confidence intervals)	Spatial error (lag 1): predicted mortality on dusty days (95% confidence intervals)	Spatial error (lag 2): predicted mortality on dusty days (95% confidence intervals)	Spatial error (lag 3): predicted mortality on dusty days (95% confidence intervals)
SVF (in 10%)	−1.8 [−2.2, −1.4]*	−2.0 [−2.5, −1.5]*	−2.0 [−2.5, −1.6]*	−1.8 [−2.2, −1.4]*
% low education (in 10%)	1.6 [0.8, 2.4]*	1.6 [0.7, 2.5]*	1.5 [0.7, 2.4]*	1.5 [0.7, 2.4]*
% low income (in 10%)	0.9 [0.2, 1.6]*	0.7 [0.0, 1.4]	0.8 [0.1, 1.5]*	0.9 [0.2, 1.6]*
% elderly (in 10%)	−2.3 [−3.5, −1.1]*	−2.1 [−0.8, −3.4]*	−2.1 [−3.3, −0.9]*	−2.2 [−3.4, −1.0]*
Lambda	N/A	0.3 [0.1, 0.4]*	0.4 [0.1, 0.6]*	0.1 [−0.2, 0.4]
AIC	1689.6	1679.97	1682.95	1689.03

* Are the results with significant p values (<0.05)

Table 3 Comparison of spatial and non-spatial models for predicting total mortality during days without prolonged dust events

Variables	Multivariate linear: predicted mortality on non-dusty days (95% confidence intervals)	Spatial error (lag 1): predicted mortality on non-dusty days (95% confidence intervals)	Spatial error (lag 2): predicted mortality on non-dusty days (95% confidence intervals)	Spatial error (lag 3): predicted mortality on non-dusty days (95% confidence intervals)
SVF (in 10%)	−1.7 [−2.1, −1.4]*	−1.9 [−2.3, −1.5]*	−2.0 [−2.4, −1.6]*	−1.8 [−2.1, −1.4]*
% low education (in 10%)	1.5 [0.8, 2.2]*	1.5 [0.7, 2.2]*	1.4 [0.7, 2.2]*	1.4 [0.7, 2.1]*
% low income (in 10%)	0.8 [0.2, 1.4]*	0.6 [0.0, 1.2]	0.7 [0.1, 0.3]*	0.8 [0.2, 1.4]*
% elderly (in 10%)	−2.1 [−3.1, −1.1]*	−1.8 [−2.9, −0.7]*	−1.9 [−2.9, −0.9]*	−1.9 [−3.0, −0.9]*
Lambda	N/A	0.3 [0.2, 0.5]*	0.4 [0.2, 0.6]*	0.2 [−0.1, 0.5]
AIC	1612.48	1582.04	1585.25	1610.28

* Are the results with significant p values (<0.05)

Table 4 Influences on excess mortality based on the best spatial regression models

Variables	Spatial error (lag 1): predicted total mortality on dusty day (95% confidence intervals)	Spatial error (lag 1): predicted total mortality on non-dusty day (95% confidence intervals)	Excess mortality (%)
SVF (in 10%)	−2.0 [−2.5, −1.5]*	−1.9 [−2.3, −1.5]*	−5.3
% low education (in 10%)	1.6 [0.7, 2.5]*	1.5 [0.7, 2.2]*	6.7
% low income (in 10%)	0.7 [0.0, 1.4]	0.6 [0.0, 1.2]	16.7
% elderly (in 10%)	−2.1 [−3.4, −0.8]*	−1.8 [−2.9, −0.7]*	−16.7

* Are the results with significant *p* values (<0.05)

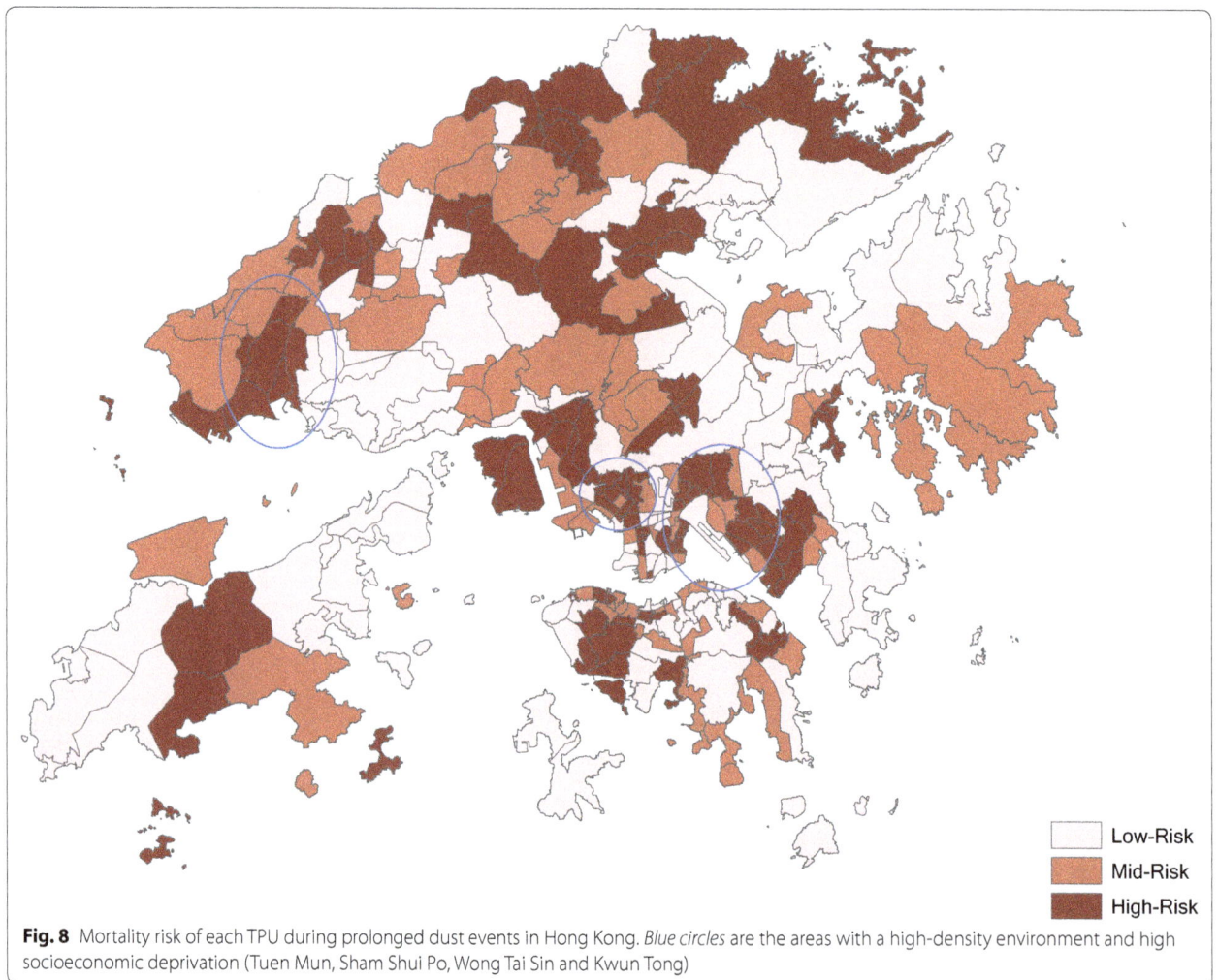

Fig. 8 Mortality risk of each TPU during prolonged dust events in Hong Kong. *Blue circles* are the areas with a high-density environment and high socioeconomic deprivation (Tuen Mun, Sham Shui Po, Wong Tai Sin and Kwun Tong)

quality, because moderate or low spatial resolution of satellite images itself may increase potential spatial biases of modelling.

Conclusion

This study applied a spatial regression approach to estimate the spatial variability of mortality during prolonged dust events. The results indicated that spatial difference in built environment (SVF) and socioeconomic status (low education and low income) will increase the mortality in a community during dust events. This study also demonstrates there is a need to include spatial autocorrelation in modelling in order to improve the accuracy of prediction. Finally, the mortality risk map can be used to locate at-risk communities and vulnerable populations for developing health protocols in Hong Kong.

Abbreviations

FAI: frontal area index (FAI); PAI: planar area index (PAI); H/W: height/width ratio; LST: land surface temperature; CI: confidence interval; AIC: Akaike information criterion; SVF: sky view factor; TPU: tertiary planning unit; VANDIX: Vancouver Area Neighborhood Deprivation Index; AOD: aerosol optical depth; AOT: aerosol optical thickness; PM: particulate matter.

Authors' contributions

HCH developed the model design. MSW, HCH and TC conducted the data analysis. YL provided input of public health analysis. JY supported the data preparation. WS provided input of spatial analysis. MSW and HCH wrote the manuscript. All authors read and approved the final manuscript.

Author details

[1] Department of Land Surveying and Geo-informatics, Hong Kong Polytechnic University, Kowloon, Hong Kong. [2] School of Nursing, Hong Kong Polytechnic University, Kowloon, Hong Kong. [3] Research Center for Humanity and Social Sciences, Academia Sinica, Taipei, Taiwan.

Acknowledgements

The authors are grateful for the mortality data from the Hong Kong Census and Statistics Department, airborne LIDAR data from the Hong Kong Civil Engineering and Development Department, land use and land cover data from the Planning Department of Hong Kong, and building GIS data from the Hong Kong Lands Department.

Competing interests

The authors declare that they have no competing interests.

Funding

This research was supported in part by a grant from the Hong Kong Polytechnic University (Grant PolyU 1-ZE24). Dr. M.S. Wong acknowledges the support in part by a grant from General Research Fund (Project ID: 15205515); Grant PolyU 1-ZVAJ from the Faculty of Construction and Environment, the Hong Kong Polytechnic University; and the Grants PolyU 1-ZVFD from the Research Institute for Sustainable Urban Development, the Hong Kong Polytechnic University.

References

1. Aminipouri M, Knudby A, Ho HC. Using multiple disparate data sources to map heat vulnerability: Vancouver case study. Can Geogr. 2016;60(3):356–68.
2. Alexeeff SE, Schwartz J, Kloog I, Chudnovsky A, Koutrakis P, Coull BA. Consequences of kriging and land use regression for PM2.5 predictions in epidemiologic analyses: insights into spatial variability using high-resolution satellite data. J Eposure Sci Environ Epidemiol. 2015;25(2):138–44.
3. Anselin L, Rey S. Properties of tests for spatial dependence in linear regression models. Geogr Anal. 1991;23(2):112–31.
4. Anselin L, Sridharan S, Gholston S. Using exploratory spatial data analysis to leverage social indicator databases: the discovery of interesting patterns. Soc Indic Res. 2007;82(2):287–309.
5. Bao J, Li X, Yu C. The construction and validation of the heat vulnerability index, a review. Int J Environ Res Public Health. 2015;12(7):7220–34.
6. Barnett AG, Fraser JF, Munck L. The effects of the 2009 dust storm on emergency admissions to a hospital in Brisbane, Australia. Int J Biometeorol. 2012;56(4):719–26.
7. Bell N, Hayes MV. The Vancouver Area Neighbourhood Deprivation Index (Vandix): a census-based tool for assessing small-area variations in health status. Can J Public Health. 2012;103:S28–32.

8. Bell ML, Zanobetti A, Dominici F. Evidence on vulnerability and susceptibility to health risks associated with short-term exposure to particulate matter: a systematic review and meta-analysis. Am J Epidemiol. 2013;178(6):kwt090.
9. Brown, M. J., Grimmond, S., & Ratti, C. (2001, December). Comparison of methodologies for computing sky view factor in urban environments. In International Society of Environmental Hydraulics Conference, Tempe, AZ.
10. Burnham KP, Anderson DR. Multimodel inference understanding AIC and BIC in model selection. Sociol Methods Res. 2004;33(2):261–304.
11. Carrier M, Apparicio P, Kestens Y, Séguin AM, Pham H, Crouse D, Siemiatycki J. Application of a Global Environmental Equity Index in Montreal: diagnostic and further implications. Ann Am Assoc Geogr. 2016;106(6):1268–85.
12. Chan CC, Ng HC. A case-crossover analysis of Asian dust storms and mortality in the downwind areas using 14-year data in Taipei. Sci Total Environ. 2011;410:47–52.
13. Chan EYY, Goggins WB, Kim JJ, Griffiths SM. A study of intracity variation of temperature-related mortality and socioeconomic status among the Chinese population in Hong Kong. J Epidemiol Community Health. 2012;66(4):322–7.
14. Chen YS, Sheen PC, Chen ER, Liu YK, Wu TN, Yang CY. Effects of Asian dust storm events on daily mortality in Taipei, Taiwan. Environ Res. 2004;95(2):151–5.
15. Chen L, Ng E, An X, Ren C, Lee M, Wang U, He Z. Sky view factor analysis of street canyons and its implications for daytime intra-urban air temperature differentials in high-rise, high-density urban areas of Hong Kong: a GIS-based simulation approach. Int J Climatol. 2012;32(1):121–36.
16. Crooks JL, Cascio WE, Percy MS, Reyes J, Neas LM, Hilborn ED. The Association between dust storms and daily non-accidental mortality in the United States, 1993–2005. Environ Health Perspect. 2016;124(11):1735–43.
17. Cutter SL. The vulnerability of science and the science of vulnerability. Ann Assoc Am Geogr. 2003;93(1):1–12.
18. Eeftens M, Beekhuizen J, Beelen R, Wang M, Vermeulen R, Brunekreef B, Hoek G. Quantifying urban street configuration for improvements in air pollution models. Atmos Environ. 2013;72:1–9.
19. Ebi KL, Kovats RS, Menne B. An approach for assessing human health vulnerability and public health interventions to adapt to climate change. Environ Health Perspect. 2006;114:1930–4.
20. Evans J, van Donkelaar A, Martin RV, Burnett R, Rainham DG, Birkett NJ, Grimmond S. Urbanization and global environmental change: local effects of urban warming. Geogr J. 2007;173(1):83–8.
21. Gal T, Lindberg F, Unger J. Computing continuous sky view factors using 3D urban raster and vector databases: comparison and application to urban climate. Theoret Appl Climatol. 2009;95(1–2):111–23.
22. Grimmond S. Urbanization and global environmental change: local effects of urban warming. Geogr J. 2007;173(1):83–8.
23. Hattis D, Ogneva-Himmelberger Y, Ratick S. The spatial variability of heat-related mortality in Massachusetts. Appl Geogr. 2012;33:45–52.
24. Health Canada. Adapting to extreme heat events: guidelines for assessing health vulnerability. 2011. https://www.canada.ca/en/health-canada/services/environmental-workplace-health/reportspublications/climate-change-health/adapting-extreme-heat-events-guidelines-assessing-healthvulnerability-health-canada-2011.html. Accessed 15 Jan 2017.
25. Ho HC, Knudby A, Sirovyak P, Xu Y, Hodul M, Henderson SB. Mapping maximum urban air temperature on hot summer days. Remote Sens Environ. 2014;154:38–45.
26. Ho HC, Knudby A, Huang W. A spatial framework to map heat health risks at multiple scales. Int J Environ Res Public Health. 2015;12(12):16110–23.
27. Ho HC, Knudby A, Walker BB, Henderson SB. Delineation of spatial variability in the temperature-mortality relationship on extremely hot days in greater Vancouver, Canada. Environ Health Perspect. 2017;125(1):66–75.
28. Hodul M, Knudby A, Ho HC. Estimation of continuous urban sky view factor from landsat data using shadow detection. Remote Sens. 2016;8(7):568.

29. Hondula DM, Davis RE, Leisten MJ, Saha MV, Veazey LM, Wegner CR. Fine-scale spatial variability of heat-related mortality in Philadelphia County, USA, from 1983–2008: a case-series analysis. Environ Health. 2012;11(1):1.

30. Jerrett M, Burnett RT, Beckerman BS, Turner MC, Krewski D, Thurston G, Gapstur SM. Spatial analysis of air pollution and mortality in California. Am J Respir Crit Care Med. 2013;188(5):593–9.

31. Johnston F, Hanigan I, Henderson S, Morgan G, Bowman D. Extreme air pollution events from bushfires and dust storms and their association with mortality in Sydney, Australia 1994–2007. Environ Res. 2011;111(6):811–6.

32. Kan H, London SJ, Chen G, Zhang Y, Song G, Zhao N, Chen B. Season, sex, age, and education as modifiers of the effects of outdoor air pollution on daily mortality in Shanghai, China: the Public Health and Air Pollution in Asia (PAPA) Study. Environ Health Perspect. 2008;116(9):1183.

33. Kandt J, Chang SS, Yip P, Burdett R. The spatial pattern of premature mortality in Hong Kong: How does it relate to public housing? Urban Stud. 2016;0042098015620341.

34. Kashima S, Yorifuji T, Tsuda T, Eboshida A. Asian dust and daily all-cause or cause-specific mortality in western Japan. Occup Environ Med. 2012;69(12):908–15.

35. Lai PC, Choi CC, Wong PP, Thach TQ, Wong MS, Cheng W, Wong CM. Spatial analytical methods for deriving a historical map of physiological equivalent temperature of Hong Kong. Build Environ. 2016;99:22–8.

36. Laaidi K, Zeghnoun A, Dousset B, Bretin P, Vandentorren S, Giraudet E, Beaudeau P. The impact of heat islands on mortality in Paris during the August 2003 heat wave. Environ Health Perspect. 2012;120(2):254.

37. Lorant V, Thomas I, Deliège D, Tonglet R. Deprivation and mortality: the implications of spatial autocorrelation for health resources allocation. Soc Sci Med. 2001;53(12):1711–9.

38. Morss RE, Wilhelmi OV, Meehl GA, Dilling L. Improving societal outcomes of extreme weather in a changing climate: an integrated perspective. Annu Rev Environ Resour. 2011;36(1):1.

39. Mueller MD, Wagner M, Barmpadimos I, Hueglin C. Two-week NO 2 maps for the City of Zurich, Switzerland, derived by statistical modelling utilizing data from a routine passive diffusion sampler network. Atmos Environ. 2015;106:1–10.

40. Neophytou AM, Yiallouros P, Coull BA, Kleanthous S, Pavlou P, Pashiardis S, Laden F. Particulate matter concentrations during desert dust outbreaks and daily mortality in Nicosia, Cyprus. J Eposure Sci Environ Epidemiol. 2013;23(3):275–80.

41. Pearce JR, Richardson EA, Mitchell RJ, Shortt NK. Environmental justice and health: a study of multiple environmental deprivation and geographical inequalities in health in New Zealand. Soc Sci Med. 2011;73(3):410–20.

42. Qi X, Hu W, Mengersen K, Tong S. Socio-environmental drivers and suicide in Australia: Bayesian spatial analysis. BMC Public Health. 2014;14(1):1.

43. Rey G, Jougla E, Fouillet A, Hémon D. Ecological association between a deprivation index and mortality in France over the period 1997–2001:

variations with spatial scale, degree of urbanicity, age, gender and cause of death. BMC Public Health. 2009;9(1):1.

44. Rinner C, Patychuk D, Bassil K, Nasr S, Gower S, Campbell M. The role of maps in neighborhood-level heat vulnerability assessment for the city of Toronto. Cartogr Geogr Inf Sci. 2010;37(1):31–44.

45. Scarano M, Sobrino JA. On the relationship between the sky view factor and the land surface temperature derived by Landsat-8 images in Bari, Italy. Int J Remote Sens. 2015;36(19–20):4820–35.

46. Shi Y, Lau KKL, Ng E. Developing street-level $PM_{2.5}$ and PM_{10} land use regression models in high-density Hong Kong with urban morphological factors. Environ. Sci. Technol. 2016;50(15):8178–87.

47. Shrestha R, Flacke J, Martinez J, Van Maarseveen M. Environmental health related socio-spatial inequalities: identifying "hotspots" of environmental burdens and social vulnerability. Int J Environ Res Public Health. 2016;13(7):691.

48. Smargiassi A, Goldberg MS, Plante C, Fournier M, Baudouin Y, Kosatsky T. Variation of daily warm season mortality as a function of micro-urban heat islands. J Epidemiol Commun Health. 2009;63(8):659–64.

49. Tobías A, Pérez L, Díaz J, Linares C, Pey J, Alastruey A, Querol X. Short-term effects of particulate matter on total mortality during Saharan dust outbreaks: a case-crossover analysis in Madrid (Spain). Sci Total Environ. 2011;412:386–9.

50. Tomlinson CJ, Chapman L, Thornes JE, Baker CJ. Including the urban heat island in spatial heat health risk assessment strategies: a case study for Birmingham, UK. Int J Health Geogr. 2011;10(1):1.

51. Tsai PJ, Lin ML, Chu CM, Perng CH. Spatial autocorrelation analysis of health care hotspots in Taiwan in 2006. BMC Public Health. 2009;9(1):1.

52. Wong CM, Ou CQ, Chan KP, Chau YK, Thach TQ, Yang L, Hedley AJ. The effects of air pollution on mortality in socially deprived urban areas in Hong Kong, China. Environ Health Perspect. 2008;116(9):1189.

53. Wong MS, Nichol JE, Holben B. Desert dust aerosols observed in a humid tropical city: Hong Kong. Int J Remote Sens. 2010;31(4):1043–51.

54. Wong MS, Xiao F, Nichol JE, Fung J, Kim J, Campbell J, Chan PW. A multi-scale hybrid neural network retrieval model for dust storm detection, a study in Asia. Atmos Res. 2015;158–159:89–106.

55. Wong MS, Peng F, Zou B, Shi WZ, Wilson GJ. Spatially analyzing the inequity of the Hong Kong urban heat island by socio-demographic characteristics. Int J Environ Res Public Health. 2016;13(3):317.

56. Yang J, Wong MS, Menenti M, Nichol J. Modeling the effective emissivity of the urban canopy using sky view factor. ISPRS J Photogramm Remote Sens. 2015;105:211–9.

57. Yang J, Wong MS, Menenti M, Nichol J, Voogt J, Krayenhoff ES, Chan PW. Development of an improved urban emissivity model based on sky view factor for retrieving effective emissivity and surface temperature over urban areas. ISPRS J Photogramm Remote Sens. 2016;122:30–40.

58. Yuan C, Ng E, Norford LK. Improving air quality in high-density cities by understanding the relationship between air pollutant dispersion and urban morphologies. Build Environ. 2014;71:245–58.

smokeSALUD: exploring the effect of demographic change on the smoking prevalence at municipality level in Austria

Melanie Tomintz[1*], Bernhard Kosar[2] and Graham Clarke[3]

Abstract

Background: Reducing the smoking population is still high on the policy agenda, as smoking leads to many preventable diseases, such as lung cancer, heart disease, diabetes, and more. In Austria, data on smoking prevalence only exists at the federal state level. This provides an interesting overview about the current health situation, but for regional planning authorities these data are often insufficient as they can hide pockets of high and low smoking prevalence in certain municipalities.

Methods: This paper presents a spatial–temporal change of estimated smokers for municipalities from 2001 and 2011. A synthetic dataset of smokers is built by combining individual large-scale survey data and small area census data using a deterministic spatial microsimulation approach. Statistical analysis, including chi-square test and binary logistic regression, are applied to find the best variables for the simulation model and to validate its results.

Results: As no easy-to-use spatial microsimulation software for non-programmers is available yet, a flexible web-based spatial microsimulation application for health decision support (called simSALUD) has been developed and used for these analyses. The results of the simulation show in general a decrease of smoking prevalence within municipalities between 2001 and 2011 and differences within areas are identified. These results are especially valuable to policy decision makers for future planning strategies.

Conclusions: This case study shows the application of *smokeSALUD* to model the spatial–temporal changes in the smoking population in Austria between 2001 and 2011. This is important as no data on smoking exists at this geographical scale (municipality). However, spatial microsimulation models are useful tools to estimate small area health data and to overcome these problems. The simulations and analysis should support health decision makers to identify hot spots of smokers and this should help to show where to spend health resources best in order to reduce health inequalities.

Keywords: Health decision support, Small area modelling, Deterministic reweighting, simSALUD, Austria, Spatial microsimulation, Web-based application, Smoking, Demographic change, Municipalities

Background

Smoking is directly responsible for many diseases, sometimes leading to death (worldwide this figure is estimated to be around 10 %). In addition, passive smokers are at high risk of also developing smoking-related diseases [1]. The Austrian Government is well known for offering a

*Correspondence: melanie.tomintz@canterbury.ac.nz
[1] GeoHealth Laboratory, Department of Geography, University of Canterbury, Private Bag 4800, Christchurch 8140, New Zealand
Full list of author information is available at the end of the article

generous social support system, including one of the best health care systems in the world. However, the topic of health inequalities has attracted growing attention, both at the European Union (EU) level and in Austria itself. This issue is especially important in the field of health promotion and prevention. An effective resource distribution strategy is required for areas with high demand (e.g. high rates of smoking, obesity, drug addiction) and poor accessibility to health care providers. Health inequalities can be addressed through government actions and policies but need to be identified first. In particular, identifying regional inequalities is essential for the future distribution of government resources. But one of the problems with the official surveys conducted by Statistics Austria is that health related data mainly exists at the federal state level only. This data provides an interesting overview of the health of the nation, but for regional planning purposes these data are often insufficient and provide no reliable estimates below state level. However, spatial microsimulation models are useful tools for estimating small area health data and thus helping to overcome these problems. Many studies have used spatial microsimulation to estimate health care demand [2–4], but in Austria little research exists to date with the exception of the research project SALUD (SpatiAL microsimUlation for Decision support) which focuses on building a spatial microsimulation model for Austria. Within this project a web-based spatial microsimulation application (simSALUD) was developed to estimate, validate and visualize smoking prevalence at the municipality level using deterministic reweighting approaches. Some microsimulation applications exist on the Web [5, 6] but an intensive literature search through current spatial microsimulation frameworks shows that at the moment no easy-to-use web-based spatial microsimulation applications, which includes spatial visualization methods for non-programmers, are available as yet.

This paper focuses on the topic of smoking because smoking is a major risk factor for poor health and premature mortality. As it is based on a poor lifestyle choice, it is in theory preventable. For effective preventive actions at the regional level, it is important to know where high numbers of smokers live and whether significant variations exist in such rates between municipalities. Recent Organisation for Economic Co-operation and Development (OECD) statistics show that 23.2 % of the adult population smoke regularly in Austria, which is 2.2 % above the average across all 41 OECD countries [1]. Austria also tends to follow the general pattern of gender differences across Europe, with higher smoking rates among men (27.3 %) in comparison to women (19.4 %) [7].

The demographic and socio-economic changes between 2001 and 2011 are shown by the census and registered-based census, respectively. According to Statistics Austria, the population count in 2015 was 8,584,926, which is an increase of 209,762 persons (2.4 %) when compared to the population count in 2011. Taking a closer look at population change between 2001 and 2011, there was an increase of 4.2 % (354,218 persons) which was mainly driven by immigration and less by an increase of births over deaths. Out of the nine provinces in Austria, only one province (Carinthia) saw a population decline (2853 persons or 0.5 %). In contrast, population

increase was seen across all other Austrian regions. Vienna had the highest increase with 8.7 % (148,899 persons), followed by Vorarlberg with 5.2 % (19,171 persons) and Tyrol with 5.1 % (36,025 persons). An increase in people aged 25–65 with a tertiary qualification was apparent, especially in the age group 27–36 (7.0 %). There was an increase of 2.4 % for the age group 0–19 years; an increase of only 0.1 % for the age group 20–64 years; but an increase of 2.2 % for the age group 65 and older [8].

The aim of this paper is to estimate changes in smoking prevalence at the municipality level between 2001 and 2011 based on population change in Austria. For this purpose, the *smokeSALUD* package is constructed using a deterministic reweighting spatial microsimulation methodology and implemented in a web-based software application called simSALUD,[1] developed within the funded research project SALUD at the Carinthia University of Applied Sciences in Austria. The simulation algorithm estimates small area data by merging individuals from the national survey data with census data at the municipality level based on common variables (e.g. age, marital status). However, these variables are limited and not comparable between both datasets without additional data processing. This requires careful data manipulation and pre-analyses are required when using survey and census data to build a spatial microsimulation model [9]. Microsimulation is excellent for estimating 'missing data', and as data on smoking prevalence is only available at province level in the health survey by Statistics Austria, this is important for estimating small-area smoking rates. The Austrian Health Surveys were conducted in 1973, 1983, 1991, 1999, 2006/07 and 2014, but with a new design making prior studies not entirely comparable. The data for the latest survey, however, was not accessible until this study was finished. With *smokeSALUD* the aim is to explore the spatial variations in smoking at the municipality level at two different points in time, i.e. 2001 and 2011. This information is highly valuable for health policy decision makers to help to understand whether government smoking prevention strategies appear to be working or not. Austria is one of the last countries that will implement a full smoking ban for cigarettes and e-cigarettes in public places from May 2018. So far, there has only been a partial implementation: dividing smoking and non-smoking rooms in bars and restaurants which has caused severe reconstruction costs for many owners in the food and drink industry. Austria also scores lowest on a tobacco control scale in 2007, 2010 and 2013, as was shown by [10]. This latter report also shows that other countries have proven the success of their smoking policy

---

[1] www.simsalud.org/simsalud.

interventions (such as the UK, Ireland or Iceland) and the model introduced in this paper can help identifying needs at a small geographical scale and to model the impact of successful interventions for Austria. In this way we hope the modelling framework has wider international appeal, providing a framework for examining smoking-related policies across the world and helping to target areas less likely to respond to current policies. But before doing so, the geography of the smoking population for small areas needs to be modelled and understood.

Methods
Methodology and workflow
Spatial microsimulation models have been built since the 1980s and there are different methods for building such models, including deterministic and probabilistic approaches [11]. There are few freely available software packages to implement spatial microsimulation. For this reason, deterministic approaches have been implemented in simSALUD, a web-based spatial microsimulation application. The advantage of using a deterministic over a probabilistic approach is that the model terminates at a unique solution each time it is run. Therefore, adjustments to the input data are immediately obvious as to whether the changes have improved the model outcome or not. *smokeSALUD* is a static model designed to match large scale survey and small area census data based on common key constraints that are most likely to predict the variable of interest; in this case the smoking population. The process can be seen as a form of cloning exercise, where persons from the survey are matched to each small area, in our study the municipality, based on the selected key constraints. A reweighting algorithm thus calculates how well a person with certain characteristics fits the characteristics of persons known to live in a certain small area [12, 13]. Given key population characteristics we can estimate whether this person is a smoker or not and this information is also reweighted to provide the results for each single municipality. The models for smokeSALUD are run using the Web application simSALUD.

The structure of the model process is shown in Fig. 1 and each step is described in detail below. The underlying algorithm is explained elsewhere [14]. The structure can be divided into five steps (data processing, pre-analyses, model execution, validation and the visualization of the simulated output) and is described according to the case study in the next subsections. Steps 3–5 can be executed directly within the simSALUD application, which has been developed by the authors as part of the research project SALUD.

Step 1: Data and data processing
Three datasets are relevant for this case study. The first dataset is the Austrian Health Interview Survey (AHIS) for 2006/07 which holds variables for demographic, socio-economic and health related information of 15,474 individuals aged 15 or above at the federal state level. The dataset also includes the variable "number of daily smokers", which is the health variable of interest and (for each person) a weight to compensate for the bias of the survey that corresponds to the total population. The second dataset is the 2001 census for municipalities and the third dataset is the registered-based 2011 census for municipalities. Both census datasets (2001 and 2011) have demographic and socio-economic information concerning the Austrian population but no health related data is included. There are 2379 municipalities in Austria and the 2001 census showed a population of 6,679,444 (people 15 years and over) and the 2011 registered-based census recorded a population of 7,174,250 persons (people 15 years and over). In this first step all datasets are tested for completeness and data cleaning is conducted if required.

Step 2: Statistical pre-analysis
Statistical analyses prior to building a spatial simulation model are important in order to identify the best predictors (i.e. characteristics of a person) of the variable being estimated—in this case the number of smokers. For this study, the chi-square test, regression analysis and t-test are applied within the statistics software IBM SPSS Statistics 21.0. In addition, an extensive literature review on the influences and characteristics of smokers was undertaken. This is necessary because creating synthetic microdata requires linking datasets based on common variables, but those variables must also be important for estimating the key 'missing data'. For a detailed discussion of the role of the constraint variables and the choice of constraints in microsimulation see [3, 15, 16]. Previous literature [2, 17, 18] indicates that smoking status is strongly predicted by variables such as age, sex and social status which are available in the AHIS. For the spatial–temporal analysis, it is also necessary to have the same variables in both census datasets (census 2001 and 2011). Otherwise adjustment procedures need to be undertaken between the datasets in order to have the same base population.

The chi-square method is chosen because it can be measured at an ordinal or nominal level (i.e. categorical data). Calculating a statistical correlation method is not possible because this would require measuring both variables at the interval or ratio level (i.e. continuous scale) which is not the case for this study. However, chi-square

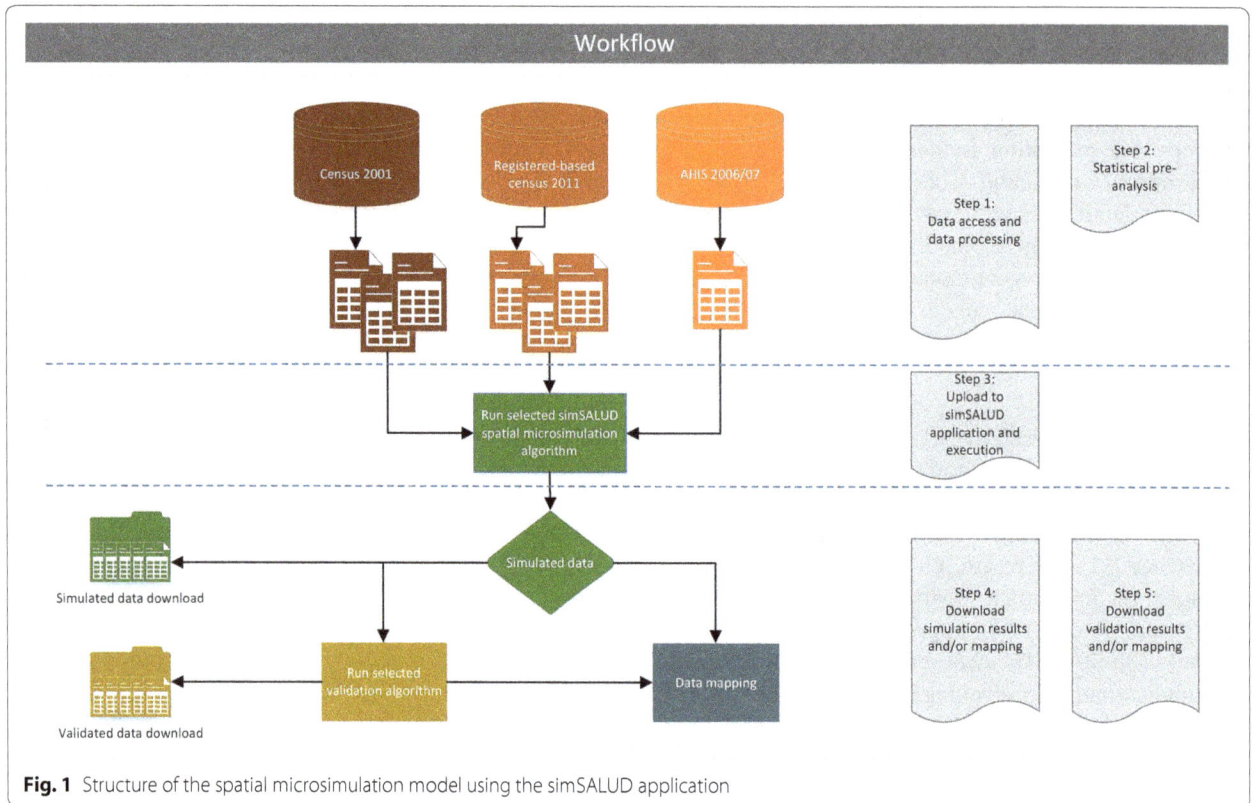

Fig. 1 Structure of the spatial microsimulation model using the simSALUD application

is used to find a possible relationship between two categorical variables. The measurement parameters for Phi and Cramer's V, which vary between 0 and 1, show the same value for all variables. The closer the value is to 1, the stronger is the relationship between the dependent and independent variable. The binary logistic regression is used to predict the probability that an observation falls into one of two categories of a dependent variable, based on one or more independent variables that can be either continuous or categorical. The output also calculates the Cox & Snell R-square and Nagelkerke R-square values, which are both methods of calculating the explained variation. Another statistical test applied is the independent samples t-test that compares the means between two unrelated groups on the same continuous, dependent variable. For example, it can be used to understand whether education level differs between smokers and non-smokers.

Tables 1 and 2 show the results for all constraints using the chi-square and binary logistic regression analyses. The values show the results for the final constraints chosen after the pre-analysis process which tested different variable combinations until the best validation results were found. The results in Table 1 show that there is a statistically significant association (p < 0.001) between daily smokers and these chosen constraints, although

the strength of association between the variables is weak (Phi/Cramer's V > 0.5 high association). Phi and Cramer's V show the highest strength of association between daily smokers and the constraint age (0.240), in contrast to education which shows the lowest value of 0.068 between the final selected constraints.

The explained variation through the binary logistic regression test ranges from 7.7 to 11.8 %. The results for each sub-constraint shown in Table 2 can be defined (one example for each constraint) as follows: by an increase of one (5 years in age), the odds of being a smoker are lower by a factor of 0.892 (ranges from 0.876 to 0.907); the likelihood of smoking decreases by a factor of 0.364 for those with a tertiary education as opposed to people without A-levels (ranges from 0.296 to 0.446); married people are 0.873 times less likely to smoke than single persons (ranges from 0.781 to 0.975); the odds of smoking are higher for females by 0.734 times (ranges from 0.676 to 0.796); and employees are 1.833 times more likely to smoke than non-employed persons (includes: retired persons, pupils, students, etc.: ranges from 1.673 to 2.007). Rows with no values are defined as reference categories.

Further, the t-test results verify the importance of the constraint "education" (i.e. the highest level of education) and "age" seen in the binary logistic regression. All other

Table 1 Summary of the chi-square analysis relating to the category "daily smokers"

Constraint	Chi square	
	Symmetric measures Phi/Cramer's V	Asymptotic significance (2-sided)
Age	0.240	$p < 0.001$
Education	0.068	$p < 0.001$
Marital status	0.180	$p < 0.001$
Sex	0.083	$p < 0.001$
Occupational status	0.186	$p < 0.001$

Table 2 Summary of the binary logistic regression analysis relating to the category "daily smokers"

Constraint	Sub-constraint	Binary logistic			95 % C.I. for EXP(B)	
		B	Significance	Expected (B)	Lower	Upper
Age	15 above	−0.115	$p < 0.001$	0.892	0.876	0.907
Education	University	−1.011	$p < 0.001$	0.364	0.296	0.446
	With A-level	−0.485	$p < 0.001$	0.616	0.548	0.691
	Without A-level					
Marital status	Single					
	Married	−0.135	$p < 0.017$	0.873	0.781	0.975
	Widowed	−0.414	$p < 0.001$	0.661	0.521	0.837
	Divorced	0.894	$p < 0.001$	2.446	2.063	2.899
Sex	Male					
	Female	−0.309	$p < 0.001$	0.734	0.676	0.796
Occupational status	Employees	0.606	$p < 0.001$	1.833	1.673	2.007
	Employer	0.188	$p < 0.030$	1.207	1.012	1.438
	Non-employed					

constraints are not applicable for the t-test because the dependent variable needs to be measured on a continuous scale (i.e. it is measured at the interval or ratio level). In this study, the level of education ranges from "university degree" to "no A-level degree", whereas the independent variable "daily smokers", consist of two groups: "daily smokers" and "never or never smoked daily". Results from the t-test show that daily smokers are statistically significant for lower educated (2.80 ± 0.476) compared to "never or never smoked daily people" (2.71 ± 0.585). Further the study found that daily smokers are statistically significant for younger persons (5.62 ± 2.88) compared to people who "never" or "never smoked daily" (7.20 ± 3.36).

The census dataset from 2001 and the register-based census dataset from 2011 include demographic and socio-economic variables for people aged 15 and above at the municipality level, but no health related data. As mentioned above, these constraints must be available in both datasets at the municipality level, as well as comparable with the survey dataset so that the deterministic reweighting methodology can be applied and the output gained from the model will be as accurate as possible [9]. Table 3 shows the demographic change between the populations for both datasets for each sub-constraint. It can be seen that the constraint 'age' (with its sub-constraints 30–34 and 35–39) shows a strong decrease of individuals in that category, whereas other sub-constraints such as 45–49, or university graduates, show a strong increase of individuals over the 10 year period.

For our final model smokeSALUD five constraint variables consisting of 23 sub-constraints (as seen in Table 3) are defined: education (3 sub-constraints), sex (2 sub-constraints), age (11 sub-constraints), marital status (4 sub-constraints), and occupational status (3 sub-constraints).

Step 3: simSALUD model execution
The first algorithm implemented within simSALUD is a deterministic combinatorial optimisation reweighting

Table 3 Comparison of all constraints of all small areas between 2001 and 2011 (age 15+)

Constraint	Sub-con-straint	2001	2011	Difference in %
Age	15–19	483,957	488,818	0.99
	20–24	472,777	527,675	10.40
	25–29	539,031	552,783	2.49
	30–34	668,281	538,307	−24.14
	35–39	704,872	564,817	−24.80
	40–44	625,783	675,242	7.32
	45–49	525,207	710,388	26.07
	50–54	514,535	626,162	17.83
	55–59	452,265	517,280	12.57
	60–64	451,057	480,665	6.16
	65 above	1,241,679	1,492,113	16.78
Education	University	497,754	831,629	40.15
	With A-level	763,430	976,652	21.83
	Without A-level	5,418,260	5,365,969	−0.97
Marital status	Single	2,060,472	2,400,266	14.16
	Married	3,527,786	3,562,949	0.99
	Widowed	573,318	573,070	−0.04
	Divorced	517,868	637,965	18.83
Sex	Male	3,195,725	3,465,023	7.77
	Female	3,483,719	3,709,227	6.08
Occupational status	Employees	3,541,877	3,801,016	6.82
	Employer	418,383	453,728	7.79
	Non-employed	2,719,184	2,919,506	6.86
Total popula-tion		6,679,444	7,174,250	6.90

approach [2, 4, 14, 19, 20], combining (non-spatial) national survey data (AHIS 2006/07) with the (spatial) census data. Model 1 uses the census data from the year 2001 based on the constraint variables selected in step 2 (age, education, marital status, sex, occupational status). The simulation for model 2 uses the same constraint variables but the population data is taken from the registered-based census data for 2011. In contrast to a probabilistic approach, this reweighing technique is an iterative process with no random sampling where the ordering of the constraints is not an issue [21]. Within the simSALUD application, the prepared.csv files can be uploaded and the simulation steps are guided through a wizard for user-friendly software handling (see Fig. 2a, b). Additionally, the application has an integerisation method implemented after [19] to only allocate whole people to the simulation output. The results of the simulation can also be exported after the model run for further spatial analyses in common geographic information software (GIS) products.

Step 4: Validation

After executing the model, the results are validated to ensure the model estimates are robust [22]. Distinguish between external and internal validation. External validation requires additional comparable external data sources which are usually not available, as the point of the simulation is to estimate 'missing data'. This was unfortunately also the case for this study. There are however exceptions to the norm. For example, the New Zealand census includes data on the number of smokers for small geographical areas and this has proved to be a great source to validate simulated data on smoking patterns and rates see

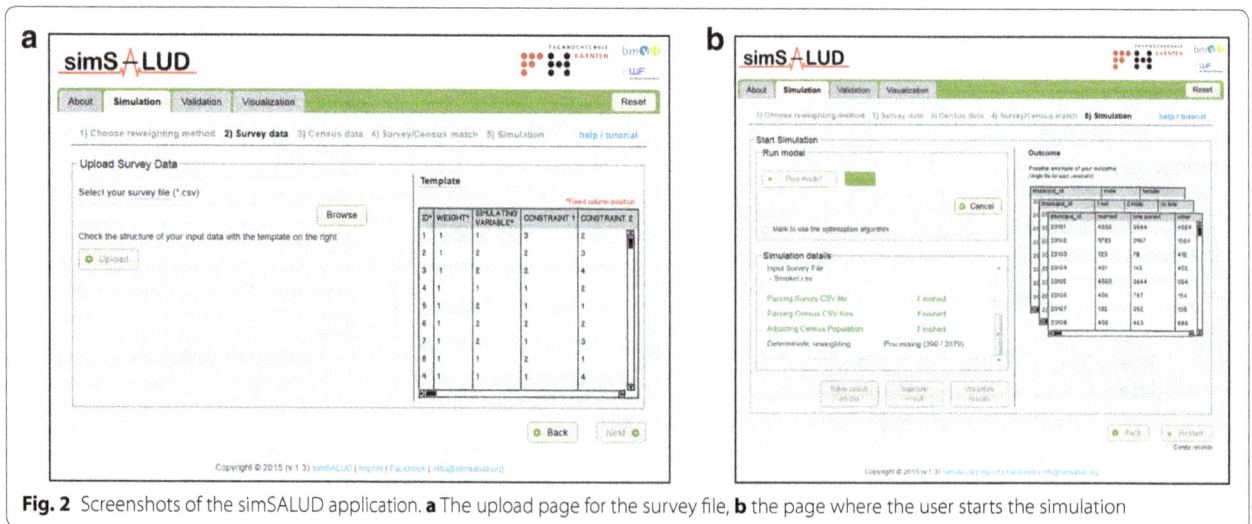

Fig. 2 Screenshots of the simSALUD application. **a** The upload page for the survey file, **b** the page where the user starts the simulation

[3]. This type of study has helped to show the validity and robustness of small-area estimation techniques.

Internal validation refers to the ability of the model to replicate census data estimated at the individual level to spatial scales where the data is available. For internal validation, different statistical methods are offered within this Web application to achieve this. Currently, seven tests (see Fig. 3) are implemented from which the user can choose from, i.e. total absolute error (TAE), total absolute error with percentage of total regions, standardized absolute error (SAE), percentage standardized absolute error (PSAE), independent samples t-test, correlation coefficient (Pearson correlation) and simple regression.

This is a major advantage of simSALUD as the modeller does not have to use an additional statistics package and, further, he/she can map the validation results immediately (see Step 5: Visualization). After finishing the validation run the user can also either save the results as a zip file for further analyses or visualize the results immediately in the application (or transfer to a common GIS package). Additionally the user can start a new simulation and validation by changing the number of constraints to see the influence that each constraint can have on the simulated results.

Step 5: Visualization

The simulation and validation outputs can be visualized in the form of a map (Fig. 4) and/or be linked with other data and external software for additional spatial analysis. The simSALUD Web-based application provides an interactive map with standard interaction controls that allows direct mapping without additional Geoinformation software or printouts. The map representation was implemented with Environmental Systems Research Institute (ESRI)'s JavaScript API (Application Programming Interface) with ArcGIS for Server. All spatial and non-spatial data (input and simulation results) are stored in a post-GIS database. The map representation allows the simulation results to be visualised according to any selected constraint. Additionally, the application provides different classification methods, i.e. equal interval, quantile and natural breaks, for mapping the results. Additional features are the resizing (maximize and minimize) of the map and the print feature.

Results

The spatial–temporal analysis estimates the change of smokers in Austria from 2001 and 2011. The following two subsections describe the model validation results, as well as the estimated smoking prevalence illustrated as a map.

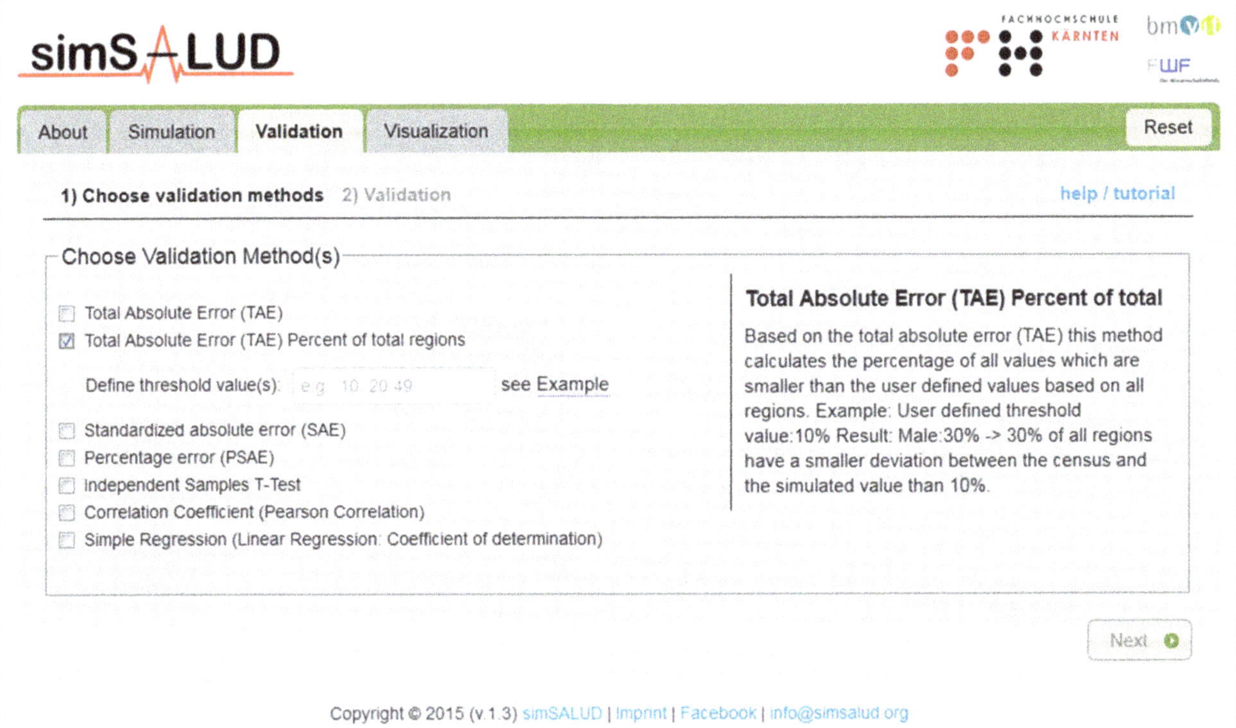

Fig. 3 Screenshots of the simSALUD application which shows the menu to select the desired validation method

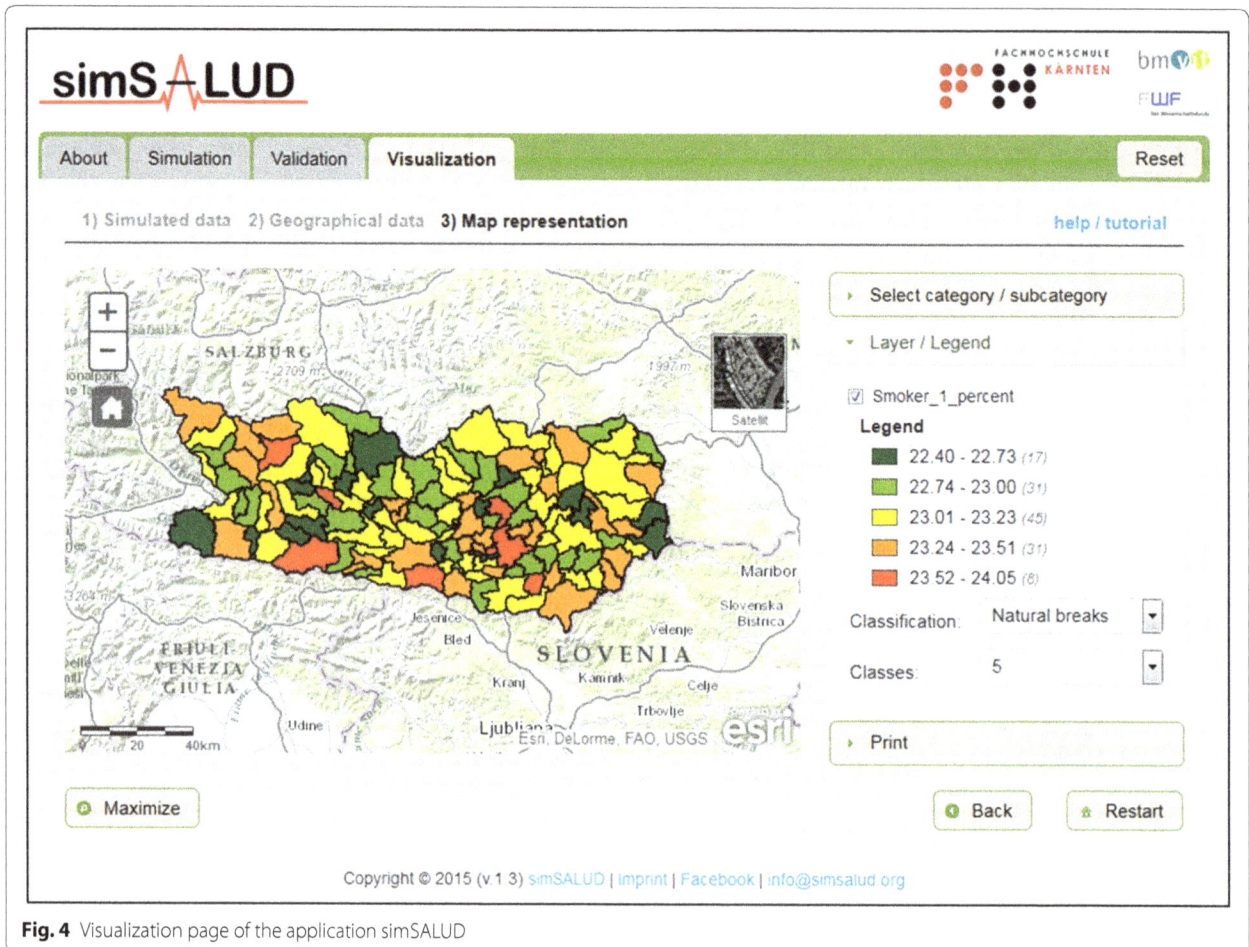

Fig. 4 Visualization page of the application simSALUD

Model validation

Model 1 (matching the 2001 census data with the AHIS 2006/07) and model 2 (matching the 2011 registered-based census data with the AHIS 2006/07) are validated using internal statistical tests. Table 4 shows the results of the PSAE and the linear regression for all sub-constraints. The PSAE shows the total under- or over-estimated values in comparison to the actual values for all sub-constraints. For 2001, the difference range from 0.4 % (sub-constraint: employer) to 6.9 % (sub-constraint: employees and non-employed) of the total population of each area. In 2011, the lowest value is 0.4 % (sub-constraint: employer) and the highest value is 8.0 % (sub-constraint: 65 above). A higher value shows a greater difference between the simulated and actual data for a particular sub-constraint.

The linear regression analyses for all constraint variables show a good fit, as an ideal fit between the simulated and census data would show a coefficient of determination very close to 1. This analysis indicates a very high coefficient of determination for all variables (0.96–0.99)

for 2001 and 2011. The lowest value (with 0.96) is seen for the sub-constraints "widowed" and "age 65 above". The variable "married" has a high coefficient for 2001 (Fig. 5a) and 2011 (Fig. 5b), where the simulated values are very close to the actual census dataset in comparison to the variable "widowed" where there is a higher variance between the simulated and the actual census data for both years 2001 (Fig. 5c) and 2011 (Fig. 5d).

Other possible constraints to predict smokers, for example "nationality", are tested but did not show a significant improvement in the fit of the model. If the constraints fit well after the pre-analyses and validation procedure, then we can be confident that the simulated health variable (in this case "daily smokers") also fits well and the results are robust.

Estimated smoking prevalence

After running the simulation model for 2001, smoking rates between 19.0 and 31.6 % were estimated and for 2011, between 14.0 and 31.2 % (at the municipality level) (Fig. 6a, b). It was found that the average number of

Table 4 Summary of the validated model outputs for all constraints between 2001 and 2011

Constraint	Sub-constraint	PSAE		R²	
		2001	2011	2001	2011
Age	15–19	0.87	0.77	0.988	0.992
	20–24	0.85	1.48	0.993	0.993
	25–29	2.57	3.76	0.991	0.988
	30–34	2.38	2.21	0.999	0.999
	35–39	1.95	1.87	0.999	0.998
	40–44	0.86	1.07	0.998	0.997
	45–49	0.63	1.01	0.998	0.996
	50–54	0.52	0.66	0.996	0.992
	55–59	0.95	1.15	0.996	0.990
	60–64	1.93	2.12	0.993	0.988
	65 above	6.17	8.01	0.984	0.977
Education	University	3.38	4.36	0.997	0.997
	With A-level	3.18	3.39	0.998	0.997
	Without A-level	6.56	7.75	0.998	0.996
Marital status	Single	5.11	4.55	0.998	0.997
	Married	2.25	2.26	0.999	0.997
	Widowed	3.49	3.11	0.973	0.962
	Divorced	0.59	0.84	0.999	0.995
Sex	Male	4.91	4.81	0.999	0.999
	Female	4.91	4.81	0.999	0.999
Occupational status	Employees	6.90	6.68	0.999	0.9989
	Employer	0.39	0.42	0.997	0.9958
	Non-employed	6.85	6.93	0.996	0.9956

people who smoke slightly decreased over time (25.4 % in 2001 and 24.7 % in 2011) based on demographic change. The province Burgenland in the east of Austria shows lower smoking rates as expected, therefore the model underestimates for this province, and after discussions with governmental tobacco control groups, reasons are not fully explained yet as to while Burgenland had such a high smoking rate in the national survey 2006/07. The geography of the results show lower smoking rates in provinces with a higher proportion of rural areas. A decrease of smoking rates in the more rural municipalities can be seen particularly in Carinthia, Styria and Lower Austria. This is likely to an increase of elderly, married or widowed, people, as it is known that birth rates reduce, young people are moving into cities and past tobacco control was not strongly availably and effective, respectively.

Figure 7 shows the spatial variation over time (between the years 2001 and 2011) for the number of estimated smokers. The map identifies a slight increase in the number of people smoking in some municipalities (with the highest values in northern parts of Styria and West Tyrol when aggregating from municipality level), but the vast majority of areas (especially in the northern parts of Carinthia and the south of Salzburg) show a decrease in the number of smokers between 2001 and 2011 (see brighter coloured municipalities). An interesting fact is that the municipalities with the highest increase (Namlos: 5.51 %) and highest decrease (Unterperfuss: 8.11 %) are both located in the province of Tyrol. Overall, the slight decrease in daily smokers based on demographic change could be due to the increase in the number of well-educated people, as education is a significant (negative) predictor of being a smoker. Further, population aging is likely to be another main reason, as there is an increase of elderly persons over time and the elderly are less likely to smoke. Both models show a west-east divide in smoking behaviour. To note is the decrease for all municipalities in Salzburg, when only with a very minor percentage. Further investigations in collaboration with governmental health departments could help to explore other possible reasons for higher and lower smoking rates in certain areas and what regional interventions these regions might benefit most.

Discussion

A limitation of the *smokeSALUD* model itself is the availability of the same variables between the census data for both 2001 and 2011. Not all variables are the same between the two data collection periods (e.g. different subclasses) and therefore restrictions have to be accepted. The reasons for the mismatch might include the change in the survey method (from paper survey to electronic registered-based survey). However, Statistics Austria plans that in future the registered-based census for certain variables will be published annually, which will be an advantage for future models. Also the forthcoming AHIS will provide further interesting results in terms of changes in the size of the smoking population.

This study also found that the choice and number of constraint variables strongly impact the simulation results for the currently implemented static deterministic reweighting approaches. The advantage of such approach is that the impact of changes relating to input variables can be immediately measured, as it is a deterministic approach. For example, does the constraint variable "nationality" have a positive or negative influence on the model output? Therefore, several tests to find the optimal model of *smokeSALUD* were conducted. Also experiments with the sub-constraints were undertaken and it was found that different age groups did not have a great impact and therefore all eleven age groups were modelled. It is important to use variables that are very strong predictors and significantly correlated with the variable being estimated. Unfortunately the number of census constraints is limited in Austria: for instance,

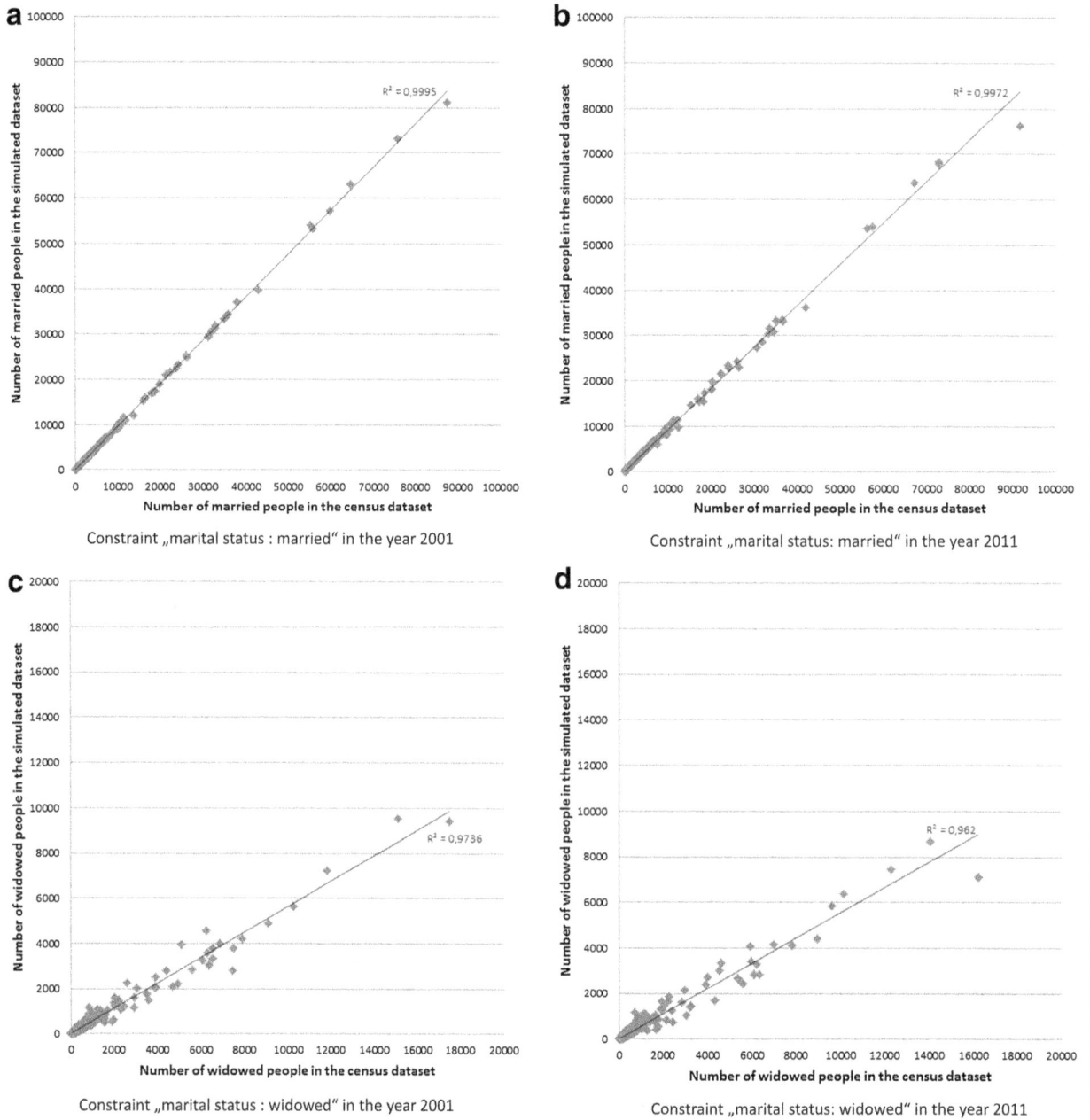

Fig. 5 Validation results as linear regression models (comparing census and simulated data) for two selected constraints in 2001 and 2011, **a** married 2001, **b** married 2011, **c** widowed 2001, **d** widowed 2011

income could be an important predictor variable, but this data is available in the health survey data only and not in the census data, and is therefore not suitable to include in the model.

The model results could also benefit from additional external model validation, in addition to internal validation. Nationwide, there is no data on smoking prevalence for municipalities available, but alternatives could

include carrying out a survey for some municipalities and potentially adjusting the model based on the results. Also, there might exist such data within an independent governmental survey for a particular region in Austria. However, the availability of such surveys is not known to the authors.

In spatial modelling, the modified area unit problem (MAUP) is a commonly discussed issue, as it can affect

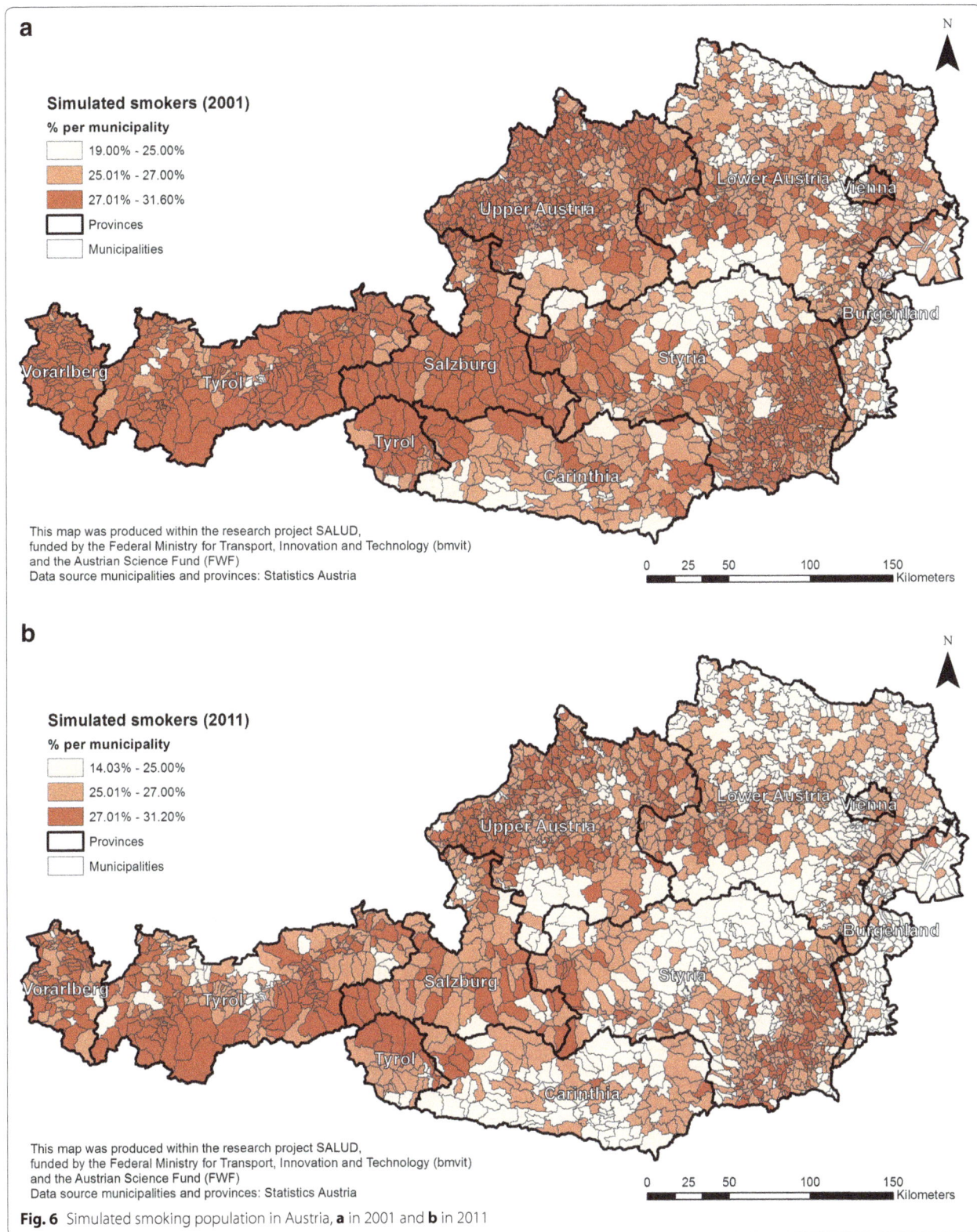

Fig. 6 Simulated smoking population in Austria, **a** in 2001 and **b** in 2011

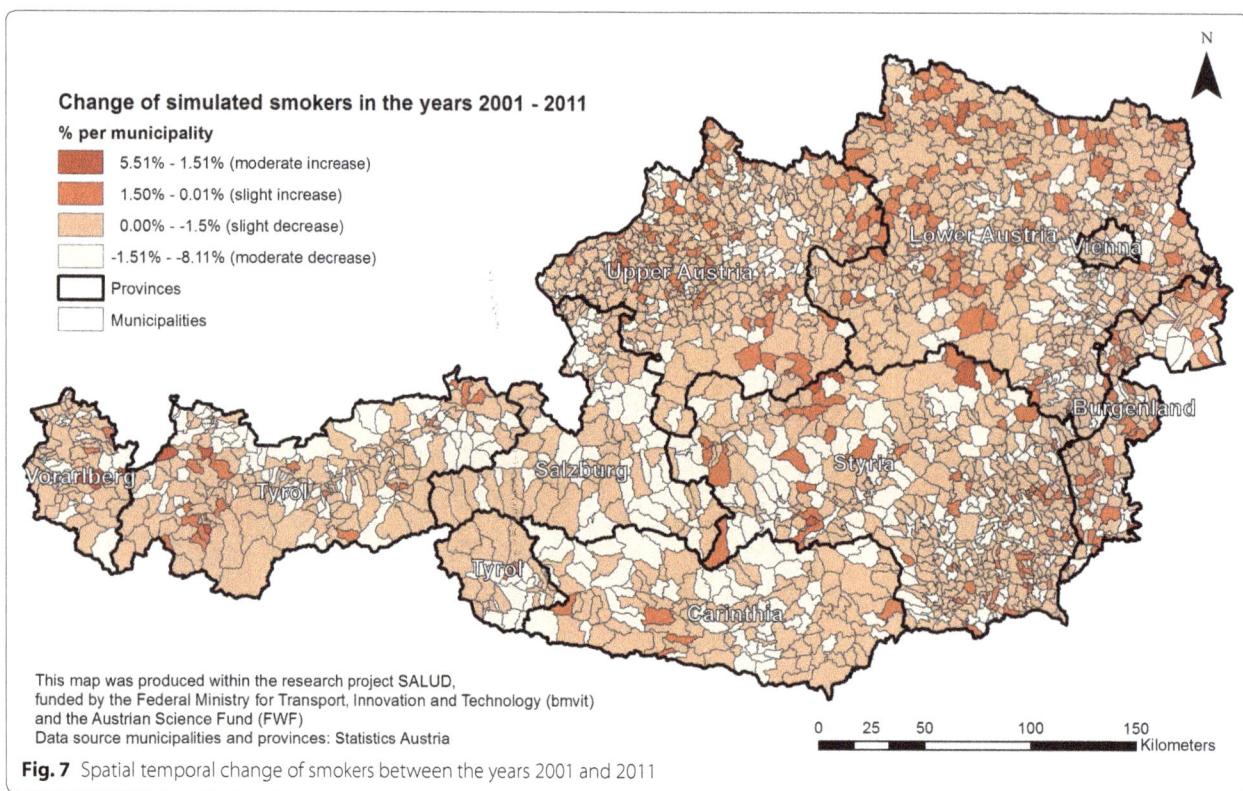

Fig. 7 Spatial temporal change of smokers between the years 2001 and 2011

the outcome depending on the spatial unit chosen. The advantage of spatial microsimulation modelling is to work with individual data that will be matched to the chosen small area level unit based on common constraints. This means that individuals that have the same constraints are allocated to the small areas. The MAUP therefore have very little effect in this case (see further discussion in [23, 24]).

In an international context, the application simSALUD is freely available to anyone and this means people from all over the world can access or install it on their machines. Further, simSALUD is not limited to health studies only, as the underlying algorithms can be applied in other disciplines, such as economics or environmental science. A main advantage of simSALUD for smoking is that it offers a framework for testing the impact of smoking policies in different parts of the world. Using simSALUD policy makers could estimate smoking rates prior to the implementation of any policy and then again some years after its introduction. Although policy makers will know national responses to the policy (in terms of the overall numbers of persons quitting smoking) they can use simSALUD to estimate small-area changes and hence allow them to rethink strategies in areas which seemed to have resisted change the most. For these regions other policies may be more appropriate, such as increasing the

price of tobacco or adding more stop-smoking clinics. Thus, it is hoped that simSALUD can be implemented worldwide in the future and not just used for Austrian data. For example, simSALUD is currently being tested in New Zealand using New Zealand census and health survey data.

Regarding policy, spatial microsimulation is very powerful as it allows to spatially model 'what-if' scenarios to identify the impact that certain interventions could have on certain population groups. Also important is the identification of areas most likely to expect highest and lowest impact of a specific intervention. An interesting future research project would be to take successfully proven interventions in other countries and apply these changes in a host country using simSALUD. For example what is the impact on the number of smokers when raising the legal age of purchasing cigarettes from 16 to 18 years and which areas would benefit most and least from this intervention (based on a region's age profile)? Further steps could then be to link this analysis to economic factors to identify the impact of the costs that this intervention involves in relation to the number of smokers quitting (a type of cost-benefit analysis). The latter is especially interesting in identifying most beneficial interventions given available public health budgets. simSALUD not only allows us to specify particular population groups that can be modelled, for example less educated women in the age of 16–24 who are regular smokers, but also to target specific regions that are of high concern of the government, especially in terms of reducing health inequalities.

Conclusions and outlook

This case study shows the application of *smokeSALUD* for modelling the spatial–temporal changes in the smoking population in Austria between 2001 and 2011. This is important as Austria has one of the highest smoking rates in Europe and no data on smoking exists at the municipality level. Policy makers can benefit from such data and spatial analysis in the future to help target specific areas of high need and hence try and reduce smoking prevalence. To build the model a deterministic reweighting algorithm was used that was implemented within the application simSALUD. This spatial simulation model matched data from the AHIS 2006/07 and the census and registered-based census data for the years 2001 and 2011 respectively. Results showed that there was a slight decrease in smoking rates of 0.6 % between the decades. This decline is thought to have been driven by the high increase (40 %) of those in tertiary education who are less likely to smoke and by the aging population, as older people are less likely to smoke. In particular, the province of Salzburg shows the highest decrease (1.6 %) of the smoking population whereas some municipalities in Tyrol show the highest increase. Not much change was seen in the existing west-east divide of the smoking prevalence. Regarding absolute numbers of smokers, all major cities have highest numbers in comparison to rural areas. This can be explained because of the high population size and contributes less to other factors. The findings of the study identified areas with slight and moderate increase of smoking prevalence and more research is needed to explore possible reasons for the increase, other than an increase in higher educated and elderly people. The model was validated using the statistical tests, the PSAE, logistic regression and the t-test, where the input constraints (census data) were compared with the simulated constraints. All three tests showed (for each model) acceptable and very good values (e.g.: high coefficients of determination) so that we can be confident that our model is robust.

The results presented in this paper are also being presented and discussed with various governmental health departments in Austria to highlight the importance of health data at the municipality level and the advantage of integrating this modelling algorithm into simSALUD. This package can help to support health care planners to identify variations in smoking rates within small areas, as such data is currently not available in health surveys. Further collaborative investigations could explore possible additional reasons for higher and lower smoking rates in certain municipalities. In addition, current policy initiatives around smoking prevention could be analysed and what-if scenarios for future modelling could be defined so that specific population groups are targeted. Possible links to the location of stop smoking services are of high interest: for instance, 'how many smokers reside within a certain distance of stop smoking services?' Where would be the optimal set of locations for the provision of such services? Non-spatial initiatives, for example increasing cigarettes prices, could also be tested to see if these would be effective, especially in localities with lower income residents (using any data which might be a good proxy for income)? see also [25, 26]. Such simulations and analysis, therefore, could give excellent support to health policy makers who are tasked to reduce smoking.

Abbreviations

AHIS: Austrian Health Interview Survey; API: Application Programming Interface; CO: Combinatorial Optimization; ESRI: Environmental Systems Research Institute; EU: European Union; GIS: Geographic Information Software; IPF: Iterative Proportional Fitting; MAUP: Modified Area Unit Problem; OECD: Organisation for Economic Co-operation and Development; PSAE: Percentage Standardized Absolute Error; SAE: Standardized Absolute Error; SALUD: SpAtiaL SimUlation for Decision support; TAE: Total Absolute Error.

Authors' contributions

MT carried out parts of the analysis, wrote certain sections of the manuscript and was responsible for the finalisation. BK designed the study, carried out parts of the analysis and drafted the manuscript. GC acted as an international collaborator and helped to write sections of the manuscript. All authors read and approved the final manuscript.

Author details

GeoHealth Laboratory, Department of Geography, University of Canterbury, Private Bag 4800, Christchurch 8140, New Zealand. [2] Geoinformation and Environmental Technologies, Carinthia University of Applied Sciences, Europastrasse 4, 9524 Villach, Austria. [3] School of Geography, University of Leeds, Leeds LS2 9JT, UK.

Acknowledgements

This Research Project SALUD is funded by the Federal Ministry for Transport, Innovation and Technology (bmvit) and the Austrian Science Fund (FWF): TRP280-G16. We would like to thank STATISTICS Austria for providing the data and Victor Garcia-Barrios for the excellent cooperation during the Project.

Competing interests

The authors declare that they have no competing interests.

Funding

This Research Project SALUD is funded by the Federal Ministry for Transport, Innovation and Technology (bmvit) and the Austrian Science Fund (FWF): TRP280-G16.

References

1. OECD Factbook 2013—statistics—OECD iLibrary [Internet]. [cited 2016Jul25]. http://www.oecd-ilibrary.org/economics/oecd-factbook-2013_factbook-2013-en.

2. Tomintz MN, Clarke GP, Rigby JE. Planning the location of stop smoking services at the local level: a geographic analysis. J Smok Cessat. 2009;4:61–73.

3. Smith DM, Pearce JR, Harland K. Can a deterministic spatial microsimulation model provide reliable small-area estimates of health behaviours? An example of smoking prevalence in New Zealand. Health Place. 2011;17:618–24.

4. Edwards KL, Clarke GP. SimObesity: combinatorial optimisation (deterministic) model. In: Tanton R, Edwards KL, editors. Spatial microsimulation: a reference guide for users. London: Springer; 2013. p. 69–85.

5. Harland K. Microsimulation Model user guide (flexible modelling framework). NCRM Working Paper. UK: NCRM; 2013.

6. Lovelace R, Dumont M. Spatial microsimulation with R. Boca Raton: Chapman & Hall CRC; 2016.

7. Statistics Austria. Jahrbuch der Gesundheitsstatistik 2011. Vienna: Statistics Austria; 2012.

8. Statistics Austria. Bevölkerung zu Jahres- und Quartalsanfang [Internet]. Bevölkerung zu Jahres-/Quartalsanfang. 2015 [cited 2016Jul25]. http://www.statistik.at/web_de/statistiken/menschen_und_gesellschaft/bevoelkerung/bevoelkerungsstand_und_veraenderung/bevoelkerung_zu_jahres-_quartalsanfang/index.html.

9. Cassells R, Miranti R, Harding A. Building a static spatial microsimulation model: data preparation. In: Tanton R, Edwards KL, editors. Spatial microsimulation: a reference guide for users. New York: Springer; 2013. p. 9–16.

10. Joossens L, Raw M. The tobacco control scale 2013 in Europe. Turkey: A report of the Association of European Cancer Leagues; 2014.

11. Tanton R. A review of spatial microsimulation methods. Int J Spat Microsimul. 2014;7(1):4–25.

12. Tanton R, Williamson P, Harding A. Comparing two methods of reweighting a survey file to small area data. Int J Microsimul. 2014;7(1):76–99.

13. Lovelace R, Birkin M, Ballas D, van Leeuwen E. Evaluating the performance of iterative proportional fitting for spatial microsimulation: new tests for an established technique. J Artif Soc Soc Simul. 2015;18(2):21.

14. Tomintz MN, Garcia-Barrios VM. simSALUD—towards a health decision support system for regional planning. In: Lombard J, Clarke GP, Stern E, editors. Applied spatial modelling and planning. London: Routledge; 2016. p. 230–48.

15. Anderson B. Estimating small-area income deprivation: an iterative proportional fitting approach. In: Tanton R, Edwards KL, editors. Spatial microsimulation: a reference guide for users. London: Springer; 2013. p. 49–67.

16. Burden S, Steel D. Constraint choice for spatial microsimulation. Popul Space Place. 2015;. doi:10.1002/psp.1942.

17. Yach D, Wipfli H, Hammond R, Glantz S. Globalization and tobacco. In: Kawachi I, Wamala S, editors. Globalization and health. New York: Oxford University Press; 2007. p. 39–67.

18. Moon G, Barnett R, Pearce J. Ethnic spatial segregation and tobacco consumption: a multilevel repeated cross-sectional analysis of smoking prevalence in Urban New Zealand, 1981–1996. Environ Plan A. 2010;42:469–86.

19. Ballas D, Clarke G, Dorling D, Eyre H, Thomas B, Rossiter D. SimBritain: a spatial microsimulation approach to population dynamics. Popul Space Place. 2005;11:13–34.

20. O'Donoghue C, Farell N, Morrissey K, Lennon J, Ballas D, Clarke G, et al. The SMILE model: construction and calibration. In: O'Donoghue C, Ballas B, editors. Spatial microsimulation for rural policy analysis. New York: Springer; 2013. p. 55–86.

21. Rahman A, Harding A, Tanton R, Shuangzhe L. Methodological issues in spatial microsimulation modelling for small area estimation. Int J Microsimul. 2010;3:3–22. http://microsimulation.org/ijm/v3_2/volume3issue2/1_ijm_47proof.pdf.

22. Edwards KL, Clarke GP, Thomas J, Forman D. Internal and external validation of spatial microsimulation models: small area estimates of adult obesity. Appl Spat Anal Policy. 2010;4:281–300.

23. Tanton R, Edwards KL, Tanton R, Harding A, McNamara J. Spatial microsimulation using a generalised regression model. In: Tanton R, Edwards KL, editors. Spatial microsimulation: a reference guide for users. New York: Springer; 2013. p. 87–104.

24. Lovelace R, Ballas D, Watson M. A spatial microsimulation approach for the analysis of commuter patterns: from individual to regional levels. J Transp Geogr. 2014;34:282–96.

25. Chaloupka FJ, Straif K, Leon ME. Effectiveness of tax and price policies in tobacco control. Tobacco Control. 2010;20:235–8.

26. Ross H, Blecher E, Yan L, Hyland A. Do cigarette prices motivate smokers to quit? New evidence from the ITC survey. Addiction. 2010;106:609–19.

12

Spatial analyzes of HLA data in Rio Grande do Sul, south Brazil: genetic structure and possible correlation with autoimmune diseases

Juliano André Boquett[1,2†] [iD], Marcelo Zagonel-Oliveira[1,3†], Luis Fernando Jobim[4], Mariana Jobim[4], Luiz Gonzaga Jr.[1,3], Maurício Roberto Veronez[1,3], Nelson Jurandi Rosa Fagundes[1,2†] and Lavínia Schüler-Faccini[1,2*]

Abstract

Background: HLA genes are the most polymorphic of the human genome and have distinct allelic frequencies in populations of different geographical regions of the world, serving as genetic markers in ancestry studies. In addition, specific HLA alleles may be associated with various autoimmune and infectious diseases. The bone marrow donor registry in Brazil is the third largest in the world, and it counts with genetic typing of HLA-A, -B, and -DRB1. Since 1991 Brazil has maintained the DATASUS database, a system fed with epidemiological and health data from compulsory registration throughout the country.

Methods: In this work, we perform spatial analysis and georeferencing of HLA genetic data from more than 86,000 bone marrow donors from Rio Grande do Sul (RS) and data of hospitalization for rheumatoid arthritis, multiple sclerosis and Crohn's disease in RS, comprising the period from 1995 to 2016 obtained through the DATASUS system. The allele frequencies were georeferenced using Empirical Bayesian Kriging; the diseases prevalence were georeferenced using Inverse Distance Weighted and cluster analysis for both allele and disease were performed using Getis-Ord Gi* method. Spearman's test was used to test the correlation between each allele and disease.

Results: The results indicate a HLA genetic structure compatible with the history of RS colonization, where it is possible to observe differentiation between regions that underwent different colonization processes. Spatial analyzes of autoimmune disease hospitalization data were performed revealing clusters for different regions of the state for each disease analyzed. The correlation test between allelic frequency and the occurrence of autoimmune diseases indicated a significant correlation between the HLA-B*08 allele and rheumatoid arthritis.

Conclusions: Genetic mapping of populations and the spatial analyzes such as those performed in this work have great economic relevance and can be very useful in the formulation of public health campaigns and policies, contributing to the planning and adjustment of clinical actions, as well as informing and educating professionals and the population.

Keywords: HLA, Autoimmune diseases, Genetic structure, Correlation, Georeferencing

*Correspondence: lavinia.faccini@ufrgs.br
†Juliano André Boquett, Marcelo Zagonel-Oliveira and Nelson Jurandi Rosa Fagundes contributed equally to this work
2 Post-Graduate Program in Genetics and Molecular Biology, Departamento de Genética, Universidade Federal do Rio Grande do Sul, Agencia Campus UFRGS, Caixa Postal 15053, Porto Alegre, RS CEP 91501-970, Brazil
Full list of author information is available at the end of the article

Background

Harboring more than 200 genes spread over a 3.6 Mb region, the Major Histocompatibility Complex (MHC) is the region of the human genome most enriched for open reading frames [1]. MHC genes, or HLA (Human Leukocyte Antigen) genes in humans, are the most polymorphic loci of the human genome [2], showing different allelic frequencies in populations from different geographic regions around the world [3–5]. Due to their high genetic variability and strong linkage disequilibrium, HLA genes have been used in studies of genetic ancestry and demography [6]. Due to their major role in immune response, the *loci* of the HLA system are the primary determinants of tolerance or rejection in organ and hematopoietic stem cell transplantation (HSCT) [7]. HSCT from bone marrow is clinically indicated for the treatment of disorders of the hematopoietic system or the immune system and in cases of malignant bone marrow diseases and disseminated solid tumors. Leukemia is the leading indication for allogeneic HSCT (72%), followed by lymphoproliferative diseases (15%), non-malignant diseases (12%) and solid tumors (0.6%) [8, 9].

In addition, specifc HLA alleles have already been associated with various autoimmune and infectious diseases [10, 11]. As a class, the overall cumulative prevalence for all autoimmune diseases (AD) is 5.0%, being 3.0% for males and 7.1% for females [12]. Rheumatoid arthritis (RA) is the most prevalent AD (0.5–1%) [13], being the HLA-DRB1 is the principal locus contributing to disease susceptibility, with an estimated contribution of 30–50% to overall susceptibility to RA [14, 15]. Other AD, such as Celiac Disease, Type 1 Diabetes Mellitus, Ankylosing spondylitis, Multiple sclerosis and Crohn's disease also presented HLA genes associated with its susceptibility [see [16] and [17] for further review]. Thus, knowledge of HLA diversity at the population level is important to guide public health policies focused on AD and to improve bone marrow transplantation programs.

The use of the geographic information system (GIS)—a toolkit for capturing, storing, transforming, analyzing and presenting spatial data—has been a powerful tool in assessing and monitoring public health in different populations around the world [18, 19]. GIS-based data contributes to the improvement of health-related services for the population, since health data combined with geographic information allow researchers to analyze the spatial variation of diseases, mortality, morbidity, access to health care systems and social or environmental determinants for health outcomes [20, 21]. The transformation of detailed data into maps can facilitate communication of the geographical distribution of health challenges in different communities and identify areas for intervention [18, 22].

The Brazilian Bone Marrow Donor Registry (REDOME, in Portuguese) is the third largest bank of bone marrow donors in the world, with more than 4 million donors registered to date. The state of Rio Grande do Sul (RS), in southern Brazil, has the fourth largest number of registered donors in Brazil, with approximately 300,000 individuals. This register contains information of HLA-A, -B and -DRB1 genotypes, city of residence of the donor as well as ethnicity by self-declaration based on skin color. In this work, we used GIS tools to evaluate the spatial correlation between immune system alleles (from HLA-A, -B and -DRB1 *loci*) and occurrence of AD in Rio Grande do Sul, based on data information available from governmental health agencies.

Methods
Sample

We analyzed a dataset containing 97,292 potential bone marrow donors residing in the state of Rio Grande do Sul who voluntarily registered in REDOME between January 2008 and December 2012. Rio Grande do Sul, the southernmost state of Brazil, is the fourth largest state of the country with more than 11 million inhabitants distributed in 497 cities [23], 439 of which are represented in the dataset. At the time of registration in REDOME, the individuals declared their ethnicity by auto-perception based on skin color, following Brazilian Institute of Geography and Statistics (IBGE) standards. Only municipalities with 50 or more registered donors were included in the analysis. For self-reported white individuals (or Euro-descendants, EURD), 120 cities distributed across all regions of the state cities met the sample size criteria (Additional file 1), totaling 86,672 individuals (Fig. 1). On the other hand, only 19 cities had more than 50 self-reported black (or Afro-descendants, AFRD) individuals, scattered across the state and, therefore, excluded from further analyses.

Genotyping for HLA-A, -B and -DRB1 *loci* was performed at the Hospital das Clínicas de Porto Alegre (HCPA) (Luminex LABType SSO system; One Lambda, Inc., Canoga Park, CA). Due to the high polymorphism of HLA genes, complete identification of each allele is only possible through sequencing-based typing. Thus, Luminex genotyping identifies only "low resolution" allelic groups. Because they are closely located on the same chromosome, HLA alleles segregate in linkage blocks, known as haplotypes.

Information on AD were available in DATASUS (Department of Informatics of the Unified Health System, in Portuguese), a database established by the Brazilian Ministry of Health since 1991 that contains health information and statistics from all municipalities in Brazil and that is publicly available through online access

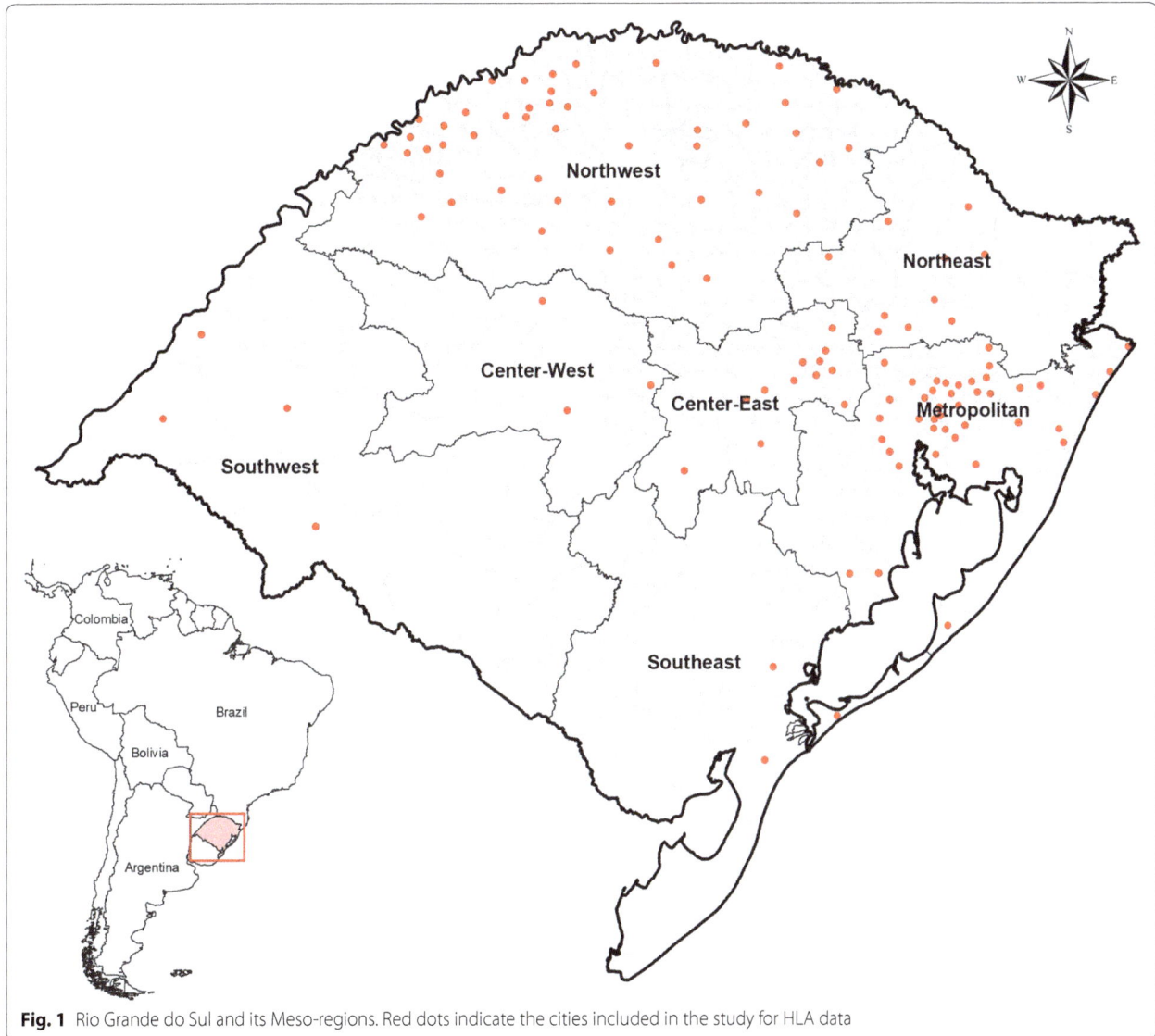

Fig. 1 Rio Grande do Sul and its Meso-regions. Red dots indicate the cities included in the study for HLA data

(datasus.saude.gov.br/datasus). In general, the DATASUS database is fed by data sent by the municipal and state health secretariats to the Ministry of Health. Of the 497 cities of Rio Grande do Sul, 496 had information about AD hospitalizations in DATASUS database.

This study was approved by the Ethics Committee of the Research and Post-Graduation Group of the Hospital de Clínicas de Porto Alegre, under number 386.216.

Statistical analyses

Allele and haplotype frequency estimations and tests of Hardy–Weinberg equilibrium (HWE) were performed using the GENE[RATE] tools as described elsewhere [7, 24–26]. Principal component analysis (PCA) was done for each *locus* using Rstudio (v0.98.1103) and the genetic

structure was measured using the synthetic genetic structure (*SPC*) measure proposed by Xue et al. [27], as follows:

$$SPC = W_1 \times PC_1 + W_2 \times PC_2 + \cdots + W_k \times PC_k$$

where *PC* is the component score and *W* is the proportion (weight) of the component contribution. All components with an eigenvalue greater than 1 were included in the *SPC* calculation, following the Kaiser criterion [28]. Hospitalization data for RA, multiple sclerosis (MS), Crohn's disease (CD) and leukemia for each city, comprising the period from January 1995 to December 2016, were obtained through the DATASUS system (tabnet.datasus.gov.br/). RA, MS and CD are the only AD recorded in DATASUS. The number of hospitalizations of each disease in each city was adjusted by the number of inhabitants and used as an indicator of disease prevalence (disease index, DI). Spearman's correlation test between each allele and each disease was performed using IBM SPSS software, Version 20.0 (IBM Corp., Armonk, NY). The result obtained in the Spearman correlation test was submitted to the multiple comparison test FDR (false discovery rate) in Rstudio (v0.98.1103) using the stats (3.3.0) package.

Allele and haplotype frequency, *SPC* data as well as positive and statistically significant alleles × diseases (hereafter A*D) in the Spearman's correlation test were spatially interpolated using the Empirical Bayesian Kriging method (EBK). For each interpolation, scatterplots were performed for the observed and predicted values and calculated their respective coefficients of determination (R^2), Spearman's correlation coefficient (ρ), Spearman's coefficient of determination (ρ^2) and the root mean square error (RMSE). The P-values were adjusted by FDR for $\alpha = 0.05$.

Cluster maps for A*D showing positive and statistically significant correlation in the Spearman test were generated through the Hot-Spot analysis using the Getis-Ord Gi* method [29, 30] based on the following formula:

$$\sqrt{\frac{DI - DImax}{DImax - DImin} \times \frac{AF - AFmax}{AFmax - AFmin}}$$

where DI is the disease index, DImax is the maximum disease index, DImin is the minimum disease index, AF is the allelic frequency, AFmax is the maximum allelic frequency and AFmin is the minimum allele frequency. All spatial analyses were performed in ArcGis v10.3.

Results

For all cities, allele frequencies did not show deviations from the Hardy–Weinberg equilibrium (Additional file 2). Considering the whole state, the most frequent alleles for each *locus* were HLA-A*02 (27.6%), HLA-B*35 (12.4) and HLA-DRB1*07 (13.4%), with substantial allele frequency variation among cities (Additional files 2, 3). Five haplotypes reached frequencies above 2% in at least one city. Haplotype A*01 ~ B*08 ~ DRB1*03 presented the highest frequency considering the entire state (3.7%). Following allele frequencies, there was substantial variation in haplotype frequencies among cities (Additional files 4, 5). Figure 2 shows the spatial HLA genetic structure based on *SPC* in Rio Grande do Sul. HLA-A and HLA-B *loci* have a very similar structure, showing a higher differentiation between the Southwest and Metropolitan regions in relation to the Central and Northwest regions. The HLA-DRB1 *locus* presents a slightly different structure, with a higher differentiation in the Northeast. The

combined data for the three *loci*, shows a very similar structure compared to HLA-A and HLA-B.

Figure 3 shows the distribution of the DI, while disease prevalence is shown, for each city, in Additional file 6. The small town of União da Serra, located in the Northeast region of the state, has a population of approximately 1500 inhabitants, which is equivalent to 0.014% of the total population of the state of Rio Grande do Sul. However, this city responded to 0.162% of all hospitalizations for RA from January 1995 to December 2016 (62 hospitalizations events). Thus, when considering the number of hospitalizations by the number of inhabitants in relation to the totals for the state, União da Serra is the municipality with the highest prevalence of RA with a DI 11.6 × higher than expected. Similarly, the town of São Sepé, in the Center-East region of the state, was the city with the highest prevalence for MS, with a DI almost 9 × higher than expected. On its turn, the town of São Pedro da Serra, in the Metropolitan region, had the highest prevalence for CD, with a DI 9.5 × higher than expected. For leukemia, the towns of Pouso Novo, in the Center-East region, Vista Alegre and Três Arroios, both in the Northwest region, had a DI 4.5 × higher than the expected. For all diseases (CD, MS, RA, and leukemia) there was strong evidence for spatial clusters in DI (Fig. 4, Additional file 7, $P < 3 \times 10^{-5}$ in all cases). Different regions appeared as hot-spots for different diseases. The Center-East and Northeast regions behaved as hot-spots for RA and MS, while the Metropolitan and the Northwest regions were cold-spots. CD had a hot-spot cluster in the Metropolitan region and in a small area in the Northeast, while for leukemia there was a hot-spot in the extreme North of the state.

Table 1 shows the Spearman correlation index (ρ) for each allele and each disease tested. Most of the statistically significant correlations found were negative. Alleles HLA-B*08 and -DRB1*03 showed a positive and significant correlation with RA; HLA-B*08 with MS; and HLA-A*29, HLA-B*38 and HLA-DRB1*01 with CD. Cluster analyses indicated a significant spatial component in A*D interaction for HLA-B*08 × RA, HLA-DRB1*03 × RA, HLA-B*08 × MS ($P < 0.01$), and HLA-A*29 × CD ($P < 0.05$), which is represented in Fig. 5 (and in Additional file 8). However, only the correlation between HLA-B*08 and RA remained significant after FDR correction. Interestingly, spatial hot-spots for A*D differ from DI hot-spots, indicating that adding genetic information on top of disease prevalence results in new insights of disease epidemiology.

The Spearman's correlation coefficient (ρ), Spearman's coefficient of determination (ρ^2) and the root mean square error (RMSE) for all observed and interpolated values of each EBK map (allelic and haplotypic frequencies, SPC

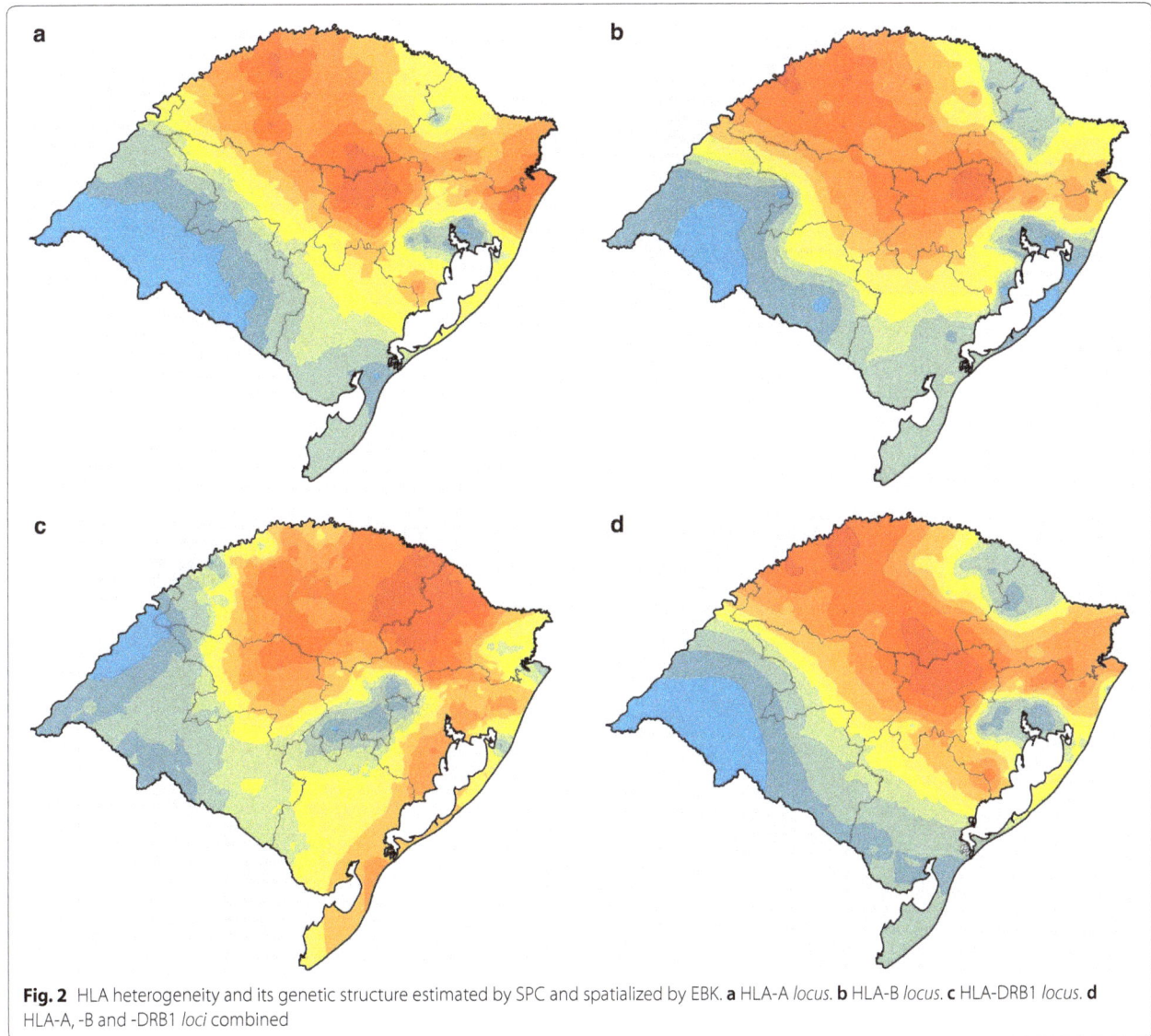

Fig. 2 HLA heterogeneity and its genetic structure estimated by SPC and spatialized by EBK. **a** HLA-A *locus*. **b** HLA-B *locus*. **c** HLA-DRB1 *locus*. **d** HLA-A, -B and -DRB1 *loci* combined

analysis and A*D correlation analysis) are presented in the Additional file 9. The lowest correlation coefficient was 0.1686 for allele HLA-B*56 and the highest was 0.9978 for HLA-A*30. The lowest RMSE found was <0.0001 for allele HLA-B*27, while the highest was 0.1628 for SPC HLA-DRB1. Except for the HLA-A*68 and HLA-B*56 allele frequency maps, all interpolations were statistically significant, even after FDR correction. Scatterplots and their respective coefficient of determination (R^2) for each interpolated map are presented in Additional file 10.

Discussion

This is the first study to perform spatial analysis of HLA genetic structure, correlating HLA population genetics data with epidemiological data on AD. Figure 1 shows

the HLA structure of the bone marrow donor population in Rio Grande do Sul based on the principal component analysis (PCA) of HLA allele frequencies. Visually, HLA-A, HLA-B and the combined data for the three *loci* showed a very similar structure, presenting a higher differentiation between the Southwest and Metropolitan regions in relation to the Central and Northwest regions.

PCA is a very useful tool in the investigation of population structure, but sampling strategy and the amount of data may impact its results [31]. In this study, only self-reported white individuals were included due to sample size limitations (only 19 cities had more than 50 self-reported black individuals, with little coverage in the state). It is unlikely that this had a major impact on the characterization of HLA genetic structure in Rio Grande

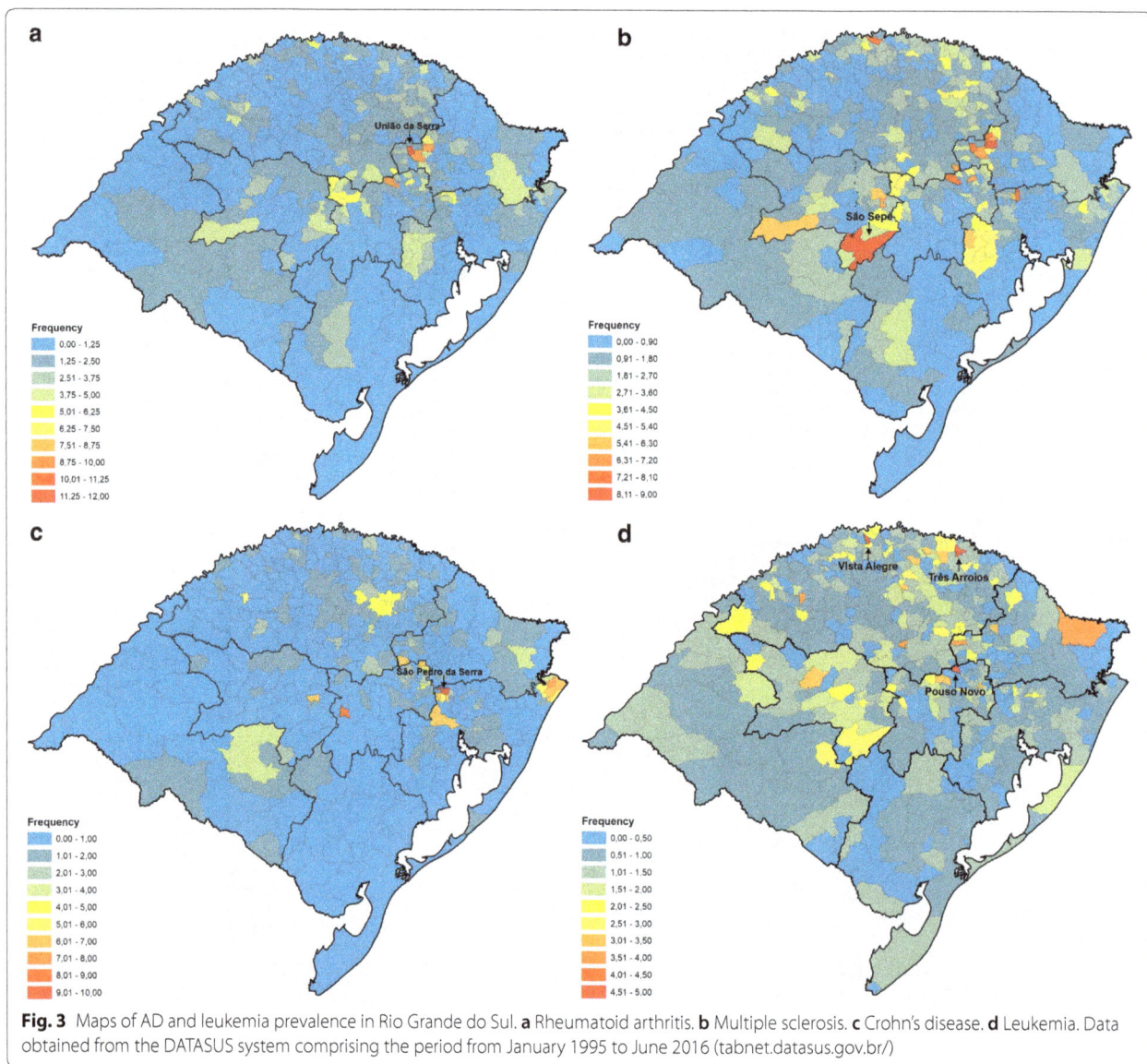

Fig. 3 Maps of AD and leukemia prevalence in Rio Grande do Sul. **a** Rheumatoid arthritis. **b** Multiple sclerosis. **c** Crohn's disease. **d** Leukemia. Data obtained from the DATASUS system comprising the period from January 1995 to June 2016 (tabnet.datasus.gov.br/)

do Sul as a whole, given that more than 80% of the population of Rio Grande do Sul is self-declared white [23], and more than 90% of REDOME donors in Rio Grande do Sul declare themselves white at the time of registration. However, given that there are differences in AD prevalence between black and white individuals [32, 33, see 34 for review], an important step forward would be characterizing geographic clusters of AD in the black population of this state and its relationship with the clusters identified in this study.

Among the classic HLA genes, HLA-A is more sensitive to demographic processes, such as genetic drift, because it is less affected by balancing selection [35, 36]. In this sense, the differentiation between the Southwest, Southeast and the Metropolitan regions, on one hand,

compared to the Central and Northwest regions, on the other hand (Fig. 1), may mirror the colonization history of Rio Grande do Sul (Additional file 11). In these former regions, Portuguese and Spanish individuals were the major settlers since the early eighteenth century, with the later arrival of African slaves, mostly in the Pelotas (Southeast) region. On the other hand, Germans (1824), Poles (1871) and Italians (1875) were major ethnicities settling the Central and Northern regions [37, 38].

Specific spatialization and interpolation techniques may influence the geographic trends shown by the data. In this study, allele and haplotype frequencies as well as A*D positive and statistically significant correlations were spatialized by the EBK method (Additional files 3, 5). This method was chosen because we had only 120

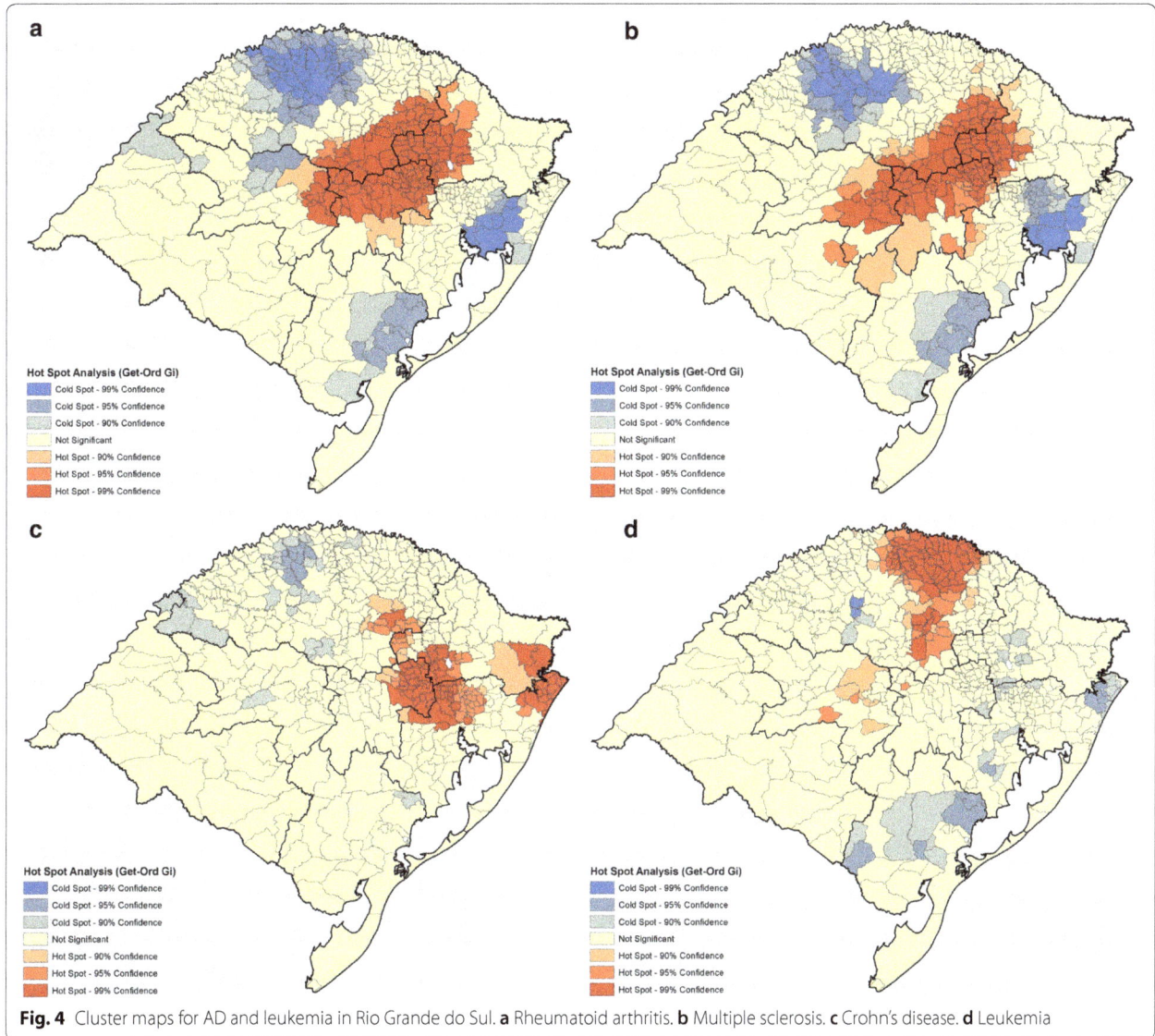

Fig. 4 Cluster maps for AD and leukemia in Rio Grande do Sul. **a** Rheumatoid arthritis. **b** Multiple sclerosis. **c** Crohn's disease. **d** Leukemia

points to represent the 496 municipalities of Rio Grande do Sul. Kriging is a probabilistic predictor, thus assuming a statistical model for the data, being able to quantify the uncertainty associated with the values predicted from the standard errors. This method uses a semivariogram—a function of distance and direction separating two locations—to quantify the spatial dependence on the data. EBK differs from classical kriging by using many semivariogram models rather than using only a single model. For each repetition, the semivariogram is used to simulate a new set of values at the input sites; then the simulated data are used to estimate a new semivariogram and its weight. Thus, predicted values and standard errors are inferred for the non-sampled regions using these weights [39].

All interpolated maps showed correlation between observed and interpolated values. The lowest correlation coefficients were typically observed in alleles with low frequencies, and where the sampling is consequently smaller. It is important to note that the alleles that showed a positive and significant correlation with AD (HLA-A*29, HLA-B*08, HLA-B*38, HLA-DRB1*01 e HLA-DRB1*03) presented a correlation coefficient for interpolation ranging from 0.513 to 0.982 and maximum RMSD of 0.017 (Additional file 9). These values indicate that the interpolation method and the analyses performed are consistent.

The Hot-Spot analysis (Getis-Ord Gi*) revealed geographic clusters of AD (RA, MS and CD) and leukemia in Rio Grande do Sul, indicating that neighbor regions

Table 1 Spearman correlation (ρ) between alleles and diseases

HLA-A	RA	MS	CD	HLA-B	RA	MS	CD	HLA-DRB1	RA	MS	CD
A*01	0.124	0.072	−0.198	B*07	0.146	0.135	−0.079	DRB1*01	0.016	−0.088	*0.187*
A*02	−0.018	−0.008	−0.125	B*08	*0.327**	*0.218*	−0.005	DRB1*03	*0.210*	0.102	0.036
A*03	0.008	0.021	−0.072	B*13	0.046	0.037	−0.143	DRB1*04	0.054	0.162	−0.249
A*11	−0.108	−0.118	−0.089	B*14	−0.077	−0.049	0.100	DRB1*07	−0.182	−0.117	0.143
A*23	−0.166	−0.255	−0.017	B*15	0.077	0.083	−0.020	DRB1*08	−0.220	−0.168	0.066
A*24	−0.059	−0.084	0.036	B*18	0.169	0.056	0.027	DRB1*09	−0.089	−0.091	−0.004
A*25	0.150	0.075	−0.113	B*27	0.094	0.067	−0.199	DRB1*10	−0.059	−0.008	0.101
A*26	0.045	0.002	0.149	B*35	0.029	−0.013	0.125	DRB1*11	0.046	0.032	0.112
A*29	−0.207	−0.203	*0.197*	B*37	−0.178	−0.157	0.028	DRB1*12	−0.121	−0.150	−0.180
A*30	−0.131	−0.055	0.172	B*38	−0.038	−0.111	*0.195*	DRB1*13	−0.115	−0.060	−0.094
A*31	−0.040	−0.085	−0.003	B*39	−0.017	−0.060	0.158	DRB1*14	−0.066	−0.077	−0.005
A*32	0.093	0.133	−0.119	B*40	−0.034	0.001	−0.248	DRB1*15	0.047	0.030	−0.015
A*33	−0.011	0.034	0.088	B*41	−0.156	−0.136	−0.096	DRB1*16	−0.230	−0.265	−0.084
A*34	−0.313	−0.229	0.065	B*42	−0.111	−0.047	0.167				
A*36	−0.149	−0.123	0.149	B*44	−0.179	−0.089	0.022				
A*43	0.020	0.073	−0.054	B*45	−0.211	−0.178	0.024				
A*66	−0.110	−0.090	0.014	B*46	0.073	0.052	0.038				
A*68	0.056	0.043	0.149	B*47	−0.155	−0.168	0.028				
A*69	−0.126	−0.120	−0.016	B*48	−0.218	−0.120	0.049				
A*74	−0.197	−0.185	0.089	B*49	−0.123	−0.148	0.004				
A*80	−0.143	−0.072	−0.016	B*50	−0.371	−0.306	0.088				
				B*51	−0.007	0.006	0.031				
				B*52	0.019	0.026	0.150				
				B*53	−0.200	−0.148	0.078				
				B*54	0.091	0.101	0.078				
				B*55	−0.120	−0.188	−0.067				
				B*56	−0.015	0.052	0.066				
				B*57	0.010	0.027	−0.077				
				B*58	−0.191	−0.182	0.076				
				B*59	−0.099	−0.083	−0.001				
				B*67	−0.010	0.004	−0.042				
				B*73	−0.106	−0.069	0.005				
				B*78	−0.050	0.002	−0.006				
				B*81	−0.289	−0.242	0.012				
				B*82	−0.098	−0.064	0.106				

RA Rheumatoid arthritis, *MS* multiple sclerosis, *CD* Crohn's disease

Italic: Positive correlation; $P \leq 0.05$

*Remained significant even after correction by FDR

should have similar disease prevalence (Additional file 7). On the other hand, our analysis also revealed spatial clusters of A*D, even though both spatial clusters had little overlap (Figs. 4, 5). A genetic cluster can be defined as a group of genetically divergent individuals that arises when gene flow is impeded by physical or cultural barriers [40]. Evolutionary forces such as the founder's effect and low immigration may reinforce genetic backgrounds that pre-dispose to some genetic conditions. One interpretation for the little overlap

between DI and A*D is that while DI spatial clustering is dominated by shared environmental and genetic (non-HLA) affecting disease status, A*D spatial clusters indicate a more important role for the common HLA genetic background (through specific "risk" alleles) for these diseases. As a result, cities having a high frequency of HLA-B*08, for example, will have a higher chance of having high DI for RA even if this city is distant from the DI spatial cluster disconsidering HLA information.

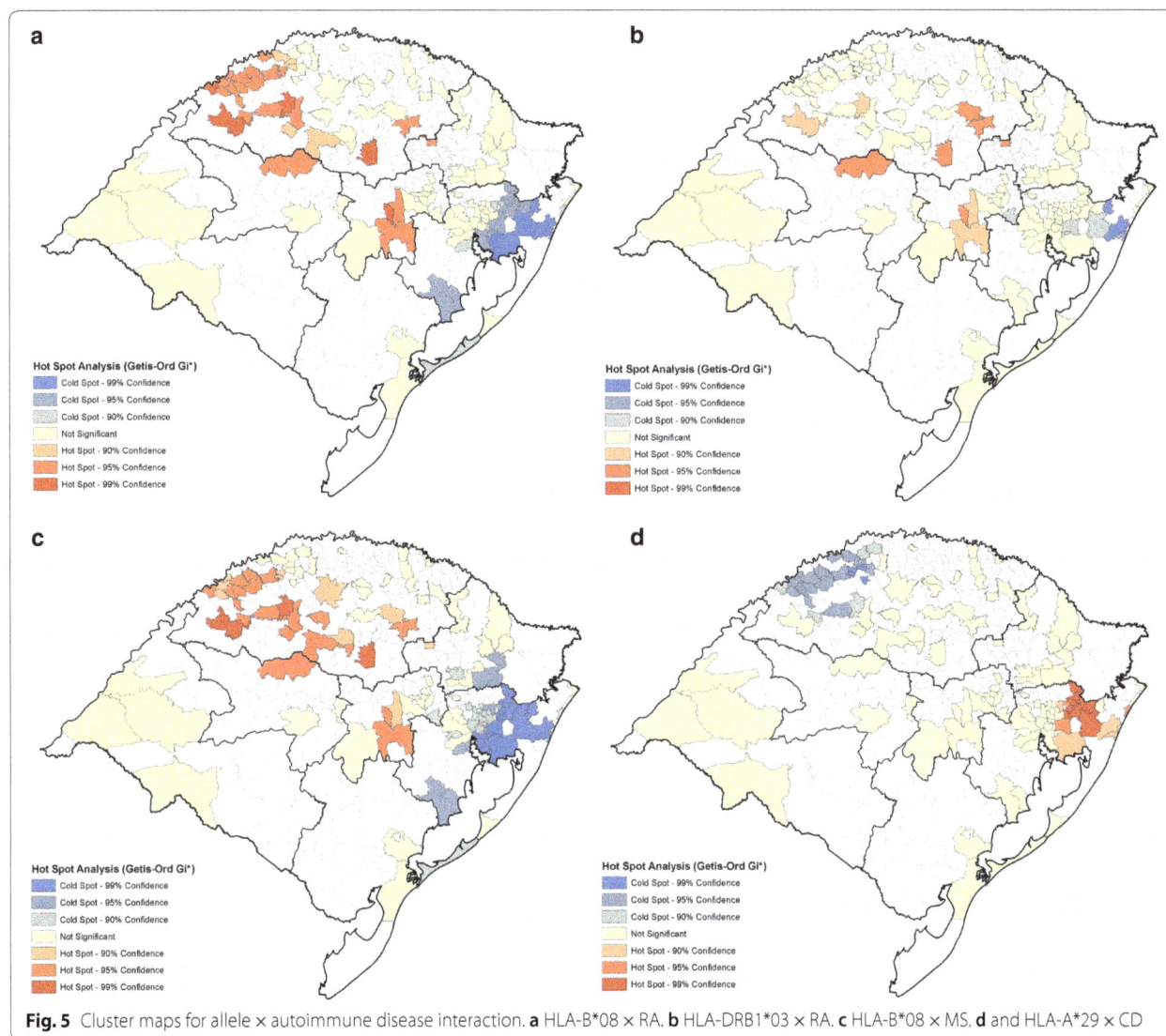

Fig. 5 Cluster maps for allele × autoimmune disease interaction. **a** HLA-B*08 × RA. **b** HLA-DRB1*03 × RA. **c** HLA-B*08 × MS. **d** and HLA-A*29 × CD

AD are heterogeneous in regard to prevalence, clinical manifestations, and pathogenesis, being caused by an immune response against constituents of the body's own tissues. Specific HLA alleles can predispose to several AD [10, 11]. Indeed, some of the positive and significant correlations between HLA alleles and AD found in our study have already been described in case–control studies. Han et al. [41] established a relationship between HLA-B*08 and RA subtype anti-citrullinated-protein-autoantibody-negative (ACPA⁻ or seronegative) in a study involving 2406 ACPA⁻ case and 13,930 control individuals. Alsaied et al. [42] found an association between HLA-DRB1*03 and juvenile RA in Kuwaiti Arab children, and Manivel et al. [43] established an association between HLA-DRB1*03 and RA subtype anti-CII (anti fibrillar collagen type II) in the Swedish population. On the contrary, Lysandropoulos et al. [44] tested the relation between MS

and HLA-B*08, but the result was inconclusive. Concerning CD, Goyette et al. [45] found a significant association with DRB1*01, but there are no other studies correlating CD and HLA-A*29 and HLA-B*38. Differently from our findings, Konda Mohan et al. [46]] and Bizzari et al. [47] indicated a protective role for HLA-DRB1*03 for RA in Indian and Arabic populations, respectively. These results may indicate that some relationships between AD and HLA background may be population-specific, which highlights the potential of spatial analyses to identify small-scale A*D clusters in populations from a similar background.

Nonetheless, some limitations of this study should be taken into account: the bone marrow donor individuals are not the same reported in the DATASUS system for the mentioned diseases, in addition to the already mentioned limiting number of cities having enough sample size for allele frequency analysis. Besides, the data used in the DATASUS system refers to the number of hospitalizations for each disease and, because we use data of chronic disease, the same person may hospitalize more than once for the same condition. However, spatially studies can serve at least as preliminary models of genetic × disease interaction to guide further investigations and promote public health actions.

Understanding the demographic processes that affect the genetic diversity of human populations at a spatial scale can be useful in public health policies in the present. The study of the HLA diversity at the population level is invaluable in disease-association studies and in the effectiveness of bone marrow transplantation programs. Thus, the results presented in this study, such as the heterogeneous genetic structure and the A*D spatial correlations, demonstrate the importance of the integrated use of large databases with spatial-specific analysis approaches, and may indicate the need to implement space-specific interventions to guide policy planning and decision making in public health.

Despite all the potential use of GIS, this tool is still underutilized in public health centers around the world. Georeferencing is an essential first step in making it possible to analyze public health data geographically [48]. Through the georeferencing of public health data it is possible to perform a spatial analysis for public health systems [49]. The correct use of GIS can inform and educate professionals and the public, give more power to decision making at all levels, assist in planning and adjusting clinical and cost-effective actions, monitor and analyze changes in health levels and exposure to disease [50].

Conclusions

In this study, we used GIS tools to evaluate the spatial correlation between HLA alleles and occurrence of AD in Rio Grande do Sul, based on data available from governmental health agencies. To the best of our knowledge, this is the first study that investigates the spatial correlation between genetic data and AD occurrence. The results presented in this study highlights the potential of spatial analyses to identify the interaction between alleles and diseases in populations from a similar background. The use of information from large databases such as REDOME and DATASUS together with georeferencing tools can help in the identification of useful markers in population genetics that may confer resistance or susceptibility to diseases. Genetic mapping of populations and the spatial analyzes such as those performed in this work have great economic relevance and can be very useful in the formulation of public health campaigns and policies, contributing to the planning and adjustment of clinical

actions, as well as informing and educating professionals and the population.

Additional files

Additional file 1. Sample size.

Additional file 2. Allelic frequencies, genetic diversity and Hardy–Weinberg equilibrium.

Additional file 3. Allelic frequency maps.

Additional file 4. Haplotype frequencies.

Additional file 5. Haplotype frequencies maps.

Additional file 6. Prevalence of hospitalizations for each disease in the cities of Rio Grande do Sul.

Additional file 7. Prevalence and cluster maps for each disease.

Additional file 8. Correlation maps between alleles and autoimmune diseases.

Additional file 9. Spearman's determination coefficient, Spearman's correlation coefficient and root mean square error for each interpolated map.

Additional file 10. Scatterplot and coefficient of determination (R^2) for each interpolated map.

Additional file 11. Meso-regions of Rio Grande do Sul and its colonization regions.

Abbreviations

MHC: Major histocompatibility complex; HLA: Human leukocyte antigen; HSCT: hematopoietic stem cell transplantation; AD: autoimmune diseases; RA: Rheumatoid arthritis; GIS: geographic information system; REDOME: Brazilian bone marrow donor registry; RS: Rio Grande do Sul; IBGE: Brazilian institute of geography and statistics; EURD: Euro-descendants; AFRD: Afro-descendants; HCPA: Hospital de Clínicas de Porto Alegre; DATASUS: Department of informatics of the unified health system; HWE: Hardy–Weinberg equilibrium; PCA: principal component analysis; SPC: synthetic genetic structure; MS: multiple sclerosis; CD: Crohn's disease; DI: disease index; FDR: false discovery ratio; EBK: Empirical Bayesian kriging.

Authors' contributions

JAB was responsible for the study concept and design, conducted the data analysis, interpreted the results and wrote the paper. MZ-O was responsible for the study concept and design, conducted the data analysis and interpreted the results. LFJ and MJ were responsible for acquisition of HLA data. MRV and LGJ conducted the data analysis and interpreted the results. NJRF and LSF were responsible for the study concept and design, interpreted the results and undertook critical revision of the manuscript. All authors read and approved the final manuscript.

Author details

[1] Instituto Nacional de Genética Médica Populacional (INaGeMP), Porto Alegre, Brazil. [2] Post-Graduate Program in Genetics and Molecular Biology, Departamento de Genética, Universidade Federal do Rio Grande do Sul, Agencia Campus UFRGS, Caixa Postal 15053, Porto Alegre, RS CEP 91501-970, Brazil. [3] Advanced Visualization and Geoinformatics Laboratory (VIZLab), Applied Computing Graduate Program, Universidade do Vale do Rio dos Sinos, São Leopoldo, RS, Brazil. [4] Department of Immunology, Hospital de Clínicas de Porto Alegre, Porto Alegre, Brazil.

Acknowledgements

We would like to thank the Brazilian funding agencies: Brazilian Ministry of Science and Technology/CNPq; INCT-INAGEMP, and CAPES by the PhD fellowship to JB. We are thankful for two anonymous reviewers for suggestions in an earlier version of the manuscript.

Competing interests

The authors declare that they have no competing interests.

Funding

This study was funded by the Conselho Nacional de Desenvolvimento Científico e Tecnológico (CNPQ), Coordenação de Aperfeiçoamento de Pessoal de Nível Superior (CAPES) and Brazilian Ministry of Science and Technology/CNPq; INCT-INAGEMP, (Grants No. 476978/2008-4).

References

1. The MHC sequencing consortium. Complete sequence and gene map of a human major histocompatibility complex. Nature. 1999;401(6756):921–3.

2. Robinson J, Halliwell JA, Hayhurst JH, Flicek P, Parham P, Marsh SGE. The IPD and IPD-IMGT/HLA Database: allele variant databases. Nucleic Acids Res. 2015;43:D423–31.

3. Middleton D, Williams F, Meenagh A, et al. Analysis of the distribution of HLA-A alleles in populations from five continents. Hum Immunol. 2000;61:1048–52.

4. Williams F, Meenagh A, Darke C, et al. Analysis of the distribution of HLA-B alleles in populations from five continents. Hum Immunol. 2001;62:645–50.

5. Solberg OD, Mack SJ, Lancaster AK, Single RM, Tsai Y, Sanchez-Mazas A, Thomson G. Balancing selection and heterogeneity across the classical human leukocyte antigen loci: a meta-analytic review of 497 population studies. Hum Immunol. 2008;69(7):443–64.

6. Sanchez-Mazas A, Fernandez-Viña M, Middleton D, et al. Immunogenetics as a tool in anthropological studies. Immunology. 2011;133:143–64.

7. Buhler S, Nunes JM, Nicoloso G, Tiercy JM, Sanchez-Mazas A. The heterogeneous HLA genetic makeup of the Swiss population. PLoS ONE. 2012;7:e41400.

8. Gratwohl A, Baldomero H, Aljurf M, Pasquini MC, Bouzas LF, Yoshimi A, et al. Hematopoietic stem cell transplantation: a global perspective. JAMA. 2010;303(16):1617–24.

9. Gratwohl A, Baldomero H, Gratwohl M, Aljurf M, Bouzas LF, Horowitz M, et al. Quantitative and qualitative differences in use and trends of hematopoietic stem cell transplantation: a Global Observational Study. Haematologica. 2013;98(8):1282–90.

10. Parham P, Lomen CE, Lawlor DA, Ways JP, Holmes N, Coppin HL, Salter RD, Wan AM, Ennis PD. Nature of polymorphism in HLA-A, -B, and -C molecules. Proc Natl Acad Sci USA. 1988;85:4005–9.

11. Trowsdale J, Knight JC. Major histocompatibility complex genomics and human disease. Annu Rev Genomics Hum Genet. 2013;14:301–23.

12. Hayter SM, Cook MC. Updated assessment of the prevalence, spectrum and case definition of autoimmune disease. Autoimmun Rev. 2012;11(10):754–65.

13. Silman AJ, Pearson JE. Epidemiology and genetics of rheumatoid arthritis. Arthritis Res. 2002;4:S265.

14. Bowes J, Barton A. Recent advances in genetics of RA susceptibility. Rheumatology. 2008;47:399.

15. Imboden JB. The immunopathogenesis of rheumatoid arthritis. Ann Rev Pathol. 2009;4:417.

16. Howell WM. HLA and disease: guilt by association. Int J Immunogenet. 2014;41(1):1–12.

17. Matzaraki V, Kumar V, Wijmenga C, Zhernakova A. The MHC locus and genetic susceptibility to autoimmune and infectious diseases. Genome Biol. 2017;18(1):76.

18. Tanser FC, Le Sueur D. The application of geographical information systems to important public health problems in Africa. Int J Health Geogr. 2002;1(1):4.

19. McLafferty SL. GIS and health care. Annu Rev Public Health. 2003;24:25–42.

20. Ricketts TC. Geographic information systems and public health. Annu Rev Public Health. 2003;24:1–6.

21. Schuurman N, Bérubé M, Crooks VA. Measuring potential spatial access to primary health care physicians using a modified gravity model. Can Geographer. 2010;54(1):29–45.

22. Chung K, Yang DH, Bell R. Health and GIS: toward spatial statistical analyses. J Med Syst. 2004;28(4):349–60.

23. IBGE: Pesquisa Nacional Por amostra de domicílios e contagem da população. Instituto Brasileiro de Geografia e Estatística, 2010.

24. Buhler S, Nunes JM, Sanchez-Mazas A, Richard L. HLA-A, B and DRB1 genetic heterogeneity in Quebec. Int J Immunogenet. 2015;42:69–77.

25. Nunes JM. Using UNIFORMAT and GENE[RATE] to analyze data with ambiguities in population genetics. Evol Bioinfor. 2015;2:19–26.

26. Boquett JA, Nunes JM, Buhler S, de Oliveira MZ, Jobim LF, Jobim M, Fagundes NJ, Schüler-Faccini L, Sanchez-Mazas A. The HLA-A, -B and -DRB1 polymorphism in a large dataset of South Brazil bone marrow donors from Rio Grande do Sul. HLA. 2017;89(1):29–38.

27. Xue FZ, Wang JZ, Hu P, Li GR. The "Kriging" model of spatial genetic structure in human population genetics. Yi Chuan Xue Bao. 2005;32(3):219–33.

28. Figueiredo Filho DB, Silva Júnior JA. Visão além do alcance: uma introdução à análise fatorial. Opinião Pública. 2010;16(1):160–85. https://doi.org/10.1590/S0104-62762010000100007.

29. Getis A, Ord JK. The analysis of spatial association by use of distance statistics. Geogr Anal. 1992;24:189–206.

30. Ord JK, Getis A. Local spatial autocorrelation statistics: distributional issues and an application. Geogr Anal. 1995;27:286–306.

31. Novembre J, Stephens M. Interpreting principal component analyses of spatial population genetic variation. Nat Genet. 2008;40(5):646–9.

32. González LA, Toloza SM, McGwin G Jr, Alarcón GS. Ethnicity in systemic lupus erythematosus (SLE): its influence on susceptibility and outcomes. Lupus. 2013;22(12):1214–24.

33. Langer-Gould A, Brara SM, Beaber BE, Zhang JL. Incidence of multiple sclerosis in multiple racial and ethnic groups. Neurology. 2013;80(19):1734–9.

34. Seldin MF. The genetics of human autoimmune disease: a perspective on progress in the field and future directions. J Autoimmun. 2015;64:1–12.

35. Sanchez-Mazas A, Buhler S, Nunes JM. A new HLA map of Europe: regional genetic variation and its implication for peopling history, disease-association studies and tissue transplantation. Hum Hered. 2013;76:162–77.

36. Inotai D, Szilvasi A, Benko S, Boros-Major A, Illes Z, Bors A, et al. HLA genetic diversity in Hungarians and Hungarian Gypsies: complementary differentiation patterns and demographic signals revealed by HLA-A, -B and -DRB1 in Central Europe. Tissue Antigens. 2015;86:115–21.

37. Neto HB, Bezzi ML. Regiões culturais: a construção de identidades culturais no Rio Grande Do Sul e sua manifestação na paisagem gaúcha. Soc Nat. 2008;20(2):135–55.

38. Neto HB, Bezzi ML. Região cultural como categoria de análise da materialização da cultura no espaço gaúcho. RA'E GA. 2009;17:17–30.

39. Krivoruchko K. Spatial statistical data analysis for GIS users. Redlands: Esri Press; 2011. p. 928.

40. Novembre J, Di Rienzo A. Spatial patterns of variation due to natural selection in humans. Nat Rev Genet. 2009;10(11):745–55.

41. Han B, Diogo D, Eyre S, Kallberg H, Zhernakova A, Bowes J, et al. Fine mapping seronegative and seropositive rheumatoid arthritis to shared and distinct HLA alleles by adjusting for the effects of heterogeneity. Am J Hum Genet. 2014;94(4):522–32.

42. Alsaeid K, Haider MZ, Kamal H, Srivastva BS, Ayoub EM. Prevalence of human leukocyte antigen (HLA) DRB1 alleles in Kuwaiti children with juvenile rheumatoid arthritis. Eur J Immunogenet. 2002;29(1):1–5.

43. Manivel VA, Mullazehi M, Padyukov L, Westerlind H, Klareskog L, Alfredsson L, Saevarsdottir S, Rönnelid J. Anticollagen type II antibodies are associated with an acute onset rheumatoid arthritis phenotype and prognosticate lower degree of inflammation during 5 years follow-up. *Ann Rheum Dis* 2017; pii: annrheumdis-2016-210873.

44. Lysandropoulos AP, Mavroudakis N, Pandolfo M, El Hafsi K, van Hecke W, Maertens A, Billiet T, Ribbens A. HLA genotype as a marker of multiple sclerosis prognosis: a pilot study. J Neurol Sci. 2017;15(375):348–54.

45. Goyette P, Boucher G, Mallon D, Ellinghaus E, Jostins L, Huang H, et al. High-density mapping of the MHC identifies a shared role for HLA-DRB1*01:03 in inflammatory bowel diseases and heterozygous advantage in ulcerative colitis. Nat Genet. 2015;47(2):172–9.

46. Konda Mohan V, Ganesan N, Gopalakrishnan R, Venkatesan V. HLA-DRB1 shared epitope alleles in patients with rheumatoid arthritis: relation to autoantibodies and disease severity in a south Indian population. Int J Rheum Dis. 2016. https://doi.org/10.1111/1756-185X.12948.

47. Bizzari S, Nair P, Al Ali MT, Hamzeh AR. Meta-analyses of the association of HLA-DRB1 alleles with rheumatoid arthritis among Arabs. Int J Rheum Dis. 2016. https://doi.org/10.1111/1756-185X.12922.

48. Vine MF, Degnan D, Hanchette C. Geographic information systems: their use in environmental epidemiologic research. Environ Health Perspect. 1997;105:598–605.

49. Lash RR, Carroll DS, Hughes CM, Nakazawa Y, Karem K, Damon IK, Peterson AT. Effects of georeferencing effort on mapping monkeypox case distributions and transmission risk. Int J Health Geogr. 2012;11:23.

50. Boulos MN. Towards evidence-based, GIS-driven national spatial health information infrastructure and surveillance services in the United Kingdom. Int J Health Geogr. 2004;3(1):1.

13

Ecological niche modeling to determine potential niche of Vaccinia virus: a case only study

Claire A. Quiner[*] ⓘ and Yoshinori Nakazawa

Abstract

Background: Emerging and understudied pathogens often lack information that most commonly used analytical tools require, such as negative controls or baseline data; thus, new analytical strategies are needed to analyze transmission patterns and drivers of disease emergence. Zoonotic infections with Vaccinia virus (VACV) were first reported in Brazil in 1999, VACV is an emerging zoonotic *Orthopoxvirus*, which primarily infects dairy cattle and farmers in close contact with infected cows. Prospective studies of emerging pathogens could provide critical data that would inform public health planning and response to outbreaks. By using the location of 87-recorded outbreaks and publicly available bioclimatic data, we demonstrate one such approach. Using an ecological niche model (ENM) algorithm, we identify the environmental conditions under which VACV outbreaks have occurred, and determine additional locations in two affected countries that may be susceptible to transmission. Further, we show how suitability for the virus responds to different levels of various environmental factors and highlight the most important factors in determining its transmission.

Methods: A literature review was performed and the geospatial coordinates of 87 molecularly confirmed VACV outbreaks in Brazil were identified. An ENM was generated using MaxENT software by combining principal component analysis results of 19 bioclim spatial layers, and 25 randomly selected subsets of the original list of 87 outbreaks.

Results: The final ENM predicted all areas where Brazilian outbreaks occurred, one out of five of the Colombian outbreak regions and identified new regions within Brazil that are suitable for transmission based on bioclimatic factors. Further, the most important factors in determining transmission suitability are precipitation of the wettest quarter, annual precipitation, mean temperature of the coldest quarter and mean diurnal range.

Conclusion: The analyses here provide a means by which to study patterns of an emerging infectious disease and identify regions that are potentially suitable for its transmission, in spite of the paucity of high-quality critical data. Policy and methods for the control of infectious diseases often use a reactionary model, addressing diseases only after significant impact on human health has ensued. The methodology used in the present work allows the identification of areas where disease is likely to appear, which could be used for directed intervention.

Keywords: Vaccinia, Emerging infectious diseases, Ecological niche model, Orthopoxvirus, Case-only study

Background

Zoonotic pathogens, including Ebola virus, H1N1, MERS and SARS [1–5], impose significant threats to human health and are projected to increase in their distribution and impact in coming years [5]. Currently, 61% of all pathogens that infect humans are zoonotic and 75% of emerging disease pathogens are zoonotic in origin [6]. This pattern is driven in part by novel interactions between humans and previously undisturbed environments, and can be attributed to human modifications,

*Correspondence: cquiner@berkeley.edu
Poxvirus and Rabies Branch, Division of High-Consequence Pathogens and Pathology (DHCPP), National Center for Emerging and Zoonotic Infectious Diseases (NCEZID), US Centers for Disease Control and Prevention, Atlanta, GA, USA

land-cover change, climate change, unplanned urbanization and human migration [5].

Vaccinia virus (VACV) is one such example of an emerging, zoonotic pathogen. VACV is an *Orthopoxvirus* and is closely related to the virus that causes smallpox (*Variola virus*). VACV was used as the vaccine against smallpox during eradication efforts, but more recently, human infections of zoonotic origin have been reported [7–9] in Brazil, India [7] and Mongolia [10]. The natural history of VACV and its transmission cycle is not known, but several wild and peri-domestic species of mammals have shown evidence of orthopoxvirus infection, including horses, coatis, opossums, monkeys and rodents, which could be involved in the maintenance of the virus in nature [11–16]. In South America, the first VACV outbreak of zoonotic origin was identified in Brazil in 1999 [17] and all documented VACV outbreaks on the continent since that year have been associated with dairy farms in Brazil [18–21] or Colombia [22]. During an outbreak, the virus is presumably spread throughout a farm by direct cow-to-cow contact or via milkers who develop lesions on their hands and spread the virus to others during milking. The virus could be transmitted to neighboring farms by sharing infected cattle for breeding practices and/or infected milkers. Secondary human cases of VACV without direct physical contact with infected cattle, have also been reported [17, 23]. VACV is not a mandatory reportable disease and the current surveillance system is not designed to capture these infections. Further, only a limited number of epidemiologic studies have been conducted, which restricts the ability to estimate the burden of the disease and the use of other analytical approaches to research transmission patterns and risk factors that would aid in its control.

VACV infection causes moderate to severe illness in humans and reduces milk production in cows; disease manifestation in humans includes pruritus at the site of infection, papules, vesicles, and pustules surrounded by erythema and induration as well as fever, headache, exhaustion, enlarged lymph nodes, and malaise; symptoms last for up to 30 days [21]. Experimentally infected cows show symptoms that last 1–32 days post inoculation (dpi), whereby vesicles, papules and ulcers form on teats, and in some cases the muzzle as well, and eventually scar. Milk production is affected by infection as mastitis begins early in infection and remains through the entirety of the disease. Milk volume drops by more than 70% by 3 dpi and milk quality, measured by somatic cell count (SSC), significantly decreases [24]. Studies of milk experimentally contaminated with VACV showed a major reduction of infective viral particles (>94%), after the pasteurization process but a few were still infective [25].

The dairy industry in Brazil is currently the world's 5th largest milk producer and is rapidly increasing. There are over 1 million dairy cattle farms in Brazil, which are heavily concentrated in the states which have experienced VACV outbreaks (Minas Gerais, São Paulo, Goiás, and Rio Grande do Sul [26]). Studies of milk experimentally contaminated with VACV showed a major, but not complete, reduction of infective viral particles (>94%) after the pasteurization process [25], this opens the possibility for viral spread through consumption of milk.

Public health control of emerging pathogens is challenging when the origin and basic risk factors for pathogen acquisition are not well understood. The mechanism by which VACV is maintained in nature, cows become infected, transmission patterns, attack rate and basic risk factors are still unknown. In lieu of opportunities to collect more data from larger outbreaks or formal epidemiological studies, this work attempts to utilize the existing and publicly available information to gain insight into this emerging threat. Based on the premise that pathogen circulation depends, in part, on certain environmental conditions, identifying and mapping those conditions can be used to hypothesize the distribution of a pathogen across the landscape [27]. Here, we aim to identify at-risk regions for VACV transmission in Brazil and Colombia by determining the environmental factors common among locations in which outbreaks have been recorded, and to identify the most relevant bioclimatic factors affecting its transmission.

Methods

Input data

Outbreak occurrence data

A literature search was performed to create a list of VACV outbreaks and their geographical coordinates. The search was conducted in PubMed, was restricted to articles in English and used the following search terms: Bovine Vaccinia, Vaccinia virus, Bovine Associated Vaccinia, or Brazilian Vaccinia. References within articles identified by this search were reviewed for other publications that were not found in the original. Results were further supplemented with publications suggested by subject matter experts including Brazilian researchers familiar with local publications. Inclusion criteria for an outbreak were (1) the outbreak occurred in Brazil, (2) the etiologic agent was confirmed as VACV via molecular diagnostics, and (3) the article noted the municipality in which the outbreak occurred. The centroid of each municipality was then used to represent the location of disease occurrence. The complete list of outbreaks used for modeling is listed in Additional file 1 and summarized by state in Table 1.

Table 1 Brazilian outbreaks of VACV by state

State	# of VACV outbreaks
Bahia	1
Espírito Santo	9
Goiás	3
Maranhão	1
Mato Grosso	2
Minas Gerais	33
Rio de Janeiro	22
Rio Grande do Sul	1
São Paulo	15

Number of recorded VACV outbreaks in each Brazilian state

Table 2 PCA results

Bio clim layer	PC 1	PC 2	PC 3	PC 4	PC 5
PWQ	*0.6356*	*0.5965*	*0.2536*	0.0680	−0.2815
MTCQ	*0.2760*	*0.2158*	−0.8614	−0.1089	*0.3413*
AP	*0.2166*	0.0951	*0.0801*	0.6262	*0.2729*
TS	0.0830	0.1829	−0.0215	−0.5473	−0.3041
PS	0.0750	0.0312	0.0203	*0.2270*	0.1051
MTWaM	0.0360	0.1909	*0.4181*	−0.4064	*0.7729*
ISO	0.0306	−0.0205	−0.0466	−0.0061	−0.0659
PDQ	0.0255	−0.0257	−0.0134	0.0306	−0.0361
PDM	0.0238	0.0547	−0.0042	−0.1760	−0.0939
MTCM	0.0236	−0.0199	−0.0302	0.0310	−0.0683
PCQ	0.0161	−0.0165	−0.0120	0.0315	−0.0308
TAR	0.0101	−0.0126	−0.0006	0.0275	−0.0036
PWaQ	0.0087	−0.0078	−0.0159	0.0340	−0.0390
MTWaQ	0.0071	−0.0047	−0.0045	−0.0161	0.0057
MTDQ	0.0066	−0.0116	−0.0029	0.0671	−0.0441
PWM	−0.0048	−0.0251	0.0070	0.0725	0.0518
AMT	−0.0069	−0.0040	0.0270	0.0338	0.0292
MTWQ	−0.0240	0.0089	0.0437	0.0732	0.0217
MDR	−0.6747	*0.7154*	−0.0722	*0.1510*	−0.0356
% of eigen values	66.9938	92.3237	97.2055	98.8945	99.6106

Eigen vectors and values

Listed are the Eigen vectors, indicating the contributions of each bioclim layer to the 5 principle component (PC) layers, used in MaxENT modeling. The three largest contributors to each layer are highlighted in italics. Eigen values listed in the last row indicate the amount of heterogeneity that each PC layer accounts for *PWQ* precipitation of wettest quarter, *MTCQ* Mean Temperature of Coldest Quarter, *AP* annual precipitation, *TS* Temperature Seasonality (standard deviation * 100), *PS* Precipitation Seasonality (Coefficient of Variation), *MTWaM* maximum temperature of the warmest month, *ISO* isothermability (Bio2/Bio7) * (100), *PDQ* Precipitation of Driest Quarter, *PDM* precipitation of the driest month, *MTCM* minimum temperature of the coldest month, *PCQ* Precipitation of Coldest Quarter, *TAR* Temperature Annual Range (MTWaM–MTCM), *PWaQ* Precipitation of Warmest Quarter, *MTWaQ* Mean Temperature of Warmest Quarter, *MTDQ* Mean Temperature of Driest Quarter, *PWM* precipitation of the wettest month, *AMT* annual mean temperature, *MTWQ* Mean Temperature of Wettest Quarter, *MDR* mean diurnal range

Information concerning reported cases of VACV in Colombia is more limited: they have occurred in the municipalities of Medina, Puerto Salgar (INS Personal Communications) and Valaparaíso [22]. Additionally, cow samples from the departments of Casanare and Santander have been found to be positive (INS Personal Communications).

Climatic data

At broad scales, climatic variables have been used in ecological niche models to find non-random associations between occurrences and environmental conditions at those locations to estimate distribution of many infectious diseases [28, 29]. Here, we used climatic datasets from WorldClim, http://www.worldclim.org/bioclim, which provide fine-scale data of various environmental factors for the entire world, including minimum, maximum, and average temperature, annual precipitation, as well as seasonal estimates for each factor. These datasets are publicly available through 19 bioclimatic spatial layers [30] and are offered in four resolutions. A visual comparison of each resolution's pixel size to the average municipality size was performed to select the most adequate spatial resolution to fit the precision of the VACV occurrence data. To reduce dimensionality and auto-correlation between variables, Principal Components (PC) were calculated based on the 19 bioclim layers in ArcMap, v. 10.3.1 over the total area of interest (Colombia and Brazil) [31] (Table 2).

Model generation

ENMs have been used to gain understanding of environmental aspects of transmission of diseases and their spatial distribution with limited amounts of available data. Maxent has been shown to be useful in its application to study infectious diseases [32], and to have a higher performance than other similar algorithms [33]. Thus, ENMs were built using MaxENT software [34], which applies the maximum entropy principle, whereby a model is constructed by fitting a probability distribution to the environmental variables, which is closest to uniform and is constrained by parameters associated with the outbreaks; by doing this, MaxENT finds non-random associations between environmental variables and VACV outbreaks via the comparison of environmental conditions at such localities and background conditions within the study area. Here, the default settings in MaxENT (i.e., regularization multiplier = 1.0, 1500 maximum iterations, 10,000 background points, convergence limit = 1025) were used.

In generating an ENM, the choice of a geographic extent in which models will be trained strongly influences the model's calibration since pseudo-absences can be selected from within this area [35]. An extent that is too large would offer the model too much area where transmission is not possible, resulting in a falsely precise model. A study area too small would not allow for sufficient environmental variability and would limit the selection of pseudo-absences (points where a case has not been reported, but cannot be ruled out) [35]. To address this, six geographic extents were tested—50, 100, 150, 200, 250 and 300 km radius (results for three of them are reported). Given that using a geographic extent that is too big would inflate AUC scores, we tested the extents iteratively, beginning with the smallest, and the one with the highest performance was chosen.

To test the ability of the ENM to predict areas suitable for VACV, the list of outbreaks was divided into two datasets—separated by whether each outbreak fell above or below the median longitude and median latitude of all outbreaks [36]. These datasets, which each contained outbreaks from different quadrants of the study area,

were then used as test and training datasets, to test and train model performance.

Mapping of VACV outbreaks (Fig. 1), identified through the literature search revealed clustering of outbreak reports in southeastern Brazil might be due to reporting bias since surveillance efforts are not uniform across the country. This clustering could interfere with the model performance metrics by means of spatial autocorrelation (i.e., nearby localities have similar environmental conditions and could predict each other) [32]. To address this bias, subsets of the outbreaks were created to generate a more homogeneous spatial representation of the distribution of the disease and correct for spatial autocorrelation. These subsets were created in R Studio, v. 0.99.849 using base packages [37]. To generate a subset, one outbreak was randomly selected as part of the subset and all points within an indicated proximity threshold [either

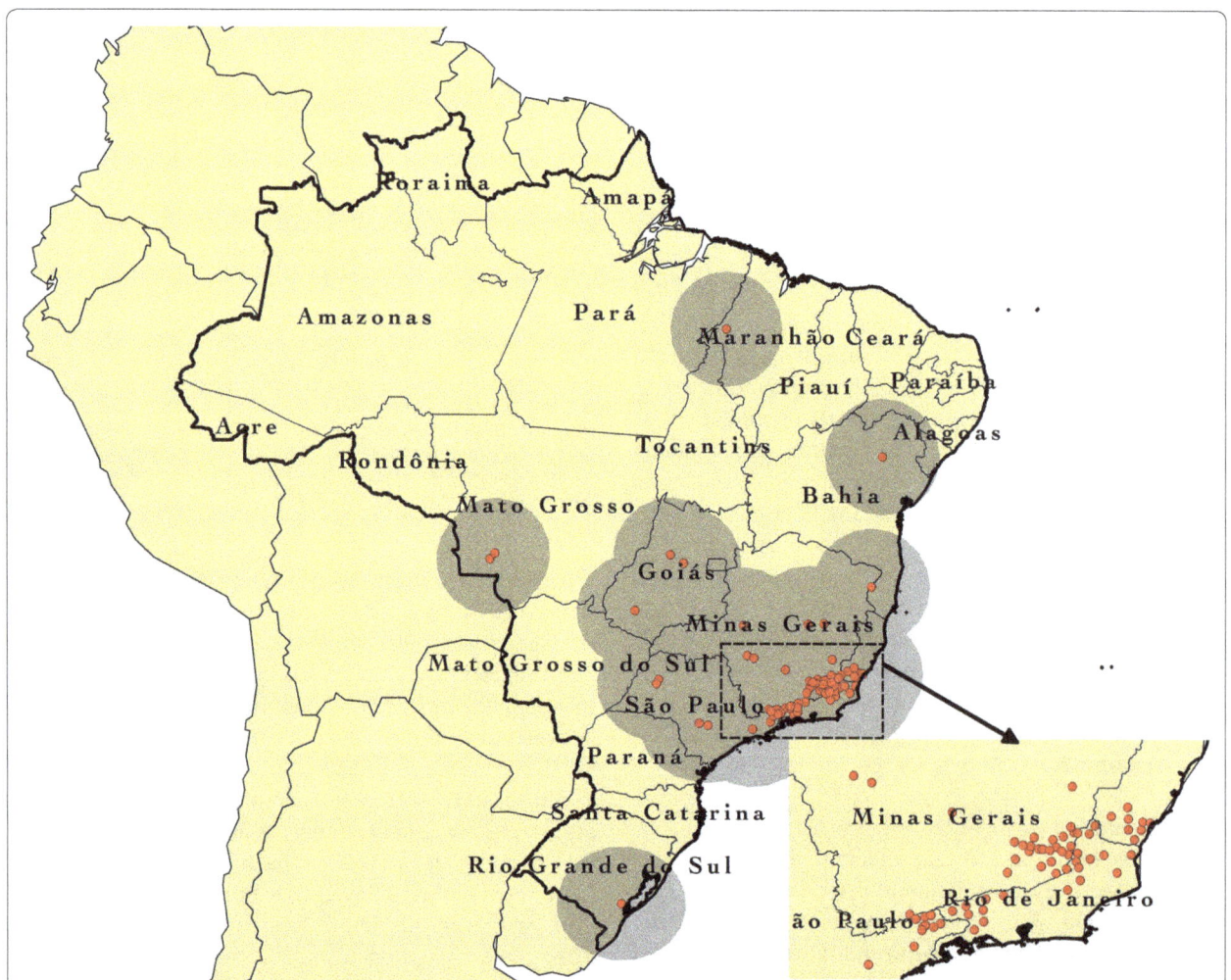

Fig. 1 VACV outbreaks in Brazil. *Red points* indicate the centroid of municipalities with confirmed VACV outbreaks. *Grey circles* show the 300 km radius from centroids, which indicates the geographic extent used in MaxENT model. *Inset* most outbreak municipalities were found in southeastern Brazil in the states of Minas Gerais, Espírito Santo, and Rio de Janeiro

33 km (0.1°) or 52 km (0.5°)] were removed. Then, a new outbreak was randomly selected from the remaining outbreaks and its neighbors (within the same proximity) were removed. This process was repeated until all outbreaks were assigned to the subset or discarded. This process was repeated 25 times to create 25 subsets with each proximity threshold, either with 33 or 52 km. The resulting subsets contained approximately 70 or 45 outbreaks, respectively. While not every outbreak was included in every subset, each outbreak was included in at least one of the subsets. Another correction for bias was applied by restricting the areas used to train the model to buffered regions around the outbreaks. Pseudo-absences were selected from within these regions, such that the selection bias of the outbreaks was applied to the environmental layers as well [38].

Models were run in MaxENT using each one of the outbreak datasets (33 km subsets, or 52 km subsets) and one set of environmental layers (PC layers clipped to either 50, 100, 150, 200, 250 or 300 km radius). Individual log probability outputs of each model were transformed into binary maps (0 = unsuitable and 1 = suitable using three probability thresholds calculated based on 0, 5, or 10% omission of the training occurrences [39]. Individual binary maps were then combined within each omission level to generate a map that represents model agreement with values ranging from 0 (all models agreed the pixel was unsuitable) to 25 (all models agreed the pixel was suitable) [39]. Finally, the model was projected onto the countries of Brazil and Colombia [40]. This projection was compared to the available geographic information of Colombian VACV outbreaks.

Model evaluation and analysis

Models were evaluated using the area under the curve (AUC) of the receiver-operating characteristic (ROC). For medical diagnostics, AUC values 0.5–0.7 are considered low accuracy, values of 0.7–0.9 are accurate and values $\geq$0.9 are highly accurate [41]. Previous studies selected an AUC of 0.85 as acceptable; given the uncertainty in the precision of the localities (municipalities) we used to generate the model, we would expect higher levels of omission, and therefore considered an AUC above 0.8 as acceptable.

A three-dimensional plot was produced using values from the first three PC layers, to visualize the climatic heterogeneity of the study area and the portions in environmental space occupied by the areas deemed suitable for transmission by the MaxENT model, as compared with the values of the actual outbreaks in Brazil and Colombia.

The PC layers used to make the ENMs contribute differentially to the final model. For each model, MaxENT provides the relative contribution of each variable. The higher the contribution, the more impact a PC layer has on predicting VACV suitability.

These values are derived by default in MaxENT. In brief, the first estimate reflects the increase in regularized gain, which is added to the contribution of the variable. Next, the values of each variable on training presence and background data are randomly permuted. The model is reevaluated on the permuted data, and the resulting drop in training AUC is shown (normalized to percentages). The average contribution of each PC layer across the 25 subsets, and the corresponding standard deviation is reported.

Values for each of the 19 bioclimatic layers were extracted from the areas identified as suitable for transmission in the final MaxENT model. Summary statistics were calculated for each layer. The same statistics are calculated at the points of outbreaks in Colombia and Brazil. These extracted values were also plotted as frequency plots.

Finally, the final model was visually compared to livestock densities as livestock is involved on the virus' transmission to humans. Estimates of livestock density are provided by the Food and Agriculture Administration of the United Nations (FAO) [42]. The density maps used here are a result of the FAO continuously collecting livestock statistics at sub-national levels. These data are then matched to their administrative boundaries and densities are calculated, accounting for suitable land (i.e., excluding lakes and cities).

Results

The literature review and selection criteria resulted in the identification of 87 Brazilian municipalities in which VACV outbreaks had occurred, mapped in Fig. 1. Most outbreaks are clustered in southeastern Brazil in the states of Rio de Janeiro, Minas Gerais and São Paulo. Some reports include multiple outbreaks that occurred over a time period [23, 43] while others reported on a single outbreak [44, 45]. Visual comparison of the four spatial resolutions of bioclim layers to the average size of VACV-affected municipalities led to the selection of the 5 arc-min resolution bioclim data for this analysis. At this resolution, pixels in bioclim layers were not considerably smaller or larger than the size of most VACV municipalities.

A principal component analysis of the 19 bioclim layers, revealed that the first five principal components account for 99.6% of the heterogeneity across Brazil and Colombia (Table 2) and were selected for use for in subsequent analyses. Among these five layers, the three largest bioclim contributors for each layer are bolded.

Precipitation of the wettest quarter (PWQ), mean temperature of the coldest quarter (MTCQ) and annual precipitation (AP) were the most important factors for PC 1. For PC 2, in addition to PWQ and MTCQ, mean diurnal range (MDR) was also identified as an important factor.

Multiple ENM models were generated using different combinations of outbreak datasets with environmental layers. These combinations and the resulting AUC values

Table 3 Summary of VACV MaxENT models

MaxENT run	Outbreak dataset	Enviro. layers (radius to centroids)	AUC (SD)	AUC (train)
1	Test v train	PC 1–5 (50 km)	0.64	0.684
2	Train v test	PC 1–5 (50 km)	0.626	0.832
3	Test v train	PC 1–5 (250 km)	0.802	0.935
4	Train v test	PC 1–5 (250 km)	0.848	0.844
5	Subsets, 52 km	PC 1–5 (250 km)	0.803 (0.007)	X
6	Subsets, 33 km	PC 1–5 (250 km)	0.861 (0.003)	X
7	Subsets, 52 km	PC 1–5 (300 km)	0.812 (0.007)	X
8	Subsets, 33 km	PC 1–5 (300 km)	0.867 (0.002)	X
9	Subsets, 52 km	BioClim 1–19 (300 km)	0.873 (0.004)	X
10	Subsets, 33 km	BioClim 1–19 (300 km)	0.907 (0.001)	X
11 (combined datasets)	Subsets, 52 km	PC 1–5 (300 km)	0.95	X

Summary, variables used and resulting AUC values, of MaxENT models run in selecting variables. Subsets had 33 or 52 km, 0.3 or 0.15 decimal degrees in between each outbreak, corresponding to ~52 and 33 km, respectively. MaxENT runs 5–7 were generated using 25 subsets of outbreaks. The AUC values reported here are averages of those AUC's from those 25 models. Standard deviations are reported in parenthesis

are summarized in Table 3. Only three of the six geographic extents tested are listed here.

MaxENT models 1–4 were run to determine the ability of an ENM to predict outbreaks by generating the model using a training dataset, which contained approximately half of the total outbreaks, and testing its ability to predict areas suitable for the other half of the outbreaks. Using a geographic extent limited to a 50 km radius surrounding outbreaks yielded models that were not accurate or predictive (Test AUC = 0.64, Train AUC = 0.684). When a buffer of 250 km was used to select the training area, the model improved considerably (Test AUC = 0.802, Train AUC = 0.935). These results indicated that the MaxENT model was capable of predicting outbreak localities by identifying environmental conditions suitable for VACV transmission.

Models were created using each set of the subsets of outbreaks and PC 1–5 layers at a 250 km radius extent. AUC values were higher for those models using subsets generated using 33 km (Model 6 AUC = 0.861) compared with the models, which used 52 km subsets (Model 5 AUC = 0.803). However, this could be due to incomplete elimination of clustering; thus, subsets generated using 52 km were used for modeling, with a slightly larger geographic extent, 300 km (Model 7 AUC = 0.812).

Models 9 and 10 were run using the 19 bioclim variables, which were not reassembled into PC layers. Each of the 19 were clipped to 300 km around each outbreak and models were generated using 52 km (Model 9) and 33 km (Model 10) outbreak subsets. As such, models 7 and 9 are comparable and models 8 and 10 are comparable. In each comparison, the AUC is slightly improved when using 19 bioclim variables, rather than PC layers 1–5. This suggests that use of PC 1–5 removed some information that describes VACV suitability. Five bioclim variables accounted for about 80% of the heterogeneity:

isothermability (26.6%), Precipitation of the coldest quarter (15.9%), mean temperature of the driest quarter (15.6%), precipitation seasonality (12.2%), and temperature seasonality (9,7%). The remaining 14 layers each contributed less than 5% each to the heterogeneity of the principle components. One of these variables, precipitation of the coldest quarter, was identified as a key environmental parameter in models, which used PC layers. That the other three variables are different may suggest that without the adjustment provided by principle components, the estimate of these variables is overly emphasized.

Final models were produced at three thresholds of omission (Fig. 2a). The 0% threshold, in addition to identifying the regions where VACV outbreaks have already occurred, uniquely highlighted new regions of the Mato Grasso, Tocantins, Rio Grande do Sul as well as several central-eastern states, as suitable for transmission. The more conservative 10% threshold identified new states and regions as suitable for transmission, including Santa Catarina, Paraná, and Mato Grosso do Sul. States which have already experienced at least one VACV outbreak, and were identified by the model as suitable to VACV transmission are: Mato Grosso, Rio Grande do Sul, Minas Gerais, Rio de Janeiro, Espírito Santo, Bahia, Goiás, and smaller portions of Maranhão and Bahia. States which have not yet experienced a VACV outbreak, yet were identified as suitable by the model were Mato Grosso do Sul, Paraná, Santa Catarina and smaller portions of Piauí, Ceará, Pernambuco, Alagoas, and Sergipe.

The final models were then projected onto Colombia (Fig. 2b). The known outbreaks that have occurred there are shown by black outline of the most granular geographic extent available: municipalities (Medina, Valaparaíso and Puerto Salgar) or departments (Casanare and

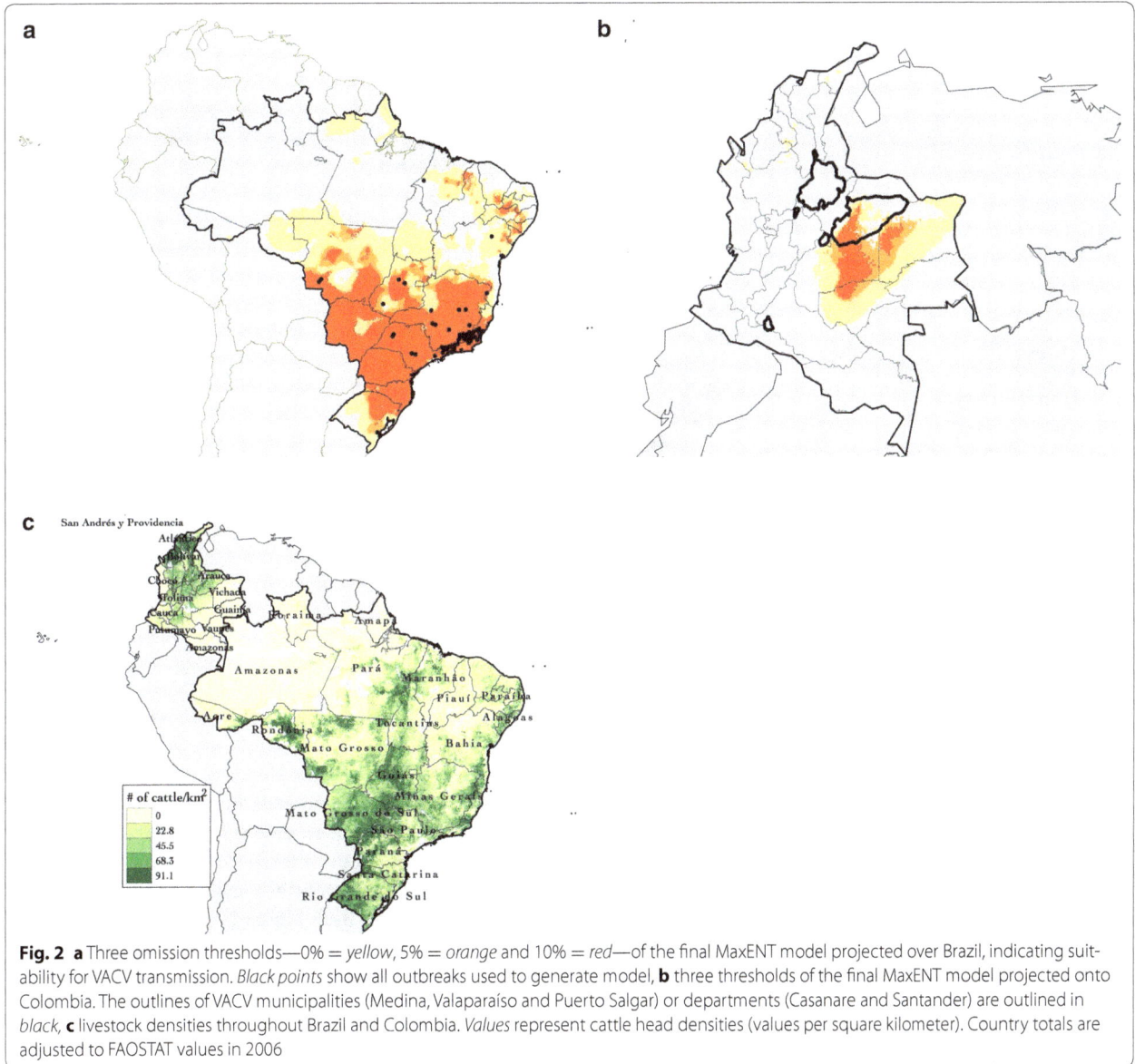

Fig. 2 a Three omission thresholds—0% = *yellow*, 5% = *orange* and 10% = *red*—of the final MaxENT model projected over Brazil, indicating suitability for VACV transmission. *Black points* show all outbreaks used to generate model, **b** three thresholds of the final MaxENT model projected onto Colombia. The outlines of VACV municipalities (Medina, Valaparaíso and Puerto Salgar) or departments (Casanare and Santander) are outlined in *black*, **c** livestock densities throughout Brazil and Colombia. *Values* represent cattle head densities (values per square kilometer). Country totals are adjusted to FAOSTAT values in 2006

Santander). Outbreaks could have occurred anywhere within the outlined regions. The model predicted part of one department, Casanare, and the model, using the 0% threshold, predicted part of one municipality, Medina, as suitable for transmission. The regions in which three of these outbreaks occurred lie outside of the predicted region.

The density of livestock [42] is mapped (Fig. 2c), and many of the Brazilian outbreaks fall within regions of Brazil that have a high density of cattle, i.e., Goiás, Rio de Janeiro, Minas Gerais, and São Paulo. Several areas with high density of livestock are predicted suitable for transmission such as Mato Grosso do Sul, and northwestern Paraná.

Figure 3a–c show several angles of the three-dimensional plot of PC 1–3 values. The MaxENT model prediction for suitable ranges for each of these variables is shown in black dots. The values for Brazil (red) fall within this range, as the model accurately predicted the majority of the outbreaks there. Some of Colombia's outbreaks fall outside of the suitable environments, as predicted by the model. One of these outbreaks is notably discordant for PC 1. Most of Colombia's outbreaks fell within Brazil's range for PC layers 2 and 3, but again, varied for PC layer 1. In Fig. 3b, c, the background and MaxENT model conditions were removed for better visualization.

The percent predictive contribution of each PC layer to the final model is listed in Table 4.

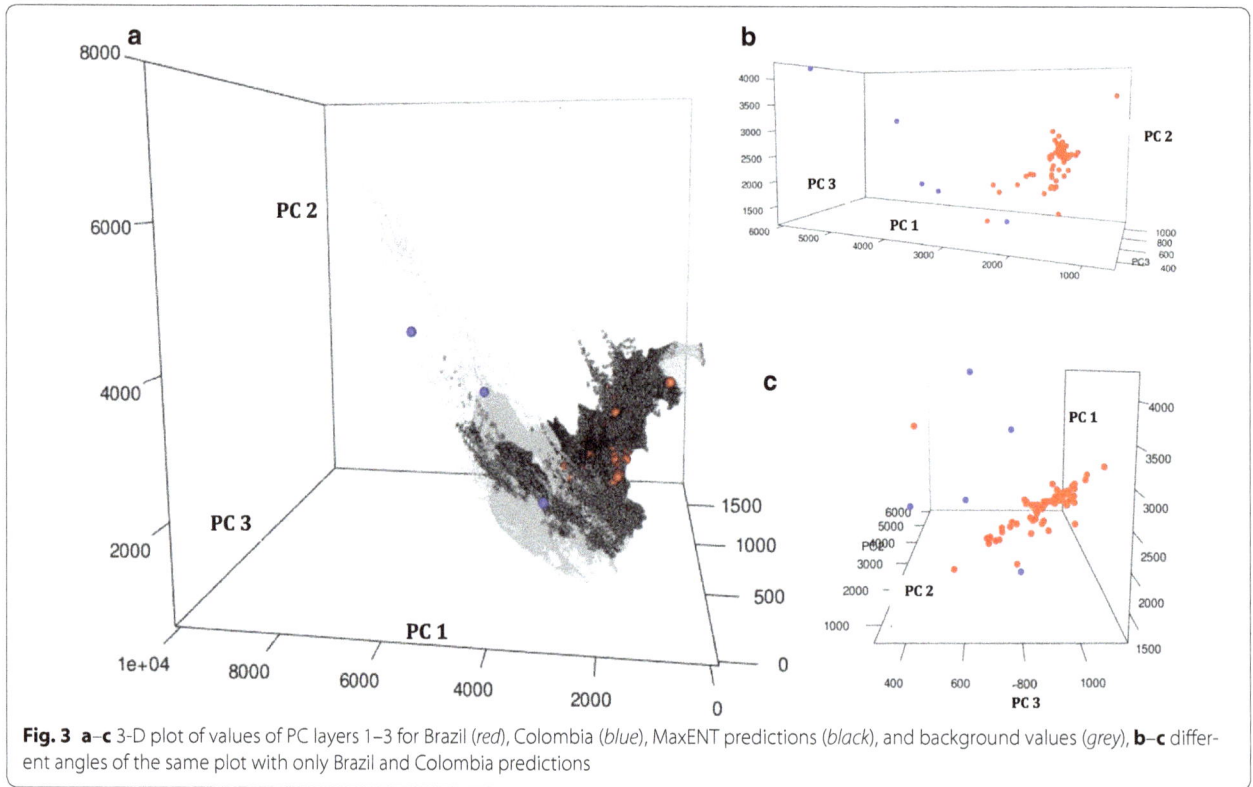

Fig. 3 a–c 3-D plot of values of PC layers 1–3 for Brazil (*red*), Colombia (*blue*), MaxENT predictions (*black*), and background values (*grey*), **b–c** different angles of the same plot with only Brazil and Colombia predictions

PC layers 1 and 2 collectively contributed over 70% to the final model. The bioclim layers with the highest contribution to PC layers 1 and 2 are precipitation of the wettest quarter (PWQ), mean temp of the coldest quarter (MTCQ), annual precipitation (AP) and mean diurnal range (MDR) and were further analyzed. Plotted in Fig. 4 is the number of pixels deemed as suitable for transmission at each value of the bioclim variable indicated: MaxENT prediction (black line), Brazilian outbreaks (red line). The range for each of these variables, as predicted by MaxENT, is as follows: PWQ (198.12–1546.86 mm), MTCQ (9.5–27.1 °C), AP (467.36–3571.24 mm), and MDR (6.6–15.7 °C). Summary statistics for each of the bioclim layers extracted from

each model can be found in Additional file 2 and pixel plots for the remaining 15 bioclim layers are provided in Additional file 3. To summarize the results of the ENM, the environmental factors associated with most of the VACV outbreaks in Brazil include an annual mean temperature of 22.5 °C, mean diurnal temperature range of 11.7 °C, and an annual precipitation of 1493.52 mm.

Discussion

Ecologic niche modeling was used to identify the actual and potential niche of VACV, an *Orthopoxvirus* which primary affects dairy cattle in Brazil. Subsets of the geographic locations of VACV cases were combined with environmental layers, condensed by a principle component analysis, and were clipped to various extents. The final extent and subset combination was selected by using the model, which produced the highest AUC value. This model was then projected onto a larger geographic range, to include neighboring Colombia, where outbreaks have also occurred. The values of each PC layer as well as the biocim values were extracted at each outbreak location. These values were compared across the two countries. Several methods were used to account for the bias inherent in the outbreak data including: using a 10% threshold of probabilistic estimates, selecting a resolution of environmental data which was not significantly more resolute

Table 4 Average contribution of each PC layer to final model

PC layer	Average	SD
PC 1	20.70	2.04
PC 2	53.16	2.82
PC 3	12.71	1.10
PC 4	9.68	1.67
PC 5	3.75	1.10

Average percent contribution of each PC layer, to the final ENM. Average of 25 subsets used to make final model is shown.

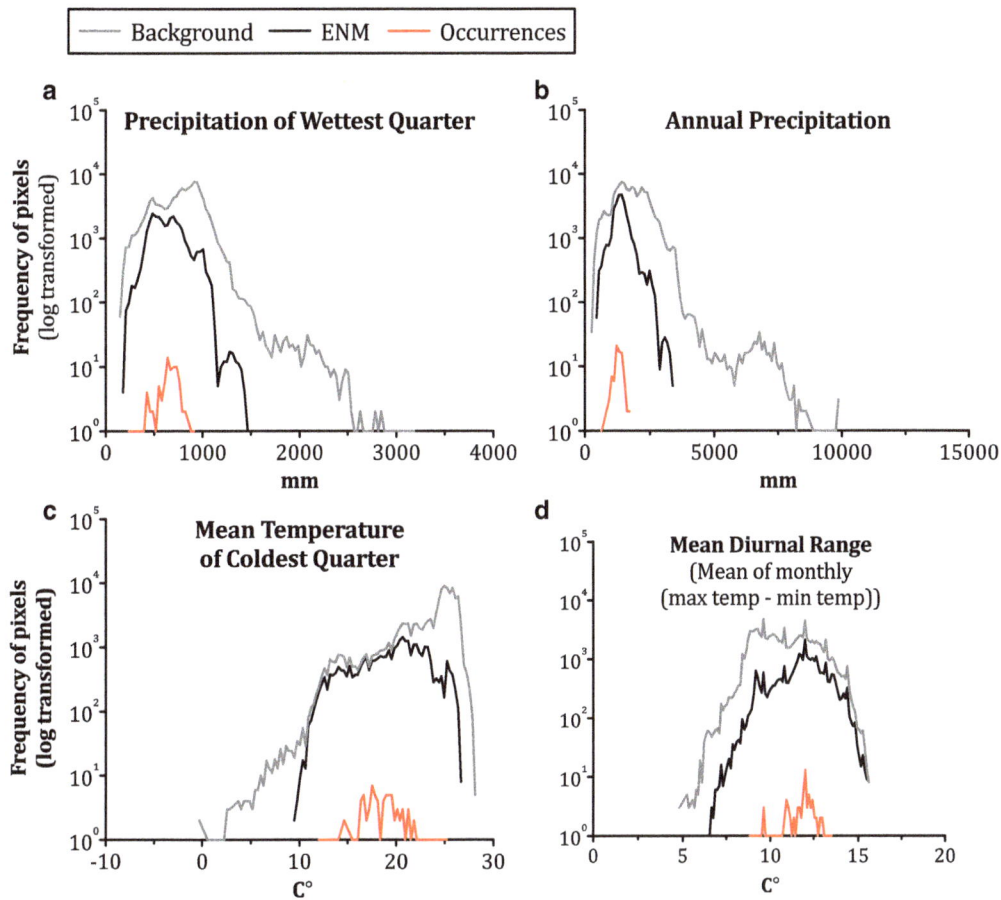

Fig. 4 Available values are plotted to demonstrate the key environmental parameters and the ecological niche occupied by VACV, according to MaxENT predictions (*black*), 87 Brazilian outbreaks (*red*), and background (*grey*). On the Y-axis is the number of pixels for each variable and the X-Axis, the bioclim variable indicated

than the available geographic granularity of the outbreaks, and creating subsets of outbreaks which reduced the effect of clustering.

The result was a model, which identified regions in Brazil where VACV outbreaks have already occurred as well as several new locations within Brazil, which could be vulnerable to a VACV outbreak. Most states identified as suitable for VACV transmission, have regions with a high density of livestock, as this industry is clustered in southern Brazil. Where high density of livestock and suitability for transmission co-localize, the risk of VACV is likely much greater.

The final model predicted a portion of one of the five regions in Colombia, which have confirmed VACV outbreaks. This prediction could be explained in several ways. For example, VACV could have different reservoirs in different regions, i.e., different mammal species maintain the virus in nature, each with different ecologic/environmental requirements. An argument for multiple reservoirs is supported given the variation in small

rodent species found to have evidence of infection with orthopoxviruses in Brazil [46]. Additionally, poxviruses can infect several species of animals i.e., *Monkeypox virus* in pouched rats, [47], prairie dogs, squirrels [48], and dormice [49], among others; *Cowpox virus* in voles [50], llamas [51], mice [52], cats [53] among other species of animals. Consistent with this is the results of the 3D graph, which allows for comparison of the ecologic niche that VACV occupies across the two countries. The discordance for PC 1 suggests that VACV occupies a different climate space in Colombia, as compared with Brazil. Further, suitable environmental conditions alone are insufficient for transmission of VACV, as the suitable area would also have to be occupied by its reservoir, and pathogen distribution is also restricted by geographic barriers, mobility, and human intervention [54]. Finally, the limited number of outbreaks that have been recorded in Colombia leaves the predictive capability of the Brazil model for Colombia, inconclusive. Only a few VACV infections in Colombia have been reported since 2014; all of which have had contact with cows. It is possible that cases are happening in areas of high livestock density in Colombia, but they go unreported since the surveillance system is not designed to capture them. Given the differences in the available data from Brazil and Colombia, (i.e., both geographically biased, but Brazil having many more years detecting and reporting) conclusions about the different niches for VACV in these places, are limited.

Key bioclimatic indicators for this disease have also been identified by the model: PWQ, MTCQ, AP and MDR.

Several limitations exist for this type of modeling. To generate the ENM reported here, the centroids of municipalities, which have experienced a VACV outbreak, not the actual farm, were used. Significant environmental heterogeneity across the municipality would reduce the precision of the final model. Further, the outbreaks used to make the model are a result of a literature review, which do not represent reports from active surveillance of disease in humans or cattle; therefore, there is an inherent bias that could over-represent the geographic areas that routinely report and test for VACV. Several measures have been taken to minimize the potential effects of these biases, including the use of subsets, limiting geographic extents, and the use of a 10% threshold to make conservative estimates. Improvements in either the specificity of coordinates used and in data collection methods would likely improve model prediction. Implementing a surveillance program for VACV would improve the precision and number of cases and outbreaks. This would, in turn, improve model accuracy and predictive capability. Additionally, overcoming barriers for reporting cases (i.e., fear of closing farms) would aid in surveillance efforts. High-quality occurrence data would also allow the use of relevant non-climatic factors such as land use, trade data, milker travel records, and other sources of environmental data (i.e., satellite imagery) at higher spatial and temporal resolutions to refine the models and broaden our understanding of the ecology of this pathogen.

Despite their limitations, the data presented here could provide valuable information to public health officials in protecting human health proactively; areas where the ecological niche predicts suitable environments for transmission could be targeted by education campaigns to inform local farmers of symptoms and warn against sharing of cows with these farms, early symptoms in cows, horses, and humans, and encourage methods to prevent its spread such as improved sanitation and ill cattle isolation. Similarly, future epidemiological and ecological studies could focus on these areas and study the local species and their potential role in the maintenance of VACV in nature. Given the prediction capabilities of the model in Brazil, in its current state, this model would be of most use in Brazil, for these purposes.

Public engagement and a participatory process, inclusive of all stakeholders: farmers, milk consumers, planning officials, public health personnel, and community organizations, would improve the quality and impact of all interventions aimed at preventing and mitigating harm from outbreaks.

This information is increasingly relevant in context of the growing dairy industry in Brazil. An estimated 30% of the total milk production in Brazil in 2014, 36 billion liters, was under informal methods, or not under the inspection of government officials [26]. Moreover, populations in VACV affected regions of Brazil practice a traditional cheese making process which uses unpasteurized milk [55], whereby virus in milk may not be entirely inactivated. There is a documented case of a human patient, without any direct contact with cows, who developed VACV lesions of the mouth [56] suggesting a potential risk for transmission via consumption of infected milk.

Most VACV publications, to date, are descriptions of outbreaks or reported cases [43, 57–61], and a few others describe controlled experiments using VACV to infect cows or mice [62]; however, to the best of our knowledge, there are no publications describing the suitable environmental conditions for the transmission of VACV. The recent VACV reports from Colombia highlights the potential for VACV, or other poxviruses, to cause human and animal disease in other countries. Further, current events have illuminated the threat of spread of infectious diseases, which in past decades may have been isolated to a certain region, but now have potential to spread globally in a relatively short period of time [63, 64]. Finally, herd immunity to poxviruses is dissipating due to smallpox vaccination no longer being routine.

Conclusions

The study of emerging diseases presents a unique set of challenges, several of which are highlighted in work presented here: selection bias, specificity of data and limited information, are among them. In addition, lack of basic information about a disease, such as a complete host range and transmission patterns, leaves prevention efforts with little direction. Finally, the lack of a surveillance, cohort or case control study, limits the analytical methods that could be used. Here, we sought to address these challenges by applying an ecological niche model as a proof of concept to demonstrate ways to spatially predict VACV outbreaks. The analyses here provide a means by which to study the patterns of an emerging infectious disease, and regions that are potentially at risk for it, in spite of the paucity of critical data and limitations described above.

Policy and methods for the control of infectious diseases often use a reactionary model, addressing diseases only after significant impact on human health has ensued. Here, we provide a means to predict where the disease is likely to appear, providing a map for effective prevention. Contemporary events [64, 65] strongly indicate the need for the study of emerging and neglected diseases despite the implicit hurdles. Global developments over the last century have given many infectious diseases a new landscape and offer them boundless immune susceptible organisms. In the pursuit to counteract these measures, current strategies will not suffice in protecting human health. We must look for novel solutions and means to prevent and mitigate infectious disease epidemics.

Additional files

> **Additional file 1.** List of Brazilian outbreaks used to generate ENM, with references.
>
> **Additional file 2.** Summary statistics of key bioclim values as predicted by MaxENT modeling, using a 10% threshold, and what is indicated at the points of VCAV occurrence in Brazil and Colombia. Temperatures are reported in degrees Fahrenheit and precipitation in mm. AMT, annual mean temperature; MDR, mean diurnal range; ISO, isothermability (Bio2/Bio7)*(100); TS, Temperature Seasonality (standard deviation *100); MTWaM; maximum temperature of the warmest month; MTCM, minimum temperature of the coldest month; TAR, Temperature Annual Range (Bio5-Bio6); MTWQ, Mean Temperature of Wettest Quarter; MTDQ, Mean Temperature of Driest Quarter; MTWaQ, Mean Temperature of Warmest Quarter; MTCQ, Mean Temperature of Coldest Quarter; AP, annual precipitation; PWM, precipitation of the wettest month; PDM, precipitation of the driest month; PS, Precipitation Seasonality (Coefficient of Variation); PWQ, Precipitation of Wettest Quarter; PDQ, Precipitation of Driest Quarter; PWaQ, Precipitation of Warmest Quarter; PWQ, Precipitation of Coldest Quarter.
>
> **Additional file 3.** Available values are plotted to demonstrate the key environmental parameters and the ecological niche occupied by VACV according to MaxENT predictions (black), 87 Brazilian outbreaks (red), and background (grey) of the remaining 15 bioclim layers not shown in Fig. 4. On the Y-axis is the number of pixels for each variable and the X-Axis, the bioclim variable indicated.

Abbreviations
VACV: Vaccinia virus; ENM: ecological niche model; DPI: days post-inoculation; PC: principal components.

Authors' contributions
CQ and YN designed the study. CQ analyzed the data and drafted the manuscript. YN oversaw data design and helped revise the manuscript. Both authors read and approved the final manuscript.

Acknowledgements
This work has benefitted from the contributions of a team of advisers including Mary Reynolds, Ben Monroe, Andrea McCollum and Ginny Emerson. A special thank you for feedback and advice to Sondra Schlesinger. The authors acknowledge to contributions of personal communications from Giliane de Souza Trindade, MC. Madureira, Galileu Barbosa Costa and Poliana de Oliveira Figueiredo; and colleagues from the Colombian National Institute of Health: Andres Paez Martinez, Jose Usme Ciro, Martha Gracia Romero, Katherine Laiton Donato. CQ thanks SD.

Competing interests
The authors declare that they have no competing interests.

Disclaimer
The findings and conclusions in this report are those of the authors and do not necessarily represent the official position of the US Centers for Disease Control and Prevention.

Funding
This work was financially supported by the Centers for Disease Control and Prevention, and Oakridge Institute for Science and Education (ORISE).

References
1. Keele BF, et al. Chimpanzee reservoirs of pandemic and nonpandemic HIV-1. Science. 2006;313(5786):523–6.
2. Centers for Disease Control and Prevention. Swine influenza A (H1N1) infection in two children—Southern California, March–April 2009. Morb Mortal Wkly Rep. 2009;58.
3. WHO Ebola Response Team. Ebola virus disease in West Africa—the first 9 months of the epidemic and forward projections. N Engl J Med. 2014;371(16):1481–95.
4. Zaki AM, van Boheemen S, Bestebroer TM, Osterhaus ADME, Fouchier RAM. Isolation of a novel coronavirus from a man with pneumonia in Saudi Arabia. N Engl J Med. 2012;367(19):1814–20.
5. Lashley FR. Emerging infectious diseases at the beginning of the 21st century. Online J Issues Nurs. 2006;11(1):2.
6. American Veterinary Medical Association. One health: A new professional imperative. One health initiative task force: final report. Schaumburg: American Veterinary Medical Association; 2008.
7. Dumbell K, Richardson M. Virological investigations of specimens from buffaloes affected by buffalopox in Maharashtra State, India between 1985 and 1987. Arch Virol. 1993;128(3–4):257–67.
8. Damaso CRA, Reis SA, Jesus DM, Lima PSF, Moussatche N. A PCR-based assay for detection of emerging vaccinia-like viruses isolated in Brazil. Diagn Microbiol Infect Dis. 2007;57(1):39–46.
9. Megid J, et al. Vaccinia virus zoonotic infection, Sao Paulo State, Brazil. Emerg Infect Dis. 2012;18(1):189–91.
10. Tulman ER, et al. Genome of horsepox virus. J Virol. 2006;80(18):9244–58.
11. Abrahao JS, et al. Vaccinia virus infection in monkeys, Brazilian Amazon. Emerg Infect Dis. 2010;16(6):976–9.
12. Peres MG, et al. Dogs and opossums positive for Vaccinia virus during outbreak affecting cattle and humans, Sao Paulo State, Brazil. Emerg Infect Dis. 2016;22(2):271–3.
13. Peres MG, et al. Serological study of Vaccinia virus reservoirs in areas with and without official reports of outbreaks in cattle and humans in Sao Paulo, Brazil. Arch Virol. 2013;158(12):2433–41.
14. Campos RK, et al. Assessing the variability of Brazilian Vaccinia virus isolates from a horse exanthematic lesion: coinfection with distinct viruses. Arch Virol. 2011;156(2):275–83.
15. Essbauer S, Hartnack S, Misztela K, Kiessling-Tsalos J, Baumler W, Pfeffer M. Patterns of orthopox virus wild rodent hosts in South Germany. Vector Borne Zoonotic Dis Larchmt N. 2009;9(3):301–11.
16. Kinnunen PM, et al. Orthopox virus infections in Eurasian wild rodents. Vector Borne Zoonotic Dis Larchmt N. 2011;11(8):1133–40.
17. Damaso CR, Esposito JJ, Condit RC, Moussatche N. An emergent poxvirus from humans and cattle in Rio de Janeiro State: Cantagalo virus may derive from Brazilian smallpox vaccine. Virology. 2000;277(2):439–49.

18. Abrahao JS, et al. One more piece in the VACV ecological puzzle: could peridomestic rodents be the link between wildlife and bovine vaccinia outbreaks in Brazil? PLoS ONE. 2009;4(10):e7428.

19. Assis FL, et al. Horizontal study of Vaccinia virus infections in an endemic area: epidemiologic, phylogenetic and economic aspects. Arch Virol. 2015;160(11):2703–08.

20. Oliveira DB, et al. Group 1 Vaccinia virus zoonotic outbreak in Maranhão State, Brazil. Am J Trop Med Hyg. 2013;89(6):1142–5.

21. de Souza Trindade G, et al. Zoonotic Vaccinia virus infection in Brazil: clinical description and implications for health professionals. J Clin Microbiol. 2007;45(4):1370–2.

22. Usme-Ciro JA, et al. Detection and molecular characterization of zoonotic poxviruses circulating in the Amazon Region of Colombia. Emerg Infect Dis. 2017;23(4):649–53.

23. Nagasse-Sugahara TK, et al. Human vaccinia-like virus outbreaks in Sao Paulo and Goias States, Brazil: virus detection, isolation and identification. Rev Inst Med Trop Sao Paulo. 2004;46(6):315–22.

24. Rehfeld IS, et al. Clinical, hematological and biochemical parameters of dairy cows experimentally infected with Vaccinia virus. Res Vet Sci. 2013;95(2):752–7.

25. de Oliveira TML, et al. Vaccinia virus is not inactivated after thermal treatment and cheese production using experimentally contaminated milk. Foodborne Pathog Dis. 2010;7(12):1491–6.

26. USDA Foreign Agricultural Service. Brazil: Dairy and products annual. Global Agricultural Information Network. 2015.

27. Peterson AT. Mapping disease transmission risk: enriching models using biogeography and ecology. 1st ed. Baltimore: Johns Hopkins University Press; 2014.

28. Soberon J, Nakamura M. Niches and distributional areas: concepts, methods, and assumptions. Proc Natl Acad Sci USA. 2009;106(Suppl 2):19644–50.

29. Blackburn JK, McNyset KM, Curtis A, Hugh-Jones ME. Modeling the geographic distribution of Bacillus anthracis, the causative agent of anthrax disease, for the contiguous United States using predictive ecological [corrected] niche modeling. Am J Trop Med Hyg. 2007;77(6):1103–10.

30. Hijmans RJ, Cameron SE, Parra JL, Jones PG, Jarvis A. Very high resolution interpolated climate surfaces for global land areas. Int J Clim. 2005;25(15):1965–78.

31. Peterson AT. Ecological niches and geographic distributions (MPB-49). Princeton: Princeton University Press; 2011.

32. Peterson AT, Moses LM, Bausch DG. Mapping transmission risk of Lassa fever in West Africa: the importance of quality control, sampling bias, and error weighting. PLoS ONE. 2014;9(8):e100711.

33. Anderson RP, et al. Novel methods improve prediction of species' distributions from occurrence data. Ecography. 2006;29(2):129–51.

34. Yates J, Chee YE, Dudík M, Hastie T, Phillips SJ, Elith J. A statistical explanation of MaxEnt for ecologists. Divers Distrib. 2011;17:43–57.

35. Barve N, et al. The crucial role of the accessible area in ecological niche modeling and species distribution modeling. Ecol Model. 2011;222(11):1810–9.

36. Peterson AT, Papeş M, Soberón J. Rethinking receiver operating characteristic analysis applications in ecological niche modeling. Ecol Model. 2008;213(1):63–72.

37. Wisz MS, et al. Effects of sample size on the performance of species distribution models. Divers Distrib. 2008;14(5):763–73.

38. Moua Y, Roux E, Girod R, Dusfour I, de Thoisy B, Seyler F, Briolant S. Distribution of the habitat suitability of the main malaria vector in French Guiana using maximum entropy modeling. J Med Entomol. 2017;54(3):606–21. doi:10.1093/jme/tjw199.

39. Pearson RG, Raxworthy CJ, Nakamura M, Peterson AT. Predicting species distributions from small numbers of occurrence records: a test case using cryptic geckos in Madagascar. J Biogeogr. 2007;34(1):102–17.

40. Anderson RP. A framework for using niche models to estimate impacts of climate change on species distributions. Ann N Y Acad Sci. 2013;1297(1):8–28.

41. Swets JA. Measuring the accuracy of diagnostic systems. Science. 1988;240(4857):1285–93.

42. Food and Agriculture Organization of the United Nations. Animal production and health. Agricultural and Consumer Protection Department; 2014.

43. Costa RVC, et al. Animal infections by vaccinia-like viruses in the state of Rio de Janeiro: 2-Paraíba river valley. Virus Rev Res. 2007;12:37–42.

44. Campos RK, et al. Assessing the variability of Brazilian Vaccinia virus isolates from a horse exanthematic lesion: coinfection with distinct viruses. Arch Virol. 2011;156(2):275–83.

45. Leite JA, et al. Passatempo virus, a Vaccinia virus strain, Brazil. Emerg Infect Dis. 2005;11(12):1935–8.

46. Miranda JB, et al. Serologic and molecular evidence of Vaccinia virus circulation among small mammals from different biomes, Brazil. Emerg Infect Dis. 2017;23(6):931–8.

47. Schwarz TF, Hassler D. Gambian giant pouched rat and prairie dogs: monkeypox outbreak in America. Dtsch Med Wochenschr 1946. 2003;128(28–29):1524.

48. Khodakevich L, Jezek Z, Kinzanzka K. Isolation of monkeypox virus from wild squirrel infected in nature. Lancet Lond Engl. 1986;1(8472):98–9.

49. Hutson CL, et al. Monkeypox zoonotic associations: insights from laboratory evaluation of animals associated with the multi-state US outbreak. Am J Trop Med Hyg. 2007;76(4):757–68.

50. Burthe S, Telfer S, Begon M, Bennett M, Smith A, Lambin X. Cowpox virus infection in natural field vole Microtus agrestis populations: significant negative impacts on survival. J Anim Ecol. 2008;77(1):110–9.

51. Cardeti G, et al. Cowpox virus in llama, Italy. Emerg Infect Dis. 2011;17(8):1513–5.

52. Chantrey J, et al. Cowpox: reservoir hosts and geographic range. Epidemiol Infect. 1999;122(3):455–60.

53. Brown A, Bennett M, Gaskell CJ. Fatal poxvirus infection in association with FIV infection. Vet Rec. 1989;124(1):19–20.

54. Phillips SJ, Anderson RP, Schapire RE. Maximum entropy modeling of species geographic distributions. Ecol Model. 2006;190(3–4):231–59.

55. Fagundes H, Barchesi L, Filho AN, Ferreira LM, Oliveira CAF. Occurrence of Staphylococcus aureus in raw milk produced in dairy farms in Sao Paulo state, Brazil. Braz J Microbiol Publ Braz Soc Microbiol. 2010;41(2):376–80.

56. Megid J. Short report: Vaccinia virus in humans and cattle in southwest region of Sao Paulo state, Brazil (vol 79, pg 647, 2008). Am J Trop Med Hyg. 2009;80(1):165–165.

57. Campos RK, et al. Assessing the variability of Brazilian Vaccinia virus isolates from a horse exanthematic lesion: coinfection with distinct viruses. Arch Virol. 2011;156(2):275–83.

58. de Souza Trindade G, et al. Zoonotic Vaccinia virus infection in Brazil: clinical description and implications for health professionals. J Clin Microbiol. 2007;45(4):1370–2.

59. Oliveira DB, et al. Group 1 Vaccinia virus zoonotic outbreak in Maranhão State, Brazil. Am J Trop Med Hyg. 2013;89(6):1142–5.

60. Abrahao JS, et al. Detection of Vaccinia virus during an outbreak of exanthemous oral lesions in Brazilian equids. Equine Vet J. 2017;49(2):221—4.

61. Schatzmayr HG, Costa RVC, Goncalves MCR, D'Andrea PS, Barth OM. Human and animal infections by vaccinia-like viruses in the state of Rio de Janeiro: a novel expanding zoonosis. Vaccine. 2011;29(Suppl 4):D65–9.

62. Rehfeld IS, et al. Clinical, hematological and biochemical parameters of dairy cows experimentally infected with Vaccinia virus. Res Vet Sci. 2013;95(2):752–7.

63. Leroy EM, et al. Multiple Ebola virus transmission events and rapid decline of central African wildlife. Science. 2004;303(5656):387–90.

64. Hennessey M, Fischer M, Staples JE. Zika virus spreads to new areas—region of the Americas, May 2015–January 2016. MMWR Morb Mortal Wkly Rep. 2016;65(3):55–8.

65. Dixon MG, Schafer IJ. Ebola viral disease outbreak—West Africa, 2014. MMWR Morb Mortal Wkly Rep. 2014;63(25):548–51.

14

Identifying youth-friendly service practices associated with adolescents' use of reproductive healthcare services in post-conflict Burundi: a cross-sectional study

Imelda K. Moise[1*], Jaclyn F. Verity[1] and Joseph Kangmennaang[2]

Abstract

Background: Very little is known about reproductive health service (RHS) availability and adolescents' use of these services in post-conflict settings. Such information is crucial for targeted community interventions that aim to improve quality delivery of RHS and outcomes in post-conflict settings. The objectives of this study therefore was to examine the density of RHS availability; assess spatial patterns of RHC facilities; and identify youth-friendly practices associated with adolescents' use of services in post-conflict Burundi.

Methods: A cross-sectional survey was conducted from a full census of all facilities (n = 892) and provider interviews in Burundi. Surveyed facilities included all public, private, religious and community association owned-centers and hospitals. At each facility efforts were made to interview the officer-in-charge and a group of his/her staff. We applied both geospatial and non-spatial analyses, to examine the density of RHS availability and density, and to explore the association between youth-friendly practices and adolescents' use of RHS in post-conflict Burundi.

Results: High spatial patterning of distances of RHC facilities was observed, with facilities clustered predominantly in districts exhibiting persistent violence. But, use of services remained undeterred. We further found a stronger association between use of RHS and facility and programming characteristics. Community outreach, designated check-in/exam rooms, educational materials (posters, print, and pictures) in waiting rooms, privacy and confidentiality were significantly associated with adolescents' use of RHS across all facility types. Cost was associated with use only at religious facilities and youth involvement at private facilities. No significant association was found between provider characteristics and use of RHS at any facility.

Conclusions: Our findings indicate the need to improve youth-friendly service practices in the provision of RHS to adolescents in Burundi and suggest that current approaches to provider training may not be adequate for improving these vital practices. Our mixed methods approach and results are generalizable to other countries and post-conflict settings. In post-conflict settings, the methods can be used to identify service availability and spatial patterns of RHC facilities to plan for targeted service interventions, to increase demand and uptake of services by youth and young adults.

Background

Access to reproductive health services (RHS) and information and by sexually active young people is

*Correspondence: moise@miami.edu
[1] Department of Geography and Regional Studies, University of Miami, 1300 Campo Sano Ave, Coral Gables, FL 33124, USA
Full list of author information is available at the end of the article

fundamental to preventing unwanted pregnancies, managing rapid population growth and improving the health and economic well-being of families and communities [1–4]. The need for reproductive health information and services is particularly dire in post-conflict settings, where the capacity to provide health services, including for sexual and reproductive health, is often limited [5–7].

In these settings, healthcare systems are fragmented and siloed, trained healthcare providers are wanting and contraceptive supply chain systems in disarray. The result is low access to RHS, increases in unwanted teen pregnancies and sexual transmitted infections (STIs) [8]. For example, in Tanzania high births rates (30%) were documented among Congolese teens(ages 14 and 18 years) [9], and in Colombia displaced young girls aged 13–19 accounted for 30% of all births in 2000 [10]. A lack of basic reproductive health information was documented among adolescents in Nepal [11]. Together, these studies highlight the need for reliable information, counseling and tailored RHS for adolescents in conflict settings.

Research to date has documented a variety of youth-friendly service (YFS) practices that are positively and negatively associated with the provision of family planning (FP) and RHS [12]. YFS practices include provider characteristics (e.g., specially trained staff, ensuring privacy and confidentiality), as well as facility characteristics, such as, convenient wait times, operating hours, locations, and maintaining comfortable surroundings. Program design characteristics include affordable cost, having a wide range of services available, teen involvement in the design and in needs identification, short wait times and provision of timely referrals [13]. The provision of YFS even after adoption of effective approaches and strategies is more likely to vary across regions, such that high and low levels of service availability and adolescents' use of FP/RH services including use of modern contraceptive methods are concentrated in specific geographic areas. Likewise, the extent to which characteristics of YFS are associated with adolescents' actual use of reproductive healthcare (RHC) services is likely to vary across space.

Therefore, there is potential to use geospatial and non-spatial analyses to better understand the RHC service availability and adolescents' use of these services. First, although research has been carried out on adolescent's use of RHC services [13], no previous study has used fine-grained geographical administrative data from a census of facilities to assess RHC service availability and adolescents' use of these services in post-conflict settings. Second, we are not aware of work that has systematically assessed whether associations between RHC service availability and areas of persistent violence vary across different geographic regions.

There remains much that we do not know about service availability and use of FP/RH services by adolescents in post-conflict settings. We have limited understanding of the ability of facilities to provide YFS to adolescents in these settings. Knowledge about the extent of RHC service availability and use of such services by adolescents in post-conflict settings could have important implications

for tailoring interventions to specific communities based on the pertinent provider, facility and program design characteristics to increase uptake of FP/RH among these individuals. The objectives of this research are (1) to examine the density of RHC service availability, (2) to assess spatial patterns of RHC facilities, and (3) to identify YFS practices associated with adolescents' use of RHC services in post-conflict Burundi. In our study, of RHC services will be used interchangeably with FP/RH services and include "family-planning, counseling services; prenatal and postnatal care and delivery; abortion services and post-abortion care; treatment and prevention of reproductive tract and sexually transmitted diseases and infections including HIV; and information and counseling about human sexuality [14]."

Methods

Study setting

The study was conducted in Burundi, an east-central African country. Burundi has an estimated population of 10.16 million as of 2013 and is one of the most densely populated countries in central Africa [15]. Although fertility rates have fallen over time, adolescent birth rates remain high. In 2011, there were 185 reported births per 1000 women aged 15–19 years [16].

Nearly 90% of Burundi's population lives in rural areas. Unfortunately, the country has been in repeated conflict since its independence in 1962. Years of continuous conflict has had an impact on the country's population such that 65% of its population is comprised of young people. Figure 1 provides a general overview of the extent of urban and rural areas in Burundi.

The Burundian healthcare system

Prolonged conflict has led to significant destruction and disruption of the healthcare system, services and quality of health. At the same time the government's capacity to invest in the health sector is limited—in 2005, just 2.7% of the total budget was dedicated to health services [17]. Ongoing insecurity in certain regions has increased the inaccessibility of healthcare for many Burundians [18]. Access to healthcare was made more difficult for many by the adoption of a cost recovery system in 2002, where all patients regardless of their socio-economic status were required to pay for all medical costs and medicines. However, in 2004, the government of Burundi institutionalized output-based financial support or performance-based financing (PBF) of the facilities.

Alike neighboring Rwanda, the roll-out of PBF to Burundi's 18 provinces between 2006 and 2010 has been seen as a way to improve quality of care, coverage of services, strengthen local facilities and to remove user fees in the health sector to children under five and pregnant

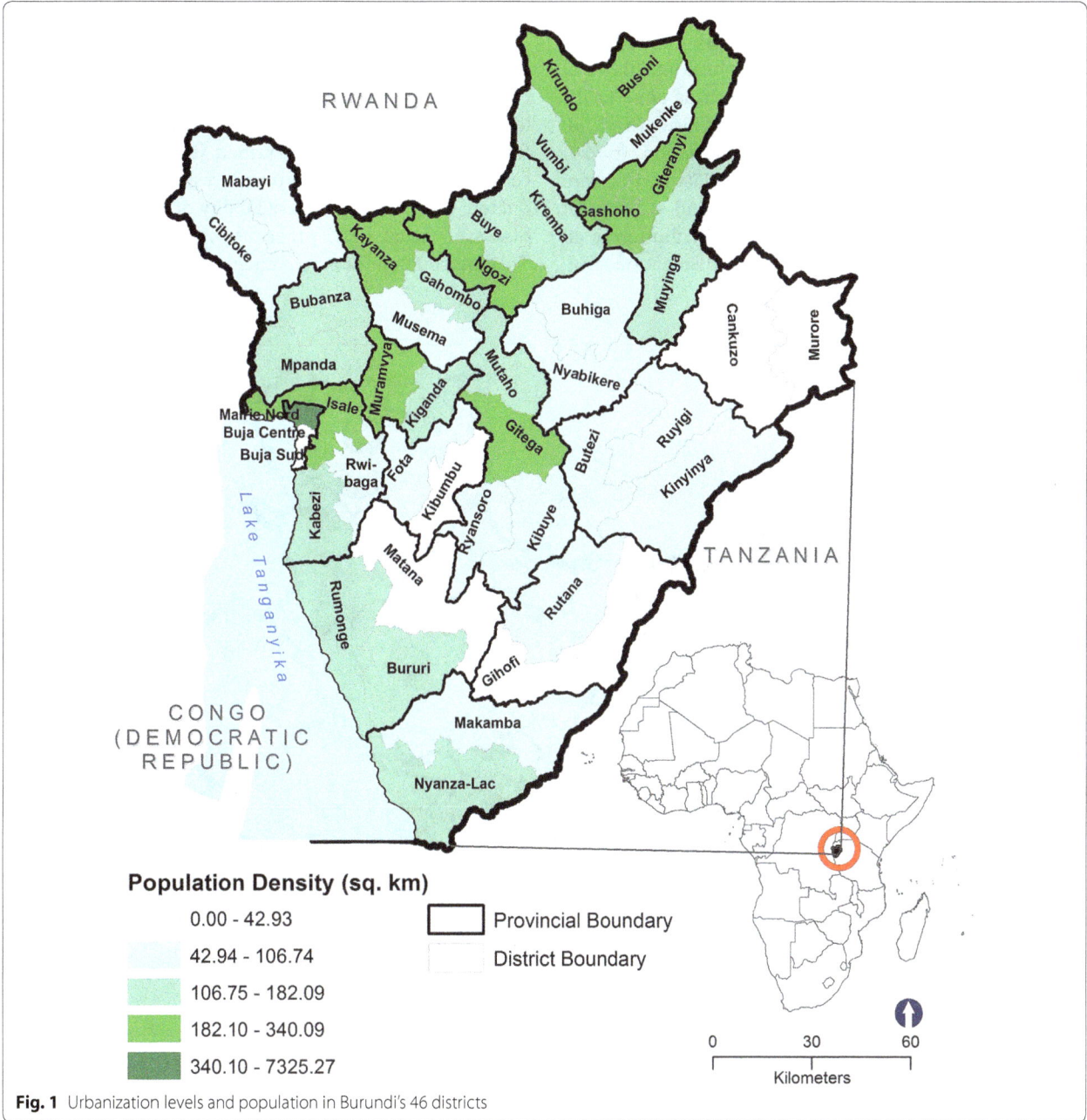

Fig. 1 Urbanization levels and population in Burundi's 46 districts

women. Facilities are free to assign their finances to different uses according to their needs (e.g., day-to-day operations, invest in small equipment, staff incentives). Likewise, primary care is provided by private and publicly operated facilities. Facilities are contracted and partially funded on the basis of their performance by a third-party agency independent of providers [i.e., NGO or Ministry of Health (MoH)]. The third-party agency is responsible for evaluating performance and providing subsidies and acting both as a purchaser and an inspector. Every time a facility (contractor) delivers a contracted service, it is eligible for a unit subsidy. Notably, more than half of the contracted indicators at the facility-level have been services for which users are not required to pay any fee.

Study design

We examined facility-based RHC services using data from the 2013 Population Services International (PSI) Burundi's Sexual and Reproductive Health Survey (SRHS).

This cross-sectional survey was designed to collect information on the landscape of sexual and reproductive health services available for adolescents across health facilities in the country [19]. PSI conducted a full census of all facilities (n = 892), including public (n=538), private (n=195), religious (n=139) and community association (n=20) owned-facilities and hospitals. At each facility efforts were made to interview the officer-in-charge and a group of his/her staff. Figure 2 shows the spatial distribution of all facilities in Burundi by facility type and urbanization level.

Health facilities data source

The 2013 SRHS data included observation data from facilities and interviews with providers. The observation data assessed the extent to which facilities practices followed standards of care that are generally recommended for the provision of YFS. Trained staff observed adolescents' visits, the use of procedures; examinations conducted, documented the availability of commodities, and discussed usual RHC practices with providers on site. This information was cross checked by reviewing records

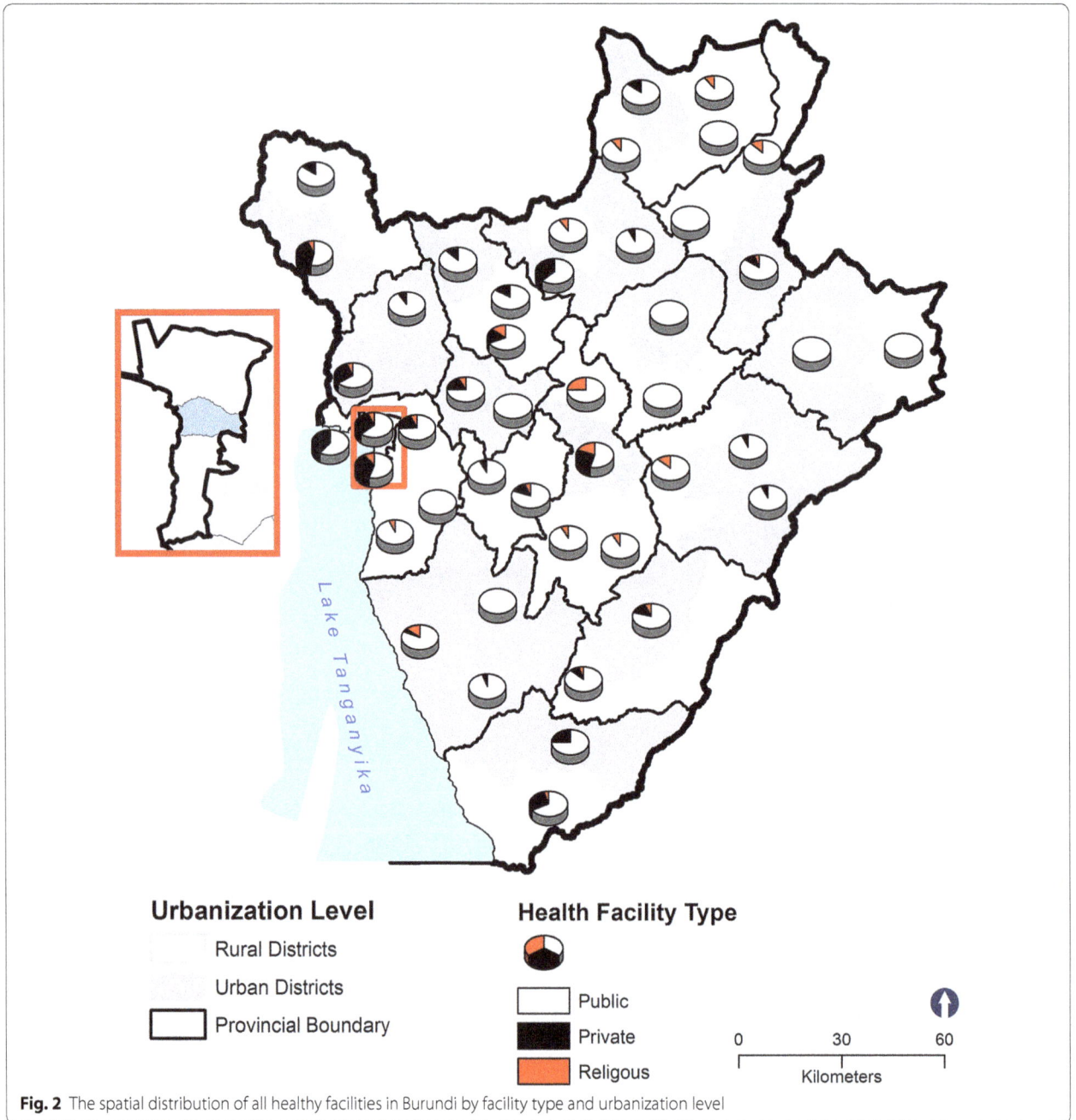

Fig. 2 The spatial distribution of all healthy facilities in Burundi by facility type and urbanization level

(e.g., registers, logbooks and monthly reports submitted to the MoH) for each facility. Interviews with providers were conducted face-to-face in the facilities to assess facility, provider and program design characteristics [19].

Measures
Response variable
Our response variable is continuous (the number of youth and young adults who visited each facility in the past 7 days for a RHC service). This variable assesses youth and young adults' use of RHS. During the survey, trained staff reviewed facilities records and noted the number of adolescents who visited each facility. Adolescents were defined as persons aged between 10 and 24 years both male and female, a definition also applied in related studies [13]. Demographic information such as gender and marital status was recorded at the aggregate-level.

Independent variables
We assessed facilities characteristics, measures of provider practices and program design factors. Facility characteristics included accessibility and environmental adaptation factors. We have chosen to group facilities into two categories (hospitals and health centers), with facility ownership (public, private, religious) used as the form of indicator variable for 'facilities'.

To assess training, providers indicated whether or not they had received specific in-service or pre-service training in relation to the care of youth and young adults and training relating to meeting the special needs of teens. Providers were also asked to indicate whether peer educators (other youth or young adults) are involved in promoting the facility's services and activities. Two other questions asked providers to indicate whether they have been informed of the rights of young people and if all providers at each facility know at least five of those rights.

To examine program design characteristics, providers reported whether or not the facility is involved in outreach efforts, has partnerships with community organizations and other sectors (e.g., schools, NGOs) to reach young people, and to indicate whether or not patient medical records are preserved to protect the privacy and confidentiality of young people. The provided facility, provider and program design information was cross checked by observations and by reviewing records, registers and logbooks for each facility. Additionally, respondents indicated whether or not the facility has educational materials and contracts for PBF.

To estimate contraceptive modern methods availability, trained staff conducted physical inventory counts, reviewed stock cards, quarterly management reports on contraceptive products and recorded the number of different types of contraceptive methods available (e.g., implants, emergency contraceptives, IUDs, injectables, condoms and pills). A contraceptive stock-out was considered if it was offered by the facility but not available for any part of the past 3 months. Table 1 shows the frequencies of variables used in the current study.

Violence and administrative boundary GIS data
At each facility, Global Positioning System (GPS) coordinates were collected to help in estimating the density of FP/RH service availability. We downloaded conflict and protest data from the Armed Conflict Location and Event Data (ACLED) project [20]. Variables in the dataset include the type of conflict, the coordinates of the incidences, estimated fatalities, warring groups, among other factors. Data from 1997 to 2013 were used to locate clusters of persistent conflict. We obtained administrative boundaries (shapefiles) districts (n = 46) and provinces (n = 18) from the Directorate of the Burundi National System of Health Information.

Geospatial analysis
Kernel density estimation and spatial proximity
We were interested in the density of RHC service availability and discrepancies in use of these services by adolescents at the facility-level unit of analysis. Therefore, we utilized geolocation facility data, and employed kernel density estimation (KDE) using the Spatial Analyst tools feature in ArcGIS version 10.3.1 [21] to estimate access to FP/RH services. The density of RHC service availability has been found to be a good proxy for access to FP/RH services than other measures of accessibility such as Euclidean distance [22].

KDE is characterized by the degree to which geographically close points (RHC facilities) that are at the center of the radius tend to be weighted higher than facilities at the margin [22, 23]. We created density variables by converting all of the geolocation facility data for each RHC facility, conflict and protest data (latitude and longitude) into continuous surfaces. This estimate gives a formal indication of areas of high RHC service availability (facilities and violent events per square kilometer) or high service use and high violence areas; and areas of low service and low violence [24]. KDE requires the user to specify the choice of circle radius. In this study, we use a radius of 4 km to represent an hour of travel time by foot as used in a previous study [22].

To measure proximity to facilities, we applied a buffer analysis. As with KDE analysis above, we used a buffer zone with radius of 4 km around all RHC facilities in Burundi. This radius reflects the localized nature of facility use in Burundi.

Table 1 Means and frequencies for all variables included in the study across Burundi, 2013

	Total N	N/(%)
Provider characteristics		
Specially trained staff		
Staff have received training in relation to the care of adolescents' RH	872	19 (2.2)
Staff have received training to meet adolescents' special RH needs	872	22 (2.5)
Facility uses peer educators/counselors	874	18 (2.1)
Ability to relate to youth in a respectful manner		
Staff have been informed of the rights of adolescents	874	92 (10.5)
All staff know at least 5 of the rights of adolescents	872	76 (8.7)
Health facility characteristics		
Accessibility		
Dedicated adolescent only hours and/or days	858	34 (3.8)
Facility hours includes evenings and/or weekend hours	865	674 (78.0)
Environmental adaptation		
Designated adolescent check-in rooms available	858	679 (79.0)
Waiting and exam rooms have pictures to appeal to adolescents	873	118 (13.5)
Waiting and exam rooms have print materials to appeal to adolescents	560	297 (53.0)
Waiting and exam rooms have posters to appeal to adolescents	557	320 (57.5)
Program design characteristics		
Adolescents are involved in the design and continuing feedback	871	16 (1.8)
Facility has a strategy to involve adolescents in planning and care provision	873	38 (4.4)
RHC services discounted to adolescents	464	52 (11.2)
Outreach		
Facility has partnerships with community organizations and other sectors, e.g., schools, NGOs to reach young people	858	94 (11.0)
Outreach and/or education provided in the community for young people	768	91 (11.8)
Facility has sign outside that states that all adolescents are welcome	516	7 (1.4)
Confidentiality		
Records are preserved to protect the privacy and confidentiality of adolescents' personal medical records and health information	868	620 (71.4)

Pictures, posters and print materials include educational materials or information relating reproductive health

RH Reproductive health, *RHC* Reproductive Health Care

Average nearest neighbor

The Average Nearest Neighbor tool was used to assess the spatial patterning of distances among RHC facilities in the country. The tools allowed us to measure the degree to which RHC facility locations cluster or are spatially near to each other. This measure gives a formal indication of clustering and dispersion [25]. Generally, the average nearest neighbor tool returns values in the final output, the "Nearest Neighbor Index (NNI)" which denotes the quotient of the Observed Mean Distance to the Expected Mean Distance. In particular, a value less than 1 suggests that the distribution pattern of the RHC facilities in Burundi is clustered, and if the index is more than 1, the trend is toward dispersion. In other words, shorter distances than would be expected under spatial randomness are interpreted as clustering, whereas longer distances are interpreted as dispersion. All geospatial analysis was done in ArcGIS, version 10.3.1 [21].

Statistical analysis

We generated descriptive statistics to describe the location of facilities, the availability of modern contraceptive methods, adolescents' use of RHS, and to describe the existence of PBF contracts in these types of care. We then investigated the associations between our response variable and the independent variables with multivariable regression models. Because our response variable is recorded as a count (the number of adolescents who visited a RHC facility for a RH service in the past 7 days), we employed a Poisson regression. Moreover, since the response variable is not normally distributed, multiple linear or logistic regressions are impossible.

Notably, the Poisson model assumes an infinitely large population from which counts are drawn, and in the case of this study, the size of the adolescent population in Burundi is large relative to the number of reported counts. Hence, the Poisson distribution can be used as an approximation to the binomial distribution, since the Poisson mean >0. In our study, the Poisson regression model expresses the log outcome rate (use of RHC services) as a linear function of a set of selected youth-friendly practices at each facility. We fit parsimonious models by removing variables one at a time (non-significant variables), beginning with the one with the largest P value until all variables included in the model were significant ($P < 0.05$). Table 3 presents the retained variables used in the study. The 'health facility' and PBF contractor as variables are used as indicator variables (e.g., Public = 1; Private = 2; Religious = 3; PBF contractor—0 = no, 1 = yes) in the regression analysis. All analyses were completed with IBM SPSS Statistics for Windows, Version 22.0 [26].

Results

Descriptive summary

A total of 24,232 adolescents aged 10–24 years visited RHC facilities in Burundi in the past 7 days prior to the survey (Table 2). Of the adolescents, 11% (2542) were male and 89% (20,821) were female, with an average gender sex ratio of 12:100. Married adolescents (72%, 16,488) were more likely to use RHC services than single adolescents (29%, 6587).

About 67% of all adolescents' visits were to public RHC facilities, for an average number of visits in the past 7 days of 147. Less than 5% adolescents visited hospitals and private centers. Additionally, of the 613 RHC facilities, most were public health centers or health posts (52.8%). Three-quarters of facilities (78%) were located in rural districts, and almost 85% of all facilities reported serving as PBF contractors.

More than 50% of public facilities reported no stock-outs of four modern contraceptive methods (oral pills, injectibles, condoms and contraception pills) at any point in the past 3-months prior to the survey. Only less than 20% of private and religious health centers reported no stock-outs of modern contraceptive methods during the same period (Fig. 3a). The availability of implants and IUDs is low across health centers regardless of facility-type. Hospitals (all ownership types) exhibited the highest stock-outs. Only 10% of hospitals reported no stock-outs of the six modern contraceptive methods (oral pills, injectibles, condoms, emergency contraception, implants and IUDs) (Fig. 3b).

Table 2 Distribution of health facilities according adolescent demographics and whether a facility offers RHC services by facility ownership, Burundi, 2013

	Facility ownership (n = 892[a])			
	Public N (%)	Private N (%)	Religious N (%)	Total N
Centers	(n = 495)	(n = 205)	(n = 125)	
Married, 10–24 years	11,130 (48.2)	1118 (4.8)	3172 (17.4)	15,420
Single, 10–24 years	4742 (20.6)	685 (3.0)	853 (13.7)	6280
Females, 10–24 years	14,371 (61.5)	1445 (6.2)	3730 (16.0)	19,546
Males, 10–24 years	1343 (5.7)	368 (1.6)	607 (2.6)	2318
Center offers RHC services	471 (57.0)	75 (9.1)	30 (3.6)	576
Center contracts with PBF	473 (54.6)	75 (8.7)	114 (13.1)	662
Center does not offer RHC services	12 (1.5)	101 (12.2)	81 (9.8)	194
% of visits in the past 7 days	67.1	3.4	18.7	
Average # of visits in the past 7 days	147.4	31.2	74.0	
Hospitals	(n = 43)	(n = 10)	(n = 14)	
Married 10–24 years	716 (3.1)	42 (0.2)	310 (1.3)	1068
Single 10–24 years	188 (0.8)	3 (0.0)	116 (0.5)	202
Females 10–24 years	888 (3.8)	58 (0.2)	329 (25.8)	1185
Males 10–24 years	165 (0.7)	2 (0.0)	57 (25.4)	224
Hospital offers RHC services	31 (3.8)	3 (0.4)	3 (0.4)	37
Hospital does not offer RHC services	9 (1.1)	3 (0.4)	7 (0.8)	19
Hospital contracts with PBF	42 (4.8)	5 (0.6)	11 (1.3)	58
% of visits in the past 7 days	4.6	4.6	1.6	
Average # of visits in the past 7 days	40.0	52.6	48.2	

The percentage (%) of adolescents' visits in the past 7 days was calculated by dividing the total number of adolescents who visited facilities that offer RHC services by total visits

[a] 66 health facilities had missing data

Number

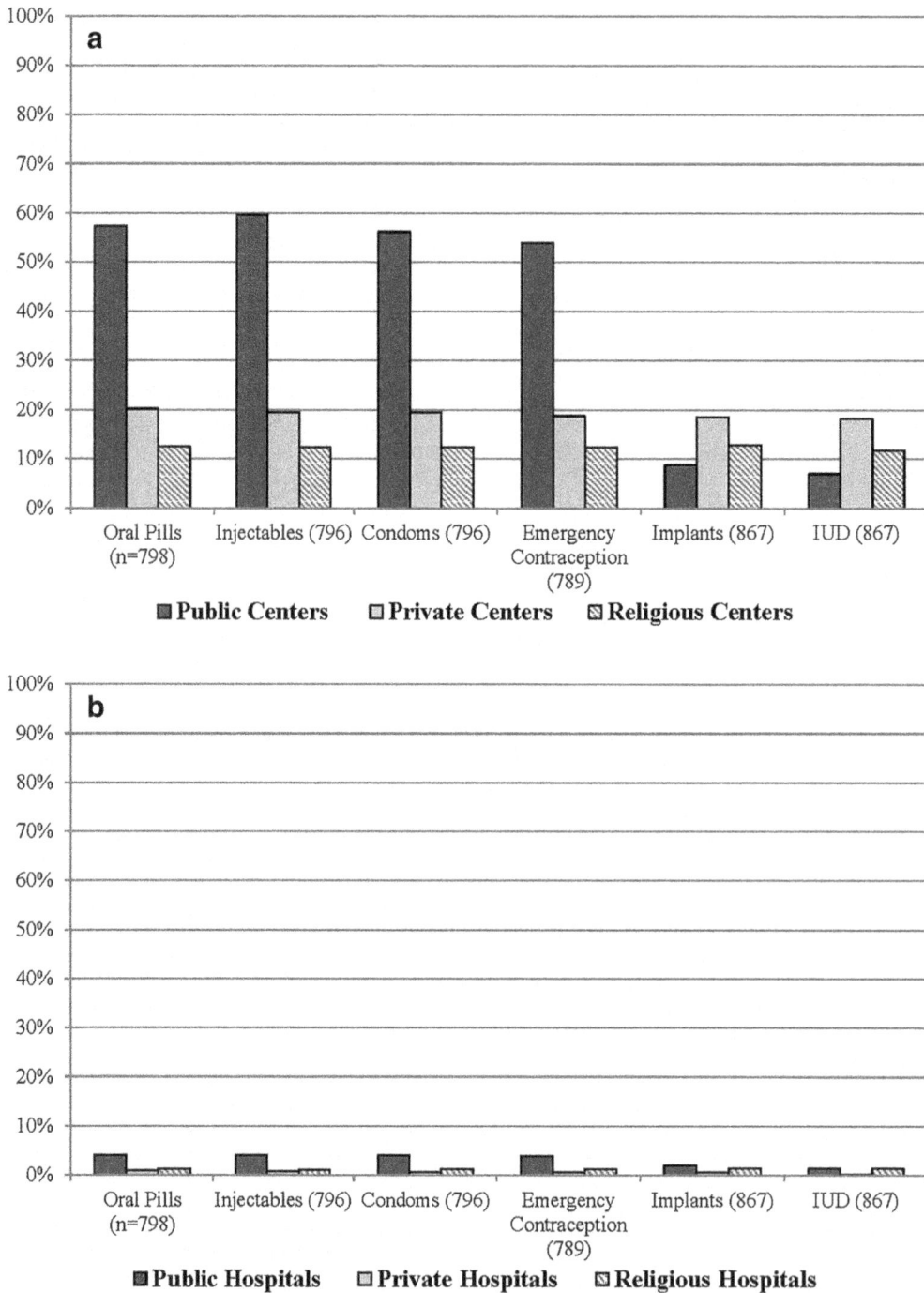

Fig. 3 Percentage of all health centers (**a**) and hospitals (**b**) with no stock-outs within min-max level in the past three-months prior to the survey. *Note*: the "Min" value represents a stock level that triggers a reorder and the "Max" value represents a new targeted stock level following the reorder

Estimating the density of RHC service availability, conflict and spatial proximity

We found high spatial patterning of distances of RHC facilities in Burundi (Z-score: −3.61, P value: .0001) (Fig. 4). Peaks were found within the 4 km radius, which represent an hour of travel time by foot. The high densities were concentrated in four districts located in two provinces of Bujumbura Mairie (Buja-Nord, Buja-Center and Buja-Sud) and Bujumbura Rural(Isale), followed by districts located in provinces of Ngozi, Kayanza, Cibitoke, Gitega, Mwaro and

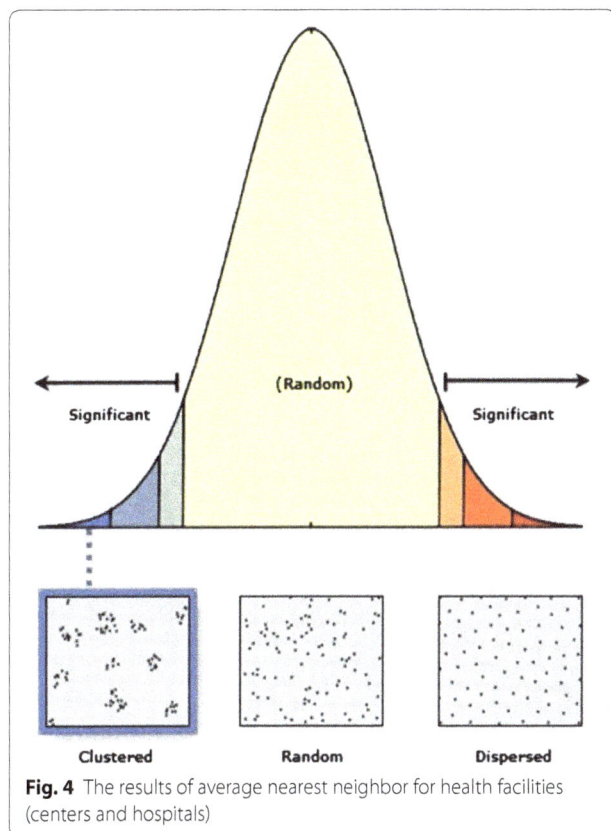

Fig. 4 The results of average nearest neighbor for health facilities (centers and hospitals)

parts of Bururi (Fig. 5). Cankuzo, a rural province located in eastern Burundi had the lowest density of RHC facilities.

We identified the districts wherein there were higher densities of persistent violence. Using the 4 km radius, we found that three urban districts of Bujumbura Mairie province (Fig. 7) exhibited persistent violence (conflict, incidences, fatalities, and warring groups). Despite this, use of RHC services by adolescents is high in these districts (Fig. 6). However, we observed low use of RHC services in less affected districts located in Cankunzo, Ruyingi, Bururi, Cibitoke and Mwaro provinces. Almost all RHC facilities in Burundi are within the 4 km catchment zone, suggesting high RHC accessibility (Fig. 7).

Youth-friendly service practices associated with use of reproductive health services

As the results in Table 3 indicate, the association between adolescents' use of RHS and each YFS practice varied between facility types. Notably, facility and program design characteristics were both positively associated with RHS use among adolescents. Across all facility types, community outreach, having designated check-in and exam rooms, educational materials (posters, print and pictures) in waiting and exam rooms that appeal to adolescents,

and privacy and confidentiality were significantly associated with adolescents' use of services ($P < 0.0001$).

Discounted services were positively associated with use of RHS ($P < 0.05$). Among religious facilities, and we found no evidence that discounted services were associated with use of services at public and private facilities. The same is true for adolescents' involvement in design and continuing feedback. The association is only with private facilities ($P < 0.01$). Provider characteristics were not statistically associated with the use of RHS at any facility type. Privacy and confidentiality, having educational pictures and posters in waiting and exam rooms to appeal to adolescents and having hours that include evenings and weekend hours were significantly associated with PBF status (Table 4).

Discussion

We sought to examine the density of RHC service availability and assess spatial patterns of these services in postconflict Burundi. We also aimed to identify YFS practices associated with adolescents' use of reproductive health services across health facility types. We found that RHC facilities were spatially clustered within three urban districts of Bujumbura Mairie province and in Isale, a district located in Bujumbura Rural province, with high densities of persistent violence acts (conflict, incidences, fatalities, and warring groups) nested within these districts. RHC facilities in Burundi show spatial patterning of distances, suggesting that most of the districts in the country (both rural and urban districts) have more than one facility located in close proximity to each other. Further, we found a stronger association between adolescents' use of RHS and YFS practices. In particular, we found significant associations with facility characteristics (e.g., designated check-in and exam rooms) and programming characteristics (e.g., community outreach, privacy and confidentiality) and adolescents' use of RHS across facility types.

Our analysis provides evidence that despite persistent violence in urban districts of Bujumbura Mairie, the administrative headquarters; adolescents' use of RHC services was high, with use of services overlapping entirely with the density of violent locations. It's possible therefore, that the recurring violence and adolescents' use of services under such circumstances, although on one hand atypical, on the other, they have become the norm. These results corroborate the ideas of Jenkins [27], who suggested that for those existing in places of recurring political violence, "the extreme and the mundane are not necessarily alternative but simultaneous states of affairs that are lived with as a persistent existential contradiction", for example, "living in a political ethos" or with respect to accessing basic needs (e.g., RHC services).

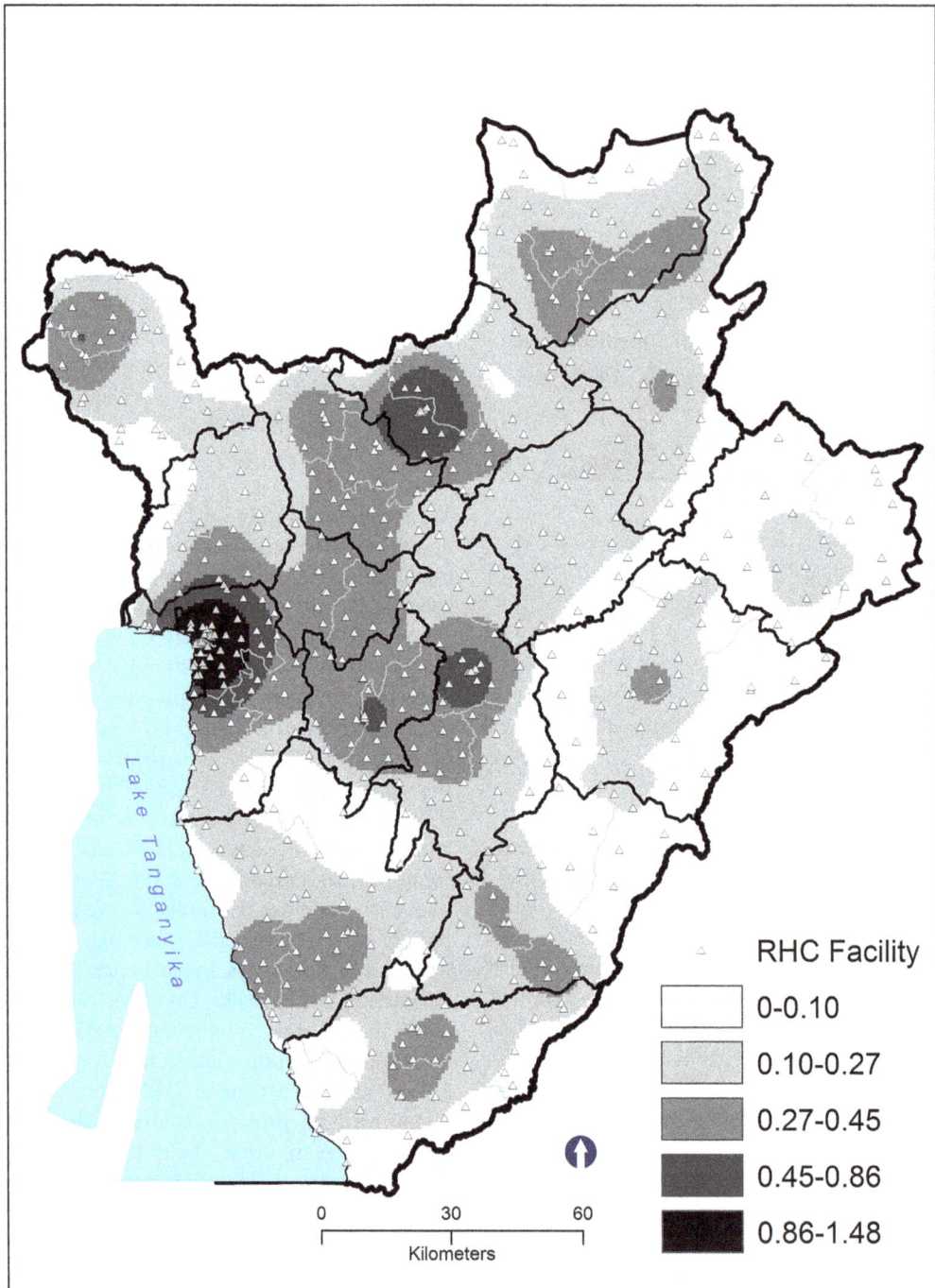

Fig. 5 Density of reproductive health service facilities (facilities per square kilometer) according to kernel estimation: Burundi, 2013. The locations of reproductive health service facilities are marked by *white triangles*

Another important finding was that the number of RHC facilities with no stock-outs of modern contraceptives in the past 3 months was high. Public centers had the highest availability of modern contraceptives than other centers and hospitals. It is possible, therefore, that a combination of government and international donors' efforts to improve the availability of family planning methods at the service delivery point is achieving intended results. Burundi has made significant progress in improving the provision of RHC services and rights.

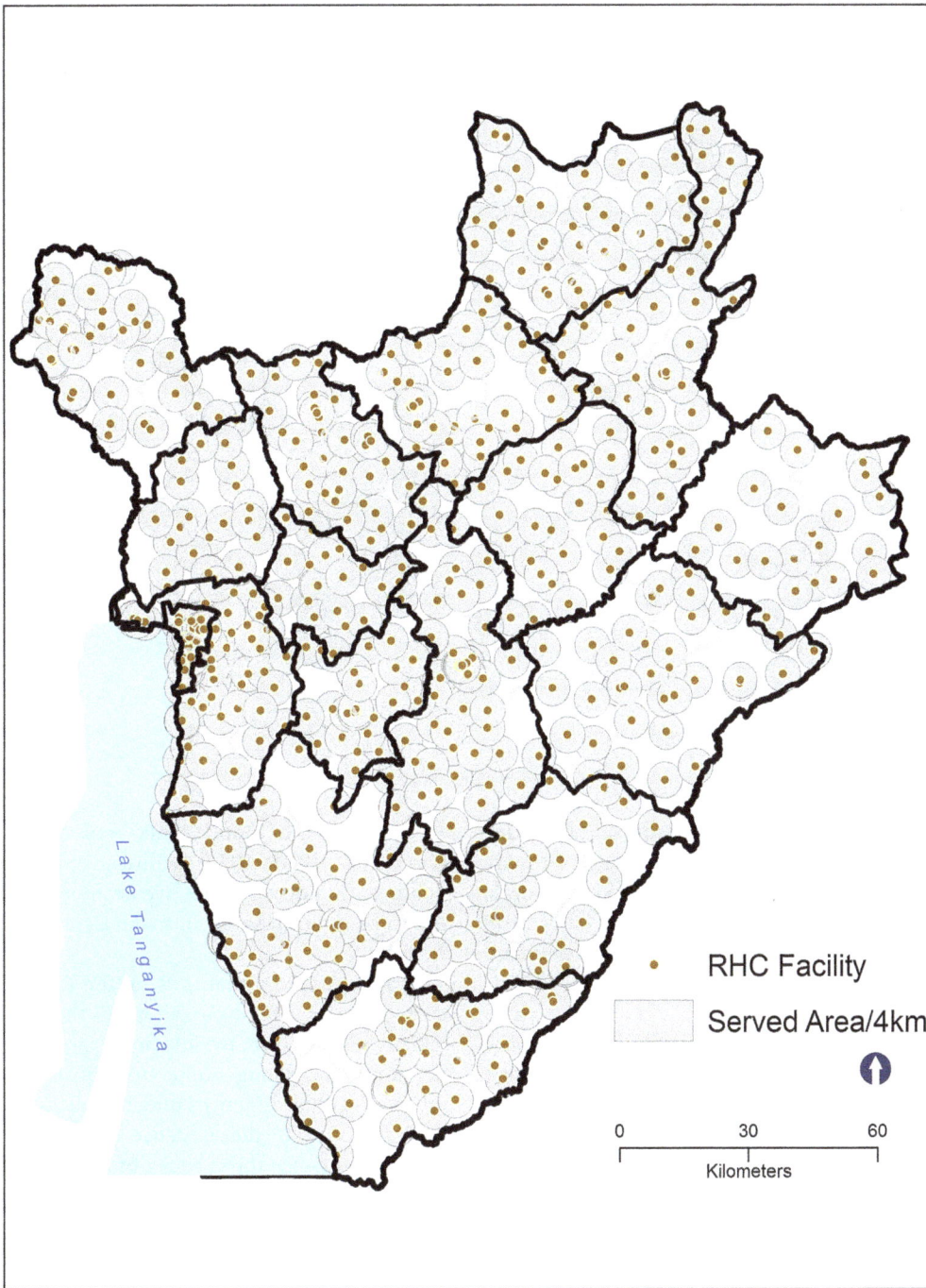

Fig. 6 Density of areas of persistent violence (violent events per square kilometer) according to kernel estimation: Burundi, 2013. Adolescents' use of services in these areas is denoted by graduated symbols in *dark green*

For example, in 2008, the MoH through the National Reproductive Health Program (PNSR) initiated an approach aimed at improving the provision of YFS planning and RHC services to adolescents. Since then, policy and strategic documents have been adopted, among which, the National Population Policy Statement (2011), the National Health Development Plan and the revised National Sexual and Reproductive Health Strategy (2013–2015). Another example illustrating efforts by the Burundian government in tackling RHC services issues

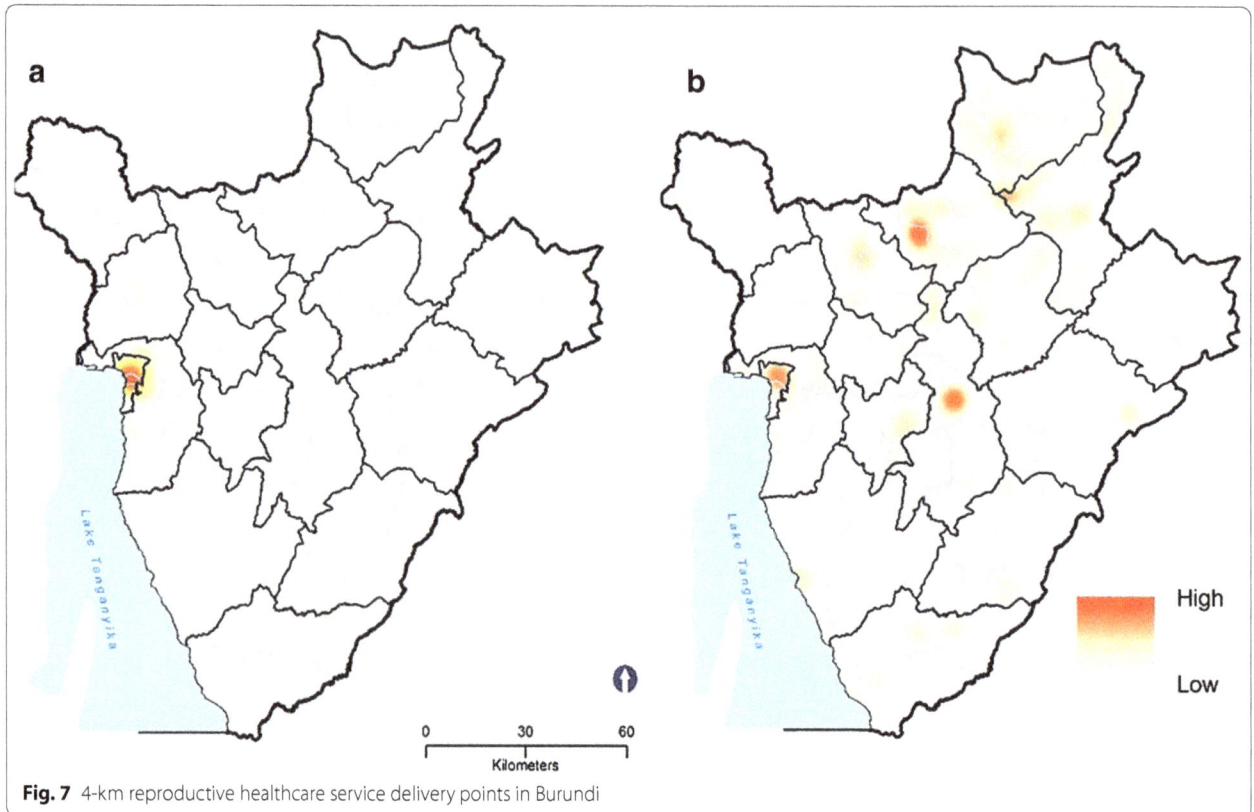

Fig. 7 4-km reproductive healthcare service delivery points in Burundi

are reflected in key development frameworks, notably the "Vision Burundi 2025", and the second Strategic Growth and Fight against Poverty (2012–2016) [18]. Burundi, therefore, provides an ideal opportunity to study how RHC services efforts made by the Burundian government to expand YFS have translated into practice at the facility level.

On the question of whether YFS practices are associated with adolescents' use of RHS, this study found that RHC service facilities across Burundi vary in their provision of youth-friendly RHS to youth and young adults. We found that of the three YFS practices (facility, provider and programming factors), the majority of facilities are making their RHC facilities youth-friendly by designating rooms for adolescent check-in and examinations as well as making educational materials (e.g., pictures and print) on sensitive topics available in examination rooms.

Facilities are also very successful at incorporating outreach in communities and schools and in ensuring privacy and confidentiality of youth and young adults. These results seem to be consistent with previous studies [13, 28–30] which found privacy and confidentiality of young people during family planning and counselling as important determinants of use of services. The lack of youth engagement strategies and low cost/discounted

RHC services to adolescents was apparent in both public and private RHC facilities. Public and religious facilities are not very effective at involving youth in the design of programs and in making decisions that affect them.

We also observed that most of the RHC facilities contracted under PBF have adopted the above program design practices (e.g., flexible hours) and practices to protect youth and young adults' privacy and confidentiality, but not the other practices under study.

Notably, despite the existence of policy documents to build and enhance the capacity of RHC facilities and providers [19, 31], we found no evidence that provider training was statistically associated with adolescents' use of RHC services. These results are in line with those of previous studies [32–34], and suggest a need for government commitment to provide tailored topical trainings to providers. These results are also likely to be related to the fact that the healthcare system in Burundi is afflicted by a lack of trained medical staff, resources to compensate them and a lack of modern equipment. This has led to an exodus of trained staff, leaving unskilled health workers to work beyond their capabilities in increasingly difficult circumstances.

This finding, while preliminary, suggests that a better understanding of the availability of youth-friendly RHS

Table 3 Association of key YFS characteristics related to adolescents' use of RHS using a Poisson regression model

Explanatory variables/youth-friendly practices	Public (n = 499)			Private (n = 215)			Religious (n = 139)		
	β	Wald 95% confidence limits		β	Wald 95% confidence limits		β	Wald 95% confidence limits	
		Confidence interval	Sig.		Confidence interval	Sig.		Confidence interval	Sig.
Intercept	94.298	80.89–109.92	***	0.005	0.005–0.005	***	26.754	17.17–41.68	***
Health facility characteristics									
Hours include evenings/weekend hours	0.739	0.698–0.781	***	1.281	0.999–1.643	*	0.824	0.704–0.965	*
Designated check-in and exam rooms available	0.113	0.068–0.187	***	.040	0.006–0.289	***	1.487	1.190–1.857	***
Waiting/exam rooms have print educational materials to appeal to adolescents	0.652	0.611–0.696	***	.124	0.057–0.271	***	0.625	0.53–0.736	***
Waiting/exam rooms have educational pictures to appeal to adolescents	0.805	0.758–0.855	***	2.819	1.822–4.363	***	0.513	0.440–0.597	***
Waiting/exam rooms have educational posters to appeal to adolescents	1.618	1.527–1.714	***	.680	0.490–0.944	*	1.445	1.273–1.640	***
Program design characteristics									
Adolescents are involved in design/feedback	~	~	~	.520	0.346–0.781	**	~	~	
Facility has strategy to involve adolescents[a]	0.939	0.838–1.052		1.970			2.663	1.983–3.576	***
Privacy and confidentiality preserved[b]	0.698	0.628–0.775	***	2.481	1.836–3.352	***	1.573	1.338–1.849	***
Outreach and/or education is provided[c]	0.889	0.841–0.939	***	.113	0.08–0.158	***	0.773	0.684–0.873	***
RHC services discounted to adolescents	1.079	0.970–1.200		~	~	~	1.399	1.069–1.830	*

β Exponential estimates

Significance level: <0.0001***; <0.01**; <0.05*

~ Model did not converge

[a] Facility has a strategy to involve adolescents in planning and in the provision of care

[b] Records are preserved to protect the privacy and confidentiality of adolescents' personal medical records and health information

[c] Outreach and/or education provided in the community for young people

in the country could help program planners increase youth uptake of such services. It can thus be suggested that geography shapes both accessibility to RHS (high densities of RHC facilities) and can have an effect on an adolescent's perception of the available services, "making contraceptives seem more common place and acceptable [22]". Future studies on the current topic in post-conflict settings are therefore recommended.

Few studies to our knowledge have used both geospatial and non-spatial methods to explore utilization of RHC services among youth and young adults in post-conflict settings. The geospatial methods used in our study can be used to delineate RHC service availability, to estimate accessibility to these services, and to develop spatially targeted RHC services. Pre-conflict, governments can use the methods used to identify

under-served or over-served areas, for example. In post-conflict settings, the methods can be used to identify and assess the availability and spatial patterns of RHC facilities to plan for targeted RHC service interventions, an important topic in the context of community recovery following civil unrest.

A limitation of this study is its cross-sectional nature, with data collected at a single point. But given the specific study objective, the study design is not a problem. The use of fine-grained geographic data from a census of facilities adds a broader, sector wide approach. Given that the census data for Burundi do not provide age specific population data, due to political reasons, it's not possible to discern the population for young people; neither for those aged 10–24 years from the general population. This fact limits the interpretation of the data,

Table 4 Association of key YFS characteristics related to performance-based financing status using a Poisson regression model

	β	Confidence interval	Sig.
Intercept	3.522	2.054–6.038	***
Program design characteristics			
Adolescents are involved in design/feedback	0.76	0.477–1.211	
Facility has strategy to involve adolescents[a]	0.906	0.743–1.107	
Privacy and confidentiality preserved[b]	1.151	1.026–1.292	*
Outreach and/or education is provided[c]	1.05	0.953–1.157	
RHC services discounted to adolescents	1.006	0.859–1.179	
Health facility characteristics			
Hours include evenings/weekend hours	1.115	1.025–1.212	**
Designated check-in and exam rooms available	0.968	0.777–1.205	
Waiting/exam rooms have print educational materials to appeal to adolescents	1.091	0.969–1.229	
Waiting/exam rooms have educational pictures to appeal to adolescents	1.101	1.002–1.209	*
Waiting/exam rooms have educational posters to appeal to adolescents	1.153	1.048–1.269	**

β Exponential estimates

Significance level: <0.0001***; <0.01**; <0.05*

N = 311

~ Model did not converge

[a] Facility has a strategy to involve adolescents in planning and in the provision of care

[b] Records are preserved to protect the privacy and confidentiality of adolescents' personal medical records and health information

[c] Outreach and/or education provided in the community for young people

particularly to the actual denominator of the population of interest. Finally, although the results are specific to the Burundi context, our mixed methods approach and results are generalizable to other countries and post-conflict settings.

Conclusion

This study demonstrated how both geospatial and non-spatial methods can be used to (1) examine the density of RHS availability, (2) assess spatial patterns of these facilities, and (3) identify youth-friendly practices associated with adolescents' use of services in post-conflict settings. The approaches used are generalizable to other post-conflict settings and to other types of interventions.

Authors' contributions

IM obtained the data, conducted the analyses, and drafted the manuscript. JV cleaned the data. JK reviewed the draft manuscript. All authors read and approved in the final version of the manuscript.

Author details

[1] Department of Geography and Regional Studies, University of Miami, 1300 Campo Sano Ave, Coral Gables, FL 33124, USA. [2] University of Waterloo, Waterloo, ON N2L 3G1, Canada.

Acknowledgements

The data for this project was made possible by Population International Services (PSI). Data obtained and analyzed with permission from Population Services International, Research & Metrics Department, Washington, D.C. (www.psi.org/research); all rights reserved by PSI.

Competing interests

The authors declare that they have no competing interests.

References

1. Kennedy E, Gray N, Azzopardi P, Creati M. Adolescent fertility and family planning in East Asia and the Pacific: a review of DHS reports. Reprod Health. 2011;8:11.

2. Crawford TV, McGrowder DA, Crawford A. Access to contraception by minors in Jamaica: a public health concern. N Am J Med Sci. 2009;1(5):247–55.

3. Braeken D, Rondinelli I. Sexual and reproductive health needs of young people: matching needs with systems. Int J Gynaecol Obstet. 2012;119(Suppl 1):S60–3.

4. Wilson S, Daniel S, Pearson J, Hopton C, Madeley R. An evaluation of a new teenage clinic and its impact on teenage conceptions in Nottingham from 1986 to 1992. Contraception. 1994;50(1):77–86.

5. Busza J, Lush L. Planning reproductive health in conflict: a conceptual framework. Soc Sci Med. 1999;49(2):155–71.

6. Roberts B, Guy S, Sondorp E, Lee-Jones L. A basic package of health services for post-conflict countries: implications for sexual and reproductive health services. Reprod Health Matters. 2008;16(31):57–64.

7. van Egmond K, Naeem AJ, Verstraelen H, Bosmans M, Claeys P, Temmerman M. Reproductive health in Afghanistan: results of a knowledge, attitudes and practices survey among Afghan women in Kabul. Disasters. 2004;28(3):269–82.

8. Cottingham J, García-Moreno C, Reis C. Sexual and reproductive health in conflict areas: the imperative to address violence against women. BJOG. 2008;115(3):301–3.

9. Takei Y, Mtalai M, Lugoi J. The cases of adolescent pregnancy and its

impact in the Congolese refugee camps in Kigoma Region, Tanzania. In: Reproductive health from disaster to development, Brussels, Belgium. 7–8 Oct 2003; 2003.

10. Profamilia: Survey National Health. In: Profamilia, editor. Bogotá, p. 48; 2008.

11. Rimal N, Bhandar D, Upreti H, Regm S. A study of the knowledge, attitude and practices (KAP) related to RH/STI/HIV/AIDS in 10–24 years youths residing in Bhutanese Refugee Camps of eastern Nepal. In: Reproductive Health From Disaster to Development: 2003; Brussels, Belgium; 2003.

12. Tylee A, Haller DM, Graham T, Churchill R, Sanci LA. Youth-friendly primary-care services: How are we doing and what more needs to be done? Lancet. 2007;369(9572):1565–73.

13. Kavanaugh ML, Jerman J, Ethier K, Moskosky S. Meeting the contraceptive needs of teens and young adults: youth-friendly and long-acting reversible contraceptive services in U.S. family planning facilities. J Adolesc Health. 2013;52(3):284–92.

14. Denno DM, Hoopes AJ, Chandra-Mouli V. Effective strategies to provide adolescent sexual and reproductive health services and to increase demand and community support. J Adolesc Health. 2015;56(1 Suppl):S22–41.

15. Moise IK, Roy SS, Nkengurutse D, Ndikubagenzi J. Seasonal and geographic variation of pediatric Malaria in Burundi: 2011 to 2012. Int J Environ Res Public Health. 2016;13(4):425.

16. The World Bank. Reproductive health at a glace: Burundi, vol. 2015. Washington: The World Bank; 2011.

17. République du Burundi MdlS: le Plan national de développement sanitaire; (2006-2010).

18. Nzokirishaka A. Burundi agenda setting for sexual and reproductive health and rights knowledge platform: mission report submitted to share-net international. In. International S-N, editor Bujumbura, Burundi: Share-Net International; 2014.

19. Kays M, Nzohabonayo J. Mapping national geo-referenced sanitary training and services of health sexual and reproductive young people from Burundi. In: International PS, editor Bujumbura, Burundi: Population Services International; 2013.

20. Raleigh C, Linke A, Hegre H, Karlsen J. Introducing ACLED: an armed conflict location and event dataset special data feature. J Peace Res. 2010;47:651–60.

21. ESRI I. In: Redlands, California; 1999.

22. Heard NJ, Larsen U, Hozumi D. Investigating access to reproductive health services using GIS: proximity to services and the use of modern contraceptives in Malawi. Afr J Reprod Health. 2004;8(2):164–79.

23. Tsui AO, Hogan DP, Teachman JD, Welti-Chanes C. Community availability of contraceptives and family limitation. Demography. 1981;18(4):615–25.

24. McLafferty S, Grady S. Immigration and geographic access to prenatal clinics in Brooklyn, NY: a geographic information systems analysis. Am J Public Health. 2005;95(4):638–40.

25. Chen D, Getis A. Point pattern analysis (PPA). San Diego, CA: Department of Geography, San Diego State University; 1998.

26. IBM Corp. IBM SPSS statistics for windows, version 22.0. In: Armonk, NY: IBM Corp.; 2013.

27. Jenkins JH. Extraordinary conditions, culture and experience in mental illness. Oakland: University of California Press; 2015.

28. Flaherty A, Kipp W, Mehangye I. 'We want someone with a face of welcome': Ugandan adolescents articulate their family planning needs and priorities. Trop Doct. 2005;35(1):4–7.

29. Soleimanpour S, Geierstanger SP, Kaller S, McCarter V, Brindis CD. The role of school health centers in health care access and client outcomes. Am J Public Health. 2010;100(9):1597–603.

30. Vahdat HL, L'Engle KL, Plourde KF, Magaria L, Olawo A. There are some questions you may not ask in a clinic: providing contraception information to young people in Kenya using SMS. Int J Gynaecol Obstet. 2013;123(Suppl 1):e2–6.

31. Falisse JB, Ndayishimiye J, Kamenyero V, Bossuyt M. Performance-based financing in the context of selective free health-care: an evaluation of its effects on the use of primary health-care services in Burundi using routine data. Health Policy Plan. 2015;30(10):1251–60.

32. Sipsma HL, Curry LA, Kakoma JB, Linnander EL, Bradley EH. Identifying characteristics associated with performing recommended practices in maternal and newborn care among health facilities in Rwanda: a cross-sectional study. Hum Resour Health. 2012;10:13.

33. Gaye PA, Nelson D. Effective scale-up: avoiding the same old traps. Hum Resour Health. 2009;7:2.

34. Rowe AK, de Savigny D, Lanata CF, Victora CG. How can we achieve and maintain high-quality performance of health workers in low-resource settings? Lancet. 2005;366(9490):1026–35.

15

Intelligent judgements over health risks in a spatial agent-based model

Shaheen A. Abdulkareem[1,2]* , Ellen-Wien Augustijn[3], Yaseen T. Mustafa[4] and Tatiana Filatova[1,5]

Abstract

Background: Millions of people worldwide are exposed to deadly infectious diseases on a regular basis. Breaking news of the Zika outbreak for instance, made it to the main media titles internationally. Perceiving disease risks motivate people to adapt their behavior toward a safer and more protective lifestyle. Computational science is instrumental in exploring patterns of disease spread emerging from many individual decisions and interactions among agents and their environment by means of agent-based models. Yet, current disease models rarely consider simulating dynamics in risk perception and its impact on the adaptive protective behavior. Social sciences offer insights into individual risk perception and corresponding protective actions, while machine learning provides algorithms and methods to capture these learning processes. This article presents an innovative approach to extend agent-based disease models by capturing behavioral aspects of decision-making in a risky context using machine learning techniques. We illustrate it with a case of cholera in Kumasi, Ghana, accounting for spatial and social risk factors that affect intelligent behavior and corresponding disease incidents. The results of computational experiments comparing intelligent with zero-intelligent representations of agents in a spatial disease agent-based model are discussed.

Methods: We present a spatial disease agent-based model (ABM) with agents' behavior grounded in Protection Motivation Theory. Spatial and temporal patterns of disease diffusion among zero-intelligent agents are compared to those produced by a population of intelligent agents. Two Bayesian Networks (BNs) designed and coded using R and are further integrated with the NetLogo-based Cholera ABM. The first is a one-tier BN1 (only risk perception), the second is a two-tier BN2 (risk and coping behavior).

Results: We run three experiments (zero-intelligent agents, BN1 intelligence and BN2 intelligence) and report the results per experiment in terms of several macro metrics of interest: an epidemic curve, a risk perception curve, and a distribution of different types of coping strategies over time.

Conclusions: Our results emphasize the importance of integrating behavioral aspects of decision making under risk into spatial disease ABMs using machine learning algorithms. This is especially relevant when studying cumulative impacts of behavioral changes and possible intervention strategies.

Keywords: Protection motivation theory, Disease diffusion, Emergent behavior, Learning, Cholera, Bayesian networks

Background

Globally, millions of individuals are regularly exposed to deadly infectious diseases. For example, news of the Zika virus outbreak was one of the main news stories of the past 2 years. Perceiving disease risk motivates people to

adapt their behavior toward a safer and more protective lifestyle. Indeed, risk perception (RP) is an integral part of the decision-making process under uncertainty and can be understood as an individual's evaluation of risk in a particular situation. This evaluation includes individual assessments of how severe and controllable a particular situation is. The reliability and effectiveness of any risk evaluation by an individual is based on the risk information available [1]. Accordingly, the availability of risk information impacts the perception of a decision

*Correspondence: s.a.abdulkareem@utwente.nl
[1] Department of Governance and Technology for Sustainability (CSTM), Faculty of Behavioral, Management, and Social Sciences (BMS), University of Twente, Enschede, The Netherlands
Full list of author information is available at the end of the article

problem, the evaluation of available options, and of any risk-coping decisions [2]. A number of factors related to the design of a risk message influence risk perception: the message, being the source of information (other people, and/or the environment), and the adaptive behavior in response to that message. These factors need to be considered in order to design effective risk communication strategies and to positively influence health-related decisions [3].

Numerous examples of human behavior influencing the spread of infectious diseases are available [4]. Namely, Manfredi and D'Onofrio (2013) refer to human behavior as to the neglected layer of complexity in current epidemiological models [5]. In the latter, the response to risk factors is fixed, and no effect of previous exposure—or learning—is incorporated in most models. This implies that a disease model may underestimate the effectiveness of preventive measures. This can lead to a higher scope of contagion compared to a real situation, consequently leading to an overestimation of the prevalence of disease cases. Instead, employing learning techniques to capture dynamics in RP and corresponding protective behavior can mimic the complex process of how human beings act upon encountering risk.

Behavioral science has developed various theories to explain, measure, and assess RP. Protection motivation theory (PMT) is one of the dominant approaches in this domain, and has already been applied to the study of health-protective behavior [6]. Originally proposed by Rogers [7], PMT has been actively applied in health research to study cognitive processes and predict health-related behavior. Behavioral aspects of decision-making under risk are active with ABMs [8–10] outside disease of research, and often without facilitating learning. In fact, ABMs are instrumental in exploring and implementing RP, such as the risk of disease diffusion. Disease ABMs have become significantly sophisticated by integrating rich GIS landscapes with detailed human activities (e.g. mobility and social networks) as well as multi-stage epidemiology models such as the SEIR (Susceptible–Exposed–Infected–Recovered) model. Moreover, ABMs are able to incorporate the social behavior of individual agents as well as the dynamics of the spatial environment, which also plays an important role in the disease diffusion process. Various infectious diseases have been modeled using ABMs [14–16]. Wise [14] provides an extensive review of disease and disaster ABMs. Although ABMs are technically suitable for incorporating agents with higher levels of intelligence, this is rarely implemented in disease models. For example, RP typically enters decision-making models either as a variable affecting a decision-making process or as a step within a rule-based procedure [15–18].

In rule–based implementations, behavior is fixed, meaning that decision-making functions and algorithms remain unchanged. While agents react to changes in their spatial and social environment, they neither adapt their rules in response nor intelligently learn from previous experiences. This is unrealistic, as human beings adjust their behavior strongly when they perceive a serious risk, which can potentially lead to disease models overestimating risk. Intelligence helps agents assess risks and potentially adapt their behavior—i.e. learn to reduce or avoid health risks—based on changes in RP.

To test the impact of adaptive RP in human decision-making, we implement PMT in a spatial disease ABM. Namely, we extend the base disease model developed by Augustijn et al. [19] to the behavioral aspects of decision-making in a risky situation using machine learning (ML) techniques. The spatial agent-based disease model—Cholera ABM—is applied to study the spread of cholera in Kumasi, Ghana. In this article, we use Bayesian Networks (BNs) as the learning method to design intelligent agents behaving according to PMT and making decisions on how to cope with cholera in a rich spatial environment. We systematically test the impact of intelligent behavior on disease spread through a series of simulation experiments: using Cholera ABM with zero-intelligent agents, agents enhanced with ML for updating their RP, and agents enhanced with ML for RP and coping appraisal behavior dynamics. BNs replace ad hoc rule-based schemes for uncertainty reasoning due to their capability for bi-directional inference combined with a strict probabilistic foundation [20]. They are capable of sensing and reacting to a stochastic environment. In addition, BNs have the ability to constantly adjust to simulate the dynamics of agents' beliefs. Therefore, BNs have been implemented in ABMs as the agents' cognitive model for different purposes, including negotiation [21], prediction [22], and adaptation [23].

Methods

We start by briefly describing the base ABM and then focus closely on the describing the learning algorithms and their stepwise implementation to support agents' intelligence.

The base cholera model and zero—intelligence agents (ZI)

The Cholera ABM is used as a testbed for this research. The model was developed to test if runoff water from open dumpsites could have been the diffusion mechanism behind the 2005 cholera outbreak in Kumasi Ghana. This ABM simulates both a hyper-infectious and a low-infectious diffusion route of cholera. It is a spatial ABM with a rich representation of GIS data, including

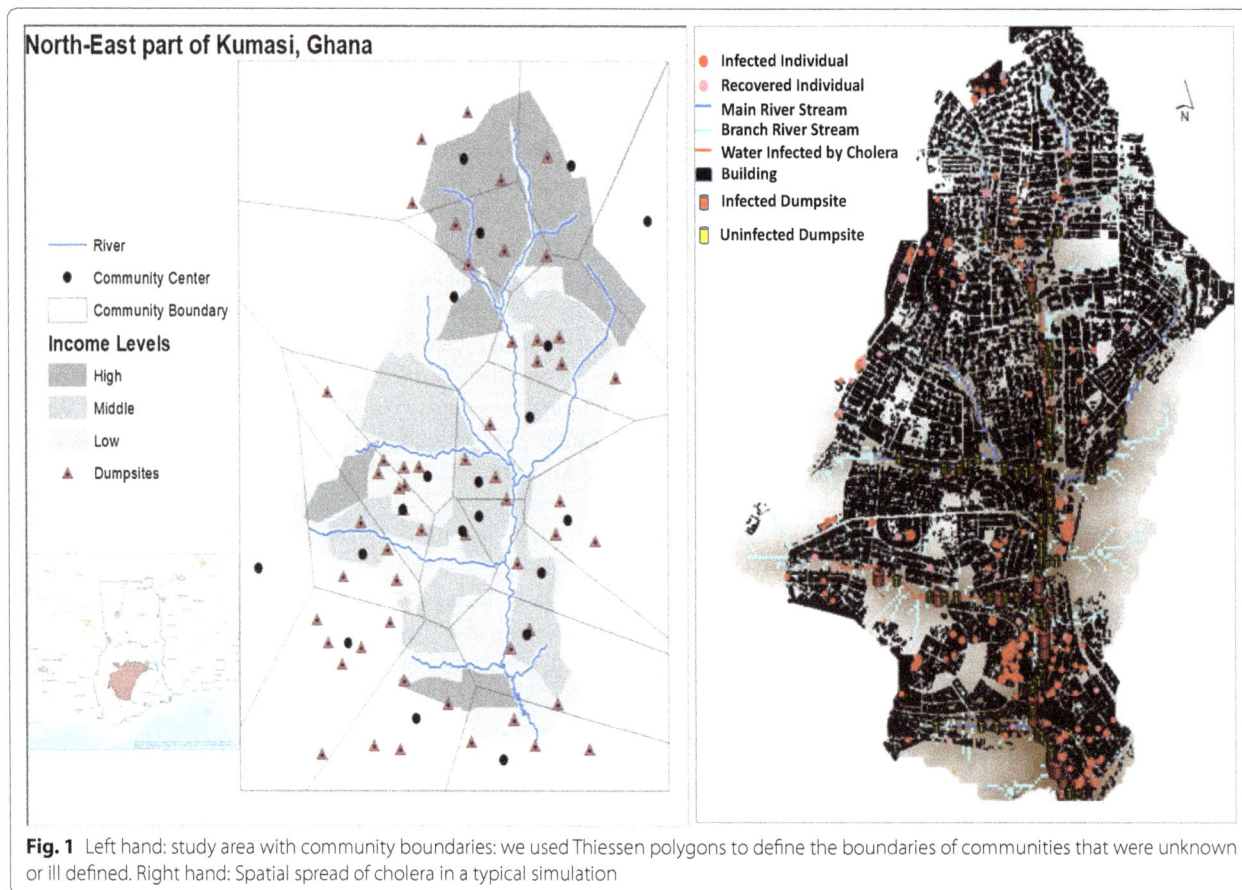

Fig. 1 Left hand: study area with community boundaries: we used Thiessen polygons to define the boundaries of communities that were unknown or ill defined. Right hand: Spatial spread of cholera in a typical simulation

elevation, the location of residential areas, river hydrology, and the location of dumpsites in the study area (Fig. 1).

The Cholera ABM contains three types of agents: households, individuals, and rain particles (Fig. 2). The model contains three sub-models: a *hydrological model*, an *activity model*, and a *disease model*. The hydrological model moves rain particles over the area. Following heavy rainfall, runoff water can become infected with cholera bacteria when passing through dumpsites, thereby transporting cholera bacteria into the river. Via the activity model, household agents will determine the type of water they should consume (tap water, bottled water, or river water).

Household agents use river water when tap water is unavailable. When a household agent uses river water, the model will choose the river location closest to agent's home and determine if the water at this location is infected. Individuals can become infected by using water polluted with cholera and will subsequently shed hyper-infectious materials that will be dumped by the household to the nearest open refuse dumpsite. This increases the infection level of this dumpsite and the probability of rain particles becoming infected. Finally, the disease

model will determine the progression of the disease in the individual and the moment of recovery. However, this Cholera ABM does not include cholera RP and behavioral change (the selection of another water source) of agents—i.e. the household agents have no intelligence. They follow the same behavior and activities during the entire simulation period. The time step of the model is 1 h, with a time horizon of 90 days.

Intelligent agents: how do intelligent households make decisions?

Protection motivation theory (PMT)

PMT is used as the theoretical framework of this paper. PMT considers that, when facing a risky situation, a person goes through two steps: "threat appraisal" and "coping appraisal" (Fig. 3). Threat appraisal in PMT is the stage at which perceptions of risk are formed. Here, a household agent assesses the probability and consequences of a risky event occurring—i.e. perceived probability and perceived severity, which in fact constitutes the agents RP. Therefore, in the proceeding sections of this paper we refer to threat appraisal as the stage at which RP is developed. The perception of severity enables households to judge how seriously the consequences could be,

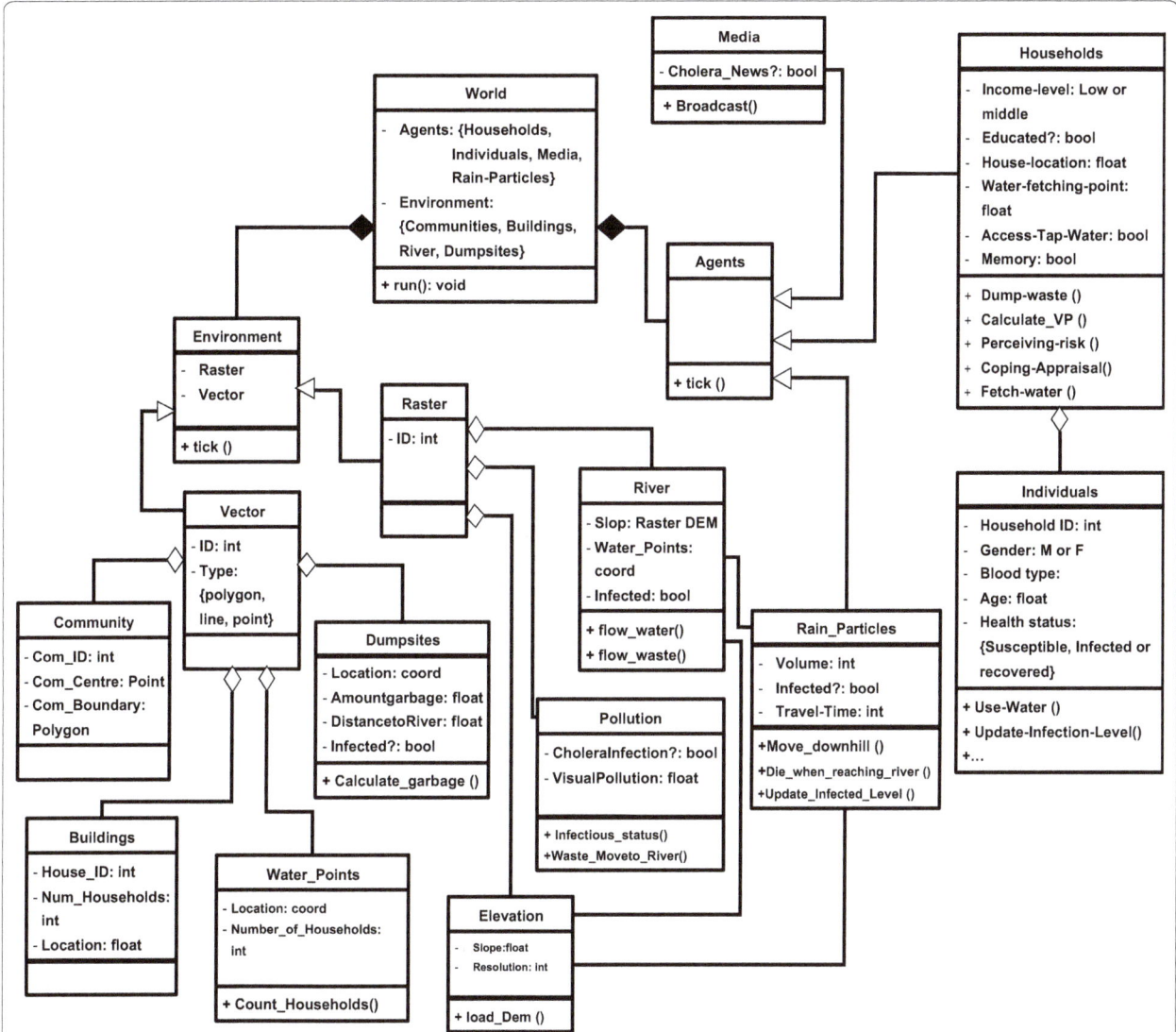

Fig. 2 The UML diagram of Cholera ABM

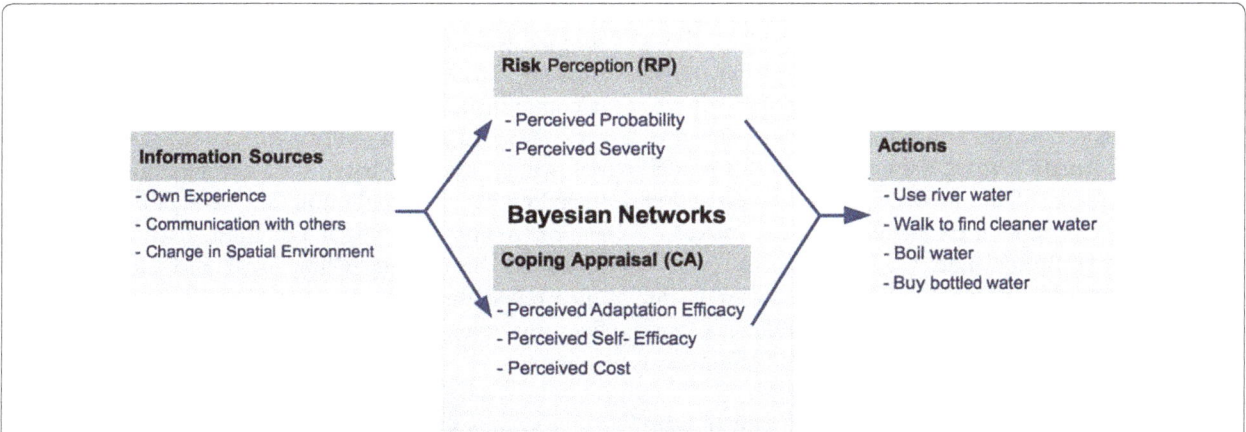

Fig. 3 Cognitive process of protection motivation theory (PMT)

should they face a threat. Perceived probability measures how susceptible a person is to a given threat. The purpose of this stage is to detect whether a risk is at an acceptable level or not.

When RP is sufficiently high, household agents consider a number of protective behaviors by passing through the coping appraisal stage. The coping stage consists of two main parts: adaptation-efficacy and self-efficacy. Adaptation-efficacy measures the effectiveness of protective behavior against a harmful situation—i.e. the beliefs of a person that the recommended behavior will protect them. Instead, self-efficacy measures the ability of a person to perform the recommended behavior. In addition, the person must evaluate the cost of coping with the threat. Hence, at this stage, households consider the psychological, physical, and economic consequences of adapting to a particular threat.

Cholera ABM—intelligent agents

In the intelligent version, the Cholera ABM is modified to simulate the RP (threat appraisal) and coping appraisal (CA) processes of household agents—i.e. including the learning technique to create intelligent agents. For this purpose, one extra agent (media) is added to the model (Fig. 2).

The state variable of the *Household agent* is the type of water they consume, and the infection level of this water. The household agent is responsible for the collection of water, and all household members will use this water for their daily consumption. Learning takes place at the level of the household, as it is directly related to the water source that the household selects. To facilitate this learning, we added memory and education level to the attributes of the household agent.

The state variable of the *Individual agent* is their health status. Individual agents can be susceptible to, infected with, or recovered from cholera.

Some studies have indicated that medical alerts do not have the impact of encouraging people to physically search for medical advice during epidemics [24]. However, information received from different media channels can prevent an epidemic from spreading [25]. Therefore, *Media* is a new agent that has been introduced to broadcast information about the epidemic in this model. The state variable of the media agent is its activation level, which determines if the media agent has started to broadcast about the epidemic.

The state variable of the *Rain particles* agent is the infection level. While flowing over the terrain, rain particles can acquire the infection (from infected dumpsites) and carry it to the nearest river or tributary.

The processes included in the original model were flow of rain particles, household fetching water, and

households dumping their waste. These processes remain unchanged in the version of the model used in the present research. However, in this version of the cholera model, we added the following processes:

1. Activation of the media agent;
2. Clearance of the dumpsites;
3. Calculations of the visual pollution (VP) level;
4. Risk perception;
5. Coping appraisal (CA).

Activation of the media agent

The media agent is deactivated in the beginning of the simulation. It is activated when the number of days exceeds a threshold value (22 days). After activation, the media agent will broadcast news about the cholera epidemic once a day, which all household agents in the simulation will receive. Once the broadcasting has begun, it will continue throughout the remaining part of the simulation. Media information is used in the risk assessment.

Clearance of the dumpsites

In the original model, dumpsites could be infected with cholera, and when the decay function was activated, this infection would gradually disappear over time. We also introduce the fact that garbage will be removed from dumpsites. This has two separate effects: it will influence the infection and will also have an impact on the visual pollution level.

Clearance of dumpsites will occur randomly. In Kumasi, 85% of household waste is collected by the municipality from the dumpsites twice per week [26]. Therefore, in this model, a random 85% of simulated dumpsites are discharged twice per week.

Calculation of the visual pollution level (VP)

Household agents fetch water from the nearest water collection point on the river, either because they do not have access to tap water, or because their tap water has stopped working due to heavy rain. Open refuse dumpsites are located at varying distances along the river. It is common in Kumasi to observe waste dumps located on riverbanks or in a river's path [27]. In the simulation, risk will be assessed based on a combination of factors, including the visual pollution (VP) level of the water collection points. The visual pollution level is calculated based on the combined link order and the number of open refuse dumpsites located within a specific distance from the river. VP is calculated based on the following equation:

$$f(VP) = \sum_{i=1}^{N} \frac{x_i g_i}{d_i} \qquad (1)$$

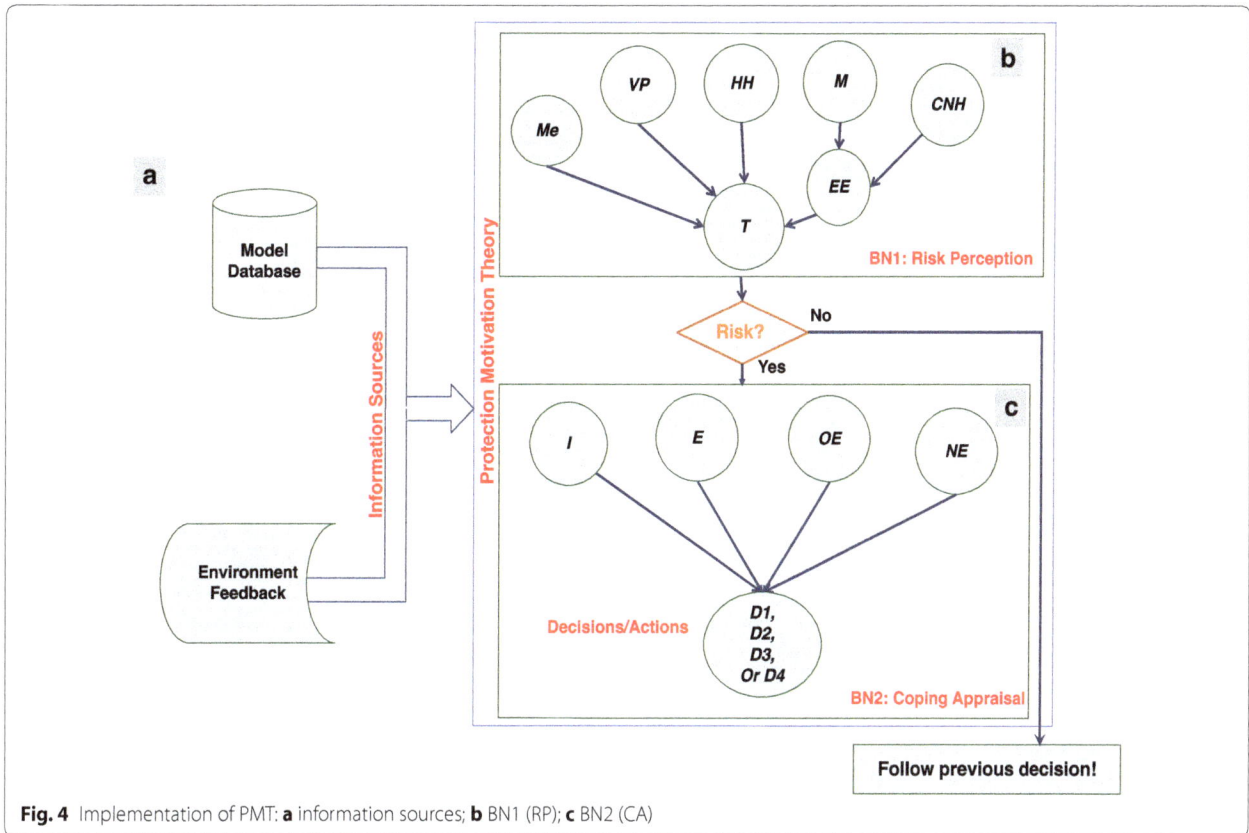

Fig. 4 Implementation of PMT: **a** information sources; **b** BN1 (RP); **c** BN2 (CA)

where N is the number of dumpsites around the water collection points; x_i is the number of households who use the dumpsite; g_i is the amount of garbage produced by each household; d_i is the distance from the dumpsites to the water collection point; and i represents all dumpsites in N (either cleared or not). Although the number of dumpsites is fixed throughout the simulation, the amount of garbage remains static, and the number of households will also remain static over a simulation run, while the visual pollution level is dynamic. This dynamic nature is due to the random selection of dumpsites that will be cleared over a simulation run.

Learning—implementation of agent's cognitive model

The PMT drives the agents' cognitive model. The information sources and the two stages of PMT are illustrated in Fig. 4. In this model, we used two BNs – BN1 to model the RP, and BN2 to model the CA.

Implementation of risk perception (RP)

At each time step, the household agent will perceive the risk of cholera infection using the BNs. The following factors are included in the RP: the number of infected individuals in the household, visual pollution level at the

water collection point, communication with other agents, media attention, and the memory of the household agent. Together, these factors and the agents' social interactions help agents to assess risk and thus select what decision they could make among several options.

Communication with other agents (social networks)

Household agents are assumed to have a total awareness of the cholera cases occurring within their neighbors' subset. A neighbor is defined as a household agent, sharing the same water collection point and living in the same community. Interaction with neighbors enables agents to perceive the infection level of the water collection point they use. In addition, household contacts help agents to gain information on adaptive decisions their neighbors took and how effective these decisions were.

No data is available on how many daily contacts Kumasi residents have. However, in a recent study by Melegaro et al. [28], they conducted a survey of daily contacts in Manicaland, Zimbabwe and reported 10.8 contacts per person/day, including contact with household members. If we consider this rate for our study and exclude the number of household members (average of 3.9), then approximately seven contacts with neighbors per day should be applied. These seven neighbors are chosen randomly every day from the agent's community.

Memory

Agents use their memory to record the RP they experienced during the previous day (the last day they fetched water) and how preventable their last decision was. The feedback of the last decision made is measured by "positive experience" if no illness was observed in the household, otherwise it is a "negative experience".

BN1: risk perception

BN1 was designed to represent the RP of PMT in such a way that it answers the question "is there risk?" In the case of a risk being present, agents will proceed to the CA.

Agents with a low or medium income level that do not have access to safe water will fetch water from the river. Therefore, they must evaluate the risk of becoming ill with cholera using BN1. In our case, BN1 is formed by the cause-and-effect concept. To design BN1, we derive five nodes from the information sources to evaluate RP (Fig. 4b). These nodes include: *memory (Me)*, *visual pollution (VP)*, *household health status (HH)*, *media (M)* and *communication with neighbor households (CNH)*. Media and communication with neighbor households are combined into "Epidemic Evidence" *(EE)*. *EE* is a binary measure that indicates to the agents if there are cholera cases outside their own households. The evaluation of infected cases differs by agent due to variations in household income and size, in the health status of different households, in their locations within the city that define VP and their selection of neighbors with whom they communicate, and in the experiences stored in their individual memories.

The reasoning and uncertainty of RP is governed by rules that can be formalized using formula (2). For example, we include the states {*yes, no*} for *memory (Me)*, {*yes, no*} for *threat (T)*, then the formula of connecting these two variables accordingly was designed as:

$$P\left(T_{\{yes,no\}}|Me_{\{yes,no\}}\right) = \frac{P\left(Me_{\{yes,no\}}|T_{\{yes,no\}}\right)P\left(T_{\{yes,no\}}\right)}{PMe_{\{yes,no\}}}$$

(2)

in such a way that each state of *Threat* is examined with each state of *memory*.

This was also applicable for computing the probability (P) of *threat* based on *visual pollution (VP)* and *household health status (HH)*, as both variables have the states {*high, low*} and {*yes, no*}, respectively.

We evaluated the epidemic evidence *(EE)* that agents record via their communication with neighbor households *(CNH)* and the media *(M)* agent.

According to Bayesian rules, the prior probabilities of the nodes should be specified in order to gain the posterior probabilities. These prior probabilities represent the integral part of human reasoning regarding certainty. The prior probabilities will be updated/changed for each agent on the basis of information being passed by each agent to BNs. In BNs, this is called evidence.

The final formula for the *threat* node *(T)* that derives the conditional probability table (CPT) will depend on *memory (Me)*, *visual pollution (VP)*, *the health status of household (HH)*, and the *severity evidence of epidemic (EE)*:

$$P(T|Me, VP, HH, EE) = \frac{P(Me, VP, HH, EE|T)P(T)}{P(Me, VP, HH, EE)}$$

(3)

Thus, intelligent agents in the Cholera ABM learn to predict health risks with the help of BN1 (Eq. 2). In BN1, the memory node feeds the network with previous information on agents' own RP. Agents learn to revise their beliefs by absorbing other factors from their environment that are updated during the simulation, e.g. currently observed visual pollution, number of illnesses among neighbors, etc. (Eqs. 2–3). Agents conclude the causal relationship between nodes in the BN1 by inference. The output of BN1 would be the probability of high or low risk perception. We consider the agent to be at risk if the probability of RP is greater than or equal to 0.5.

Coping appraisal (CA)

BN2 was designed to represent the coping appraisal of PMT in such a way that it answers the question "what to do?" In the case of perceiving risk, an agent may either: use the polluted water anyway, walk (find another location to fetch water), boil the fetched water (to increase safety), or purchase bottled water. To select one of these four decisions, a number of variables (nodes) affecting this process were identified and used. These variables include: the income level of the agents (medium or low); their education level (educated or uneducated); and the feedback of their previous and their neighbors' previous action (positive or negative). Agents cannot learn from their own experience unless they have a feedback on their previous actions [29]. Together, all of these dynamics guide the decision-making process.

BN2: coping appraisal

BN2 represents the structure of the CA (Fig. 4c). The probability of which decision might be chosen by the agent is computed via BN2. The perceived adaptation efficacy will differ per decision. Walking to another location to collect water has a lower efficacy compared to boiling the water, and this has a lower efficacy compared to buying bottled water. Also, perceived self-efficacy (i.e.

Table 1 Cholera ABM new parameters

New parameters	Value	Description
Literacy rate	74.1%	[30]
Media	Activation day 22	During the 2005 outbreak, newspapers and TV channels published news about the cholera in the region after about 3 weeks of epidemic started (visit: Ghana News Archive)
Waste collection	85% of dumpsites	85% of waste is collected by Kumasi municipality [26]. The rest remain uncollected for a week or more
Amount of garbage	2.925 kg/household/day	Derived from literature [31]
Number of contacts with neighbors	7 neighbors	Derived from literature [28]

Table 2 Model settings varied across the three experiments

Model settings	Exp1	Exp2	Exp3
Threat appraisal	None	BN1	BN1
Initial weights[a]	n.a.	(0.1; 0.2; 0.01; 0.01; 0.2)	(0.1; 0.2; 0.01; 0.01; 0.2)
Me, VP, HH, M, CNH	n.a.	Change as agents learn	Change as agents learn
Weights during a simulation	n.a.	RP, (0;1)	RP, (0;1)
Outcome			
Coping appraisal	None	Deterministic	BN2
Initial weights	n.a.	Rule based, Table 3	(0.52; 0.74; 0.9; 0.6)
I, E, OE, NE	n.a.	Static	Change as agents learn
Weights during a simulation	D1	D1–D4: fixed population share	D1–D4: adaptive, based on previous experience
Outcome			

[a] To elicit the factors that may play a role in the context of a water-spread disease in a developing country as well as their relative importance we ran a survey among students. We approached the participants of the Massive Open Online Course (MOOC) on GeoHealth run at ITC (authors host institute) in Sep, 2016. Majority of the participants of this course are from developing countries. Ideally, one would survey real citizens in the case-study area. This was not possible due to the lack of funds and access to the potential respondents

perceived effectiveness enabling an agent to perform the preventive measure) is varied for each decision. In addition, the perceived costs of the options differ, as river water is free of cost, boiling water has a price tag, and so does the purchase of bottled water. Here, the agents' income level determines which decision is more likely to be taken.

The formula of BN2 for computing the CPT of a decision can be expressed as:

$$P(D|I,E,OE,NE) = \frac{P(I,E,OE,NE|D)P(D)}{P(I,E,OE,NE)} \quad (4)$$

where D stands for decision, which can take the form (state) of 'use water from the same fetching point' ($D1$), 'walk to another fetching point' ($D2$), 'boil water' ($D3$), and 'buy water' ($D4$); I denotes an income level, what can be middle or low; E is the education level (educated or not); OE is an agent's own experience with cholera, which can be either positive (no household member is ill) or negative (at least one household member is ill); and NE is the neighbor's experience with cholera [anyone ill (negative) or not (positive)].

Model parameterization

The probability values of both networks variables are derived from the existing literature and census data for Kumasi. The census data of Kumasi, Ghana includes income distribution. The distribution of the three levels is 19% (low), 52% (medium), and 29% (high). However, we exclude high level incomes since they will not use river water. Therefore, by scaling both medium and low-income levels, we get 73 and 27%, respectively (which represents 71% of the number of simulated households). Additionally, 14% of low and middle-income level households do not have access to tap water. Table 1 presents the additional parameters of this cholera model. Naturally, for real policy application, the quality of data regarding initial weights in BN1 (Table 2) and the frequency and the extent of information delivery, either via media or through the word-of-mouth across social networks, is essential. We run a sensitivity analysis of final outcomes on the initial weights of both BNs ("Appendix 1"). The results indicate that the model is rather robust, with minimal impact on the final outcomes.

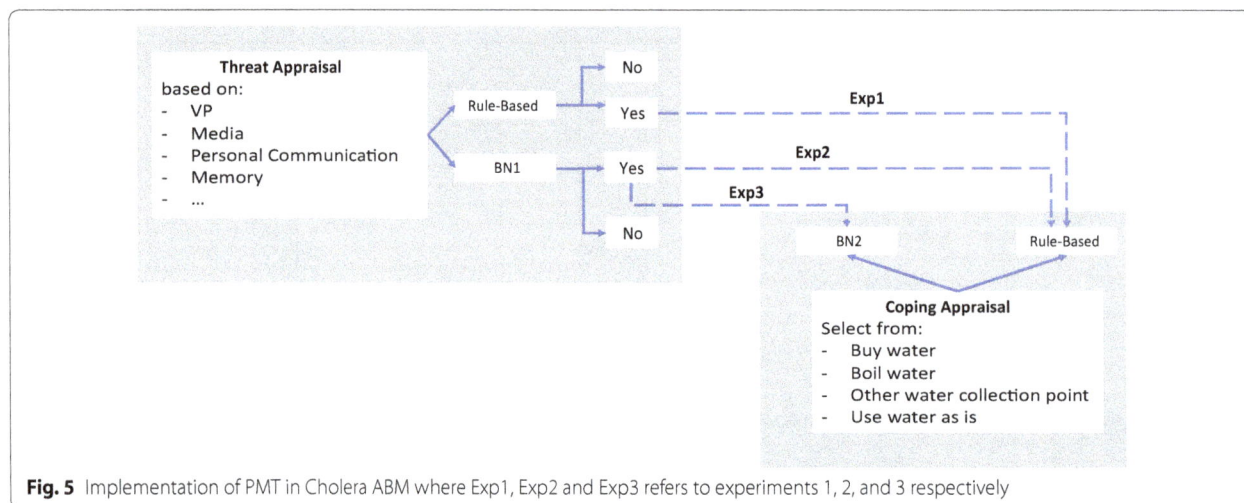

Fig. 5 Implementation of PMT in Cholera ABM where Exp1, Exp2 and Exp3 refers to experiments 1, 2, and 3 respectively

Simulation results

Experiment setup

To answer the research questions, we have designed three experiments. We systematically vary the cognitive abilities of agents by gradually adding intelligence by means of the two BNs (Fig. 5). In particular, the first experiment (Exp1) presents a benchmark case to study disease diffusion patterns in a spatial landscape with a population of zero-intelligence agents. Agents are heterogeneous in income, education, and household size but have no cognitive abilities to either perceive risk or act upon it. In the second experiment (Exp2), agents are enhanced with the BN that represents the first stage of decision-making in a risky context: the risk appraisal (BN1). As agents learn and interact with each other, the probabilities of specific factors influencing risk appraisal change. The second stage of decision-making in Exp2 is modeled in a simplistic manner by adopting a rule-based algorithm, which deterministically guides an agent to a specific action if its RP is high. Finally, the third experiment (Exp3) adopts intelligent decision making at both stages of decision making under risk: the risk appraisal (BN1) and the coping appraisal (BN2) both supported by BNs learning algorithms. Thus, if agents begin to perceive risk as an outcome of BN1, they employ BN2 to decide how to act upon it. As agents learn from their own experience and others' through interaction, the probabilities of specific actions to be chosen through BN2 evolve. All other settings among the three experiments remain static (Table 2). Each of the experiments is run 100 times to assure the robustness of the results.

We report the results per experiment in terms of several macro metrics of interest: epidemic curve, RP curve, and decision type curve. An *epidemic curve* is a graphical description of the number of illness cases by date during an outbreak. It illustrates the temporal trend and periods of disease incubation. A *RP curve* is a graphical description of a number of agents that perceive disease threat, i.e. have their RP equal to 1 in a specific time step. A *decision types curve* counts the number of agents following a particular decision when deciding on how to cope with cholera risk. In addition, we show several maps illustrating the spatial patterns of RP (Decisions: D1-D4).

Disease diffusion in a population of zero-intelligent agents

The temporal patterns of a cholera epidemic given a population of zero-intelligent (ZI) agents neither perceiving risk nor pursuing any protective measures is presented in Fig. 6a. It is evident that, even if a household member becomes ill, media broadcasts cholera being present, and some visual pollution is observed at a water fetching point, a ZI agent will still continue to collect water for its daily needs at the same water fetching point and will use it without precautionary measures. The number of infected agents reaches a maximum between day 28 and day 40 before gradually decreasing towards the end of the epidemic. In total, 81% of the simulation population (27,000 out of 34,000 individuals) is infected with cholera in Exp1. While the ZI Cholera ABM succeeds in reproducing the qualitative pattern of this Cholera epidemic, it largely overestimates the number of infected individuals. A simulation with non-adaptive ZI agents misrepresents reality, since even middle income and educated people continue to consume potentially contaminated water: 28.6, 64.7, and 6.5% in the low, middle, and high-income categories, respectively.

When agents have no cognitive abilities, and are not reactive, then the probability of becoming infected during a rainy period depends on the concentration of

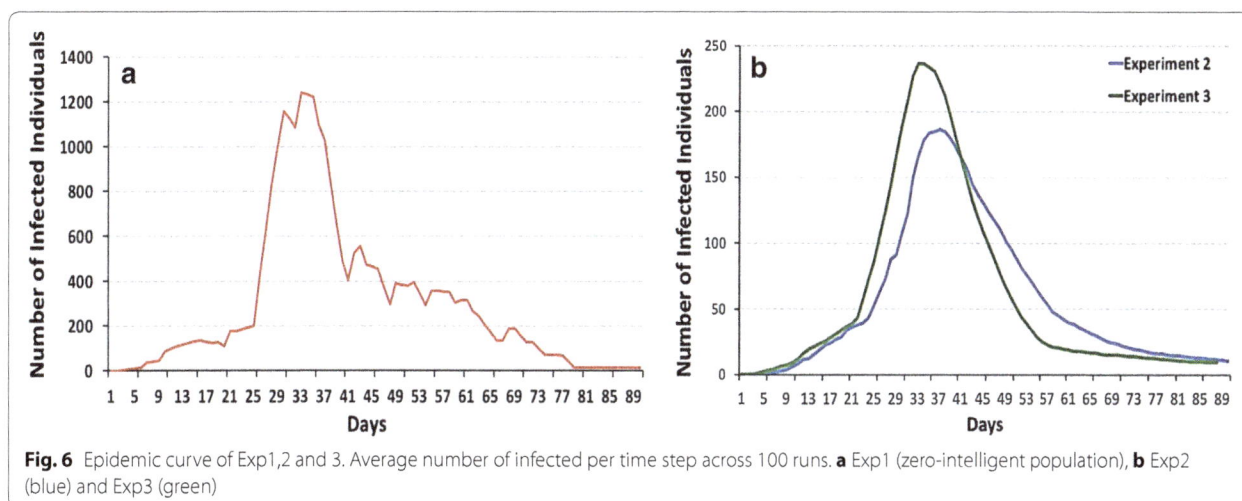

Fig. 6 Epidemic curve of Exp1,2 and 3. Average number of infected per time step across 100 runs. **a** Exp1 (zero-intelligent population), **b** Exp2 (blue) and Exp3 (green)

Table 3 Rule-based algorithm (CA) for Experiment 2 where agents select a static decision to take based on their characteristics

Household characteristics				Decision
Income	Educated	Infection in household	Infection in neighbor households	
Low	No	No	No	D1 (same)
Low	No	No	Yes	D1
Low	No	Yes	No	D2 (walk)
Low	No	Yes	Yes	D2
Low	Yes	No	No	D1
Low	Yes	No	Yes	D2
Low	Yes	Yes	No	D2
Low	Yes	Yes	Yes	D2
Middle	No	No	No	D1
Middle	No	No	Yes	D2
Middle	No	Yes	No	D4 (buy)
Middle	No	Yes	Yes	D4
Middle	Yes	No	No	D1
Middle	Yes	No	Yes	D3 (boil)
Middle	Yes	Yes	No	D3
Middle	Yes	Yes	Yes	D4

infected agents, which may dump infected waste on a dumpsite, leading to flow of cholera-infected rainwater into the river.

Intelligent risk perception

From a psychological perspective, to be able to act upon risk, people—i.e. agents in the Cholera ABM—must first be aware of a risk. Experiment 2 presents the case when intelligence is added in the threat appraisal (BN1) stage. When being aware of risk while fetching water, agents in Exp2 may change their behavior using a deterministic rule-based algorithm (Table 3). Thus, actions that agents select in this CA stage are based on current information, ignoring any previous experiences. Enhancing agents with cognitive abilities for threat appraisal (BN1) reduces the total number of infected agents by 90%. In Exp2, the total number of cholera-infected agents decreases (see the blue epidemic curve of Exp2 in Fig. 6b). In other words, information about a disease spreads through different channels—media, own observations, the experience of others, while a simple set of precautionary actions give rise to a steadier epidemic curve. Following the epidemic peak, agents are risk-aware and take a variety of precautionary actions based on their income class and education, ill individuals in their own and/or their neighbors' households; thus, fewer infections occur at the later stages of epidemics. Therefore, the BN1 epidemic curve (in Fig. 6b) has a lower peak and a steeper, vanishing tail compared to the ZI epidemic curve (Fig. 6a). The first heavy rainfall boosts the spread of cholera and can be detected in the shape of this curve at approximately day 23 in Exp2. Then, the effect of new disease exposure on the number of infected is counterbalanced by the activated risk awareness within the BN1 population. New exposure occurs when agents either lack infection experience in their social network or choose to ignore risks at the coping stage. The Cholera ABM enhanced with BN1 for the threat appraisal may be used to explore the spatial and temporal patterns of disease spread depending on varying risk communication strategies. To demonstrate this notion, we run a sensitivity analysis on the main communication channels.

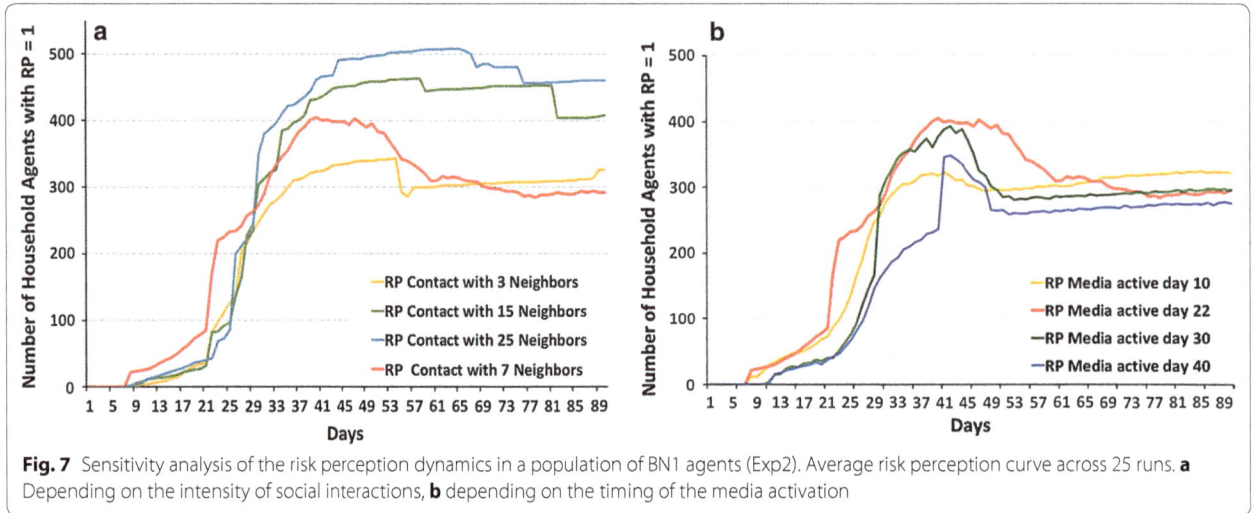

Fig. 7 Sensitivity analysis of the risk perception dynamics in a population of BN1 agents (Exp2). Average risk perception curve across 25 runs. **a** Depending on the intensity of social interactions, **b** depending on the timing of the media activation

Sensitivity analysis on the number of social interactions

A diffusion of information about disease risk and the effectiveness of risk-coping measures occur through social interactions. Their intensity impacts the spread of awareness about cholera risk in the study area as well as the number of infected individuals. Following Melegaro et al. [28], the base scenario of Exp2 (and Exp3) assumes that when fetching water, agents exchange information daily with seven agents from their social network. These social links are set up randomly among households in the same community using the same water collection point. In addition, we run sensitivity analysis considering 3, 15, and 25 unique social interactions with individuals outside their own household per day. Figure 7a and Table 4 illustrate the sensitivity of the number of individuals perceiving cholera risk and the resulting number of infections under various assumptions regarding social interaction.

All curves in Fig. 7a demonstrate a steep increase in risk perception around day 23 of the simulations. This point indicates the first heavy rainfall, when the population of agents depending on river water increases, and the disease diffusion via the dumpsites begins. During this first period, all scenarios exhibit the same pattern. However, after day 40, a clear difference is observed between the four scenarios. As expected, the higher the number of daily contacts (with which intelligent BN1-agents exchange information), the higher the number of households who perceived risk. Higher levels of cholera risk awareness trigger agents to make alternative decisions regarding water use (D2-D4 instead of D1), following the deterministic rule-based algorithm, and thus leads to a reduction in the number of infected individuals (Table 4).

With fewer social interactions, BN1-agents are less likely to be aware of any cholera cases in their neighborhood. Therefore, they will use the usual water fetching point, causing more individuals to be infected with cholera. As the speed of information exchange increases, agents learn from the experience of a larger group of individuals with respect to safety of alternative water fetching points and potential preventive behaviors. Since communication with neighbors is not the sole information source influencing the formation of RP in intelligent BN1-agents, the relation between the number of daily contacts and the resulting number of infected is non-linear: when interaction intensity changes from 7 to 15 people, the number of disease cases decreases by only 25% (Table 4).

Sensitivity analysis with respect to the timing of media broadcasting

During the 2005 cholera epidemic in Kumasi, the media began to widely broadcast epidemic information 21 days after the first infected case. We test the sensitivity of risk perception dynamics and the number of infected in response to the different media broadcasting timings. Thus, we ran the Cholera ABM with different media

Table 4 Sensitivity of the extent of an epidemic on the intensity of social interactions and information exchange among intelligent agents (Exp2)

No. of contacts	RP peak day	Epidemic peak day	Percentage of total population infected from the base (%)
Three	83	35	103
Seven (base)	40	36	100
Fifteen	71	35	75
Twenty-Five	66	36	74

Table 5 Sensitivity of the extent of an epidemic on the timing of media broadcasting in the population of intelligent agents (Exp2)

Day of media activation	Percentage of total population perceived risk (%)	Epidemic peak day	Percentage of total population infected from the base (%)
Tenth	83.7	36	89.4
Twenty second (base)	100	36	100
Thirtieth	87.8	35	106.1
Fortieth	75.2	35	108.3

activation dates—10, 30, and 40 days post-infection—in addition to day 22 (the base case of Exp2). Figure 7b illustrates that, generally, when the media reports on the cholera outbreak, the number of BN1-agents perceiving risk increases abruptly. This is true for the media activation scenarios on day 22, 30, and 40; however, this does not hold true for early activation (at day 10). The BN learning algorithm considers several factors at the threat appraisal stage. Thus, although BN1-agents have been alerted about cholera by the media on day 10, they did not yet observe any cholera cases in their household or neighborhood. In addition, depending on the rainfall intensity, they may still have access to safe tap water that will only stop working following heavy rainfall on day 23. This combination of observations within their household and social network triggers BN1-agents to discard media messages and conclude BN1 simulations with low RP.

The timing of media messages does not affect the peak day of an epidemic, but impacts the resulting number of infected individuals (Table 5). It seems that early media attention (day 10) increases public awareness, resulting in individuals taking precautionary measures at a later stage, when other factors contributing to thread appraisal become evident (the yellow RP curve above others at the second half of the epidemics in Fig. 7b). Yet, the relationship is non-linear: the later the announcement, the smaller the marginal impact. Namely, postponing the broadcast for 10 additional days (e.g. day 22 vs. day 30) results in 6% more infected individuals, while another 10 days of delay results in only 2% more infected (day 30 vs. day 40). It is evident that announcing the epidemic 10 days earlier than the base scenario (day 22) reduces infections by over 10%.

Disease coping strategies: rule-based vs. intelligent risk protection

According to PMT, when individuals are aware of risks, they choose actions based on their response efficacy and

self-efficacy (positive influence) and the response costs (negative influence). The population of agents in Exp2 is intelligent in their risk appraisal, but pursue simple, rule-based decision- making (Table 3) at the CA stage.

Following the heavy rainfall (between days 23 and 50), BN1 agents begin to explore alternative options to drawing water from their normal nearest fetching point (D1). The latter is almost equally chosen by low and middle-income households throughout the entire simulation (Fig. 8a). As cholera risk awareness spreads, the proportion of agents deciding to walk to an alternative fetching point (D2, only low-income households) and to boil water (D3, only middle-income households) increases. Some middle-income households also decide to purchase water (D4). However, since all three alternatives—walk, boil, and purchase—infer additional costs, households shift back to the default D1 option as soon as heavy rainfall ceases, and the number of disease cases decreases. As Fig. 8a. illustrates, a difference also exists in the distribution of preventive actions across income classes. However, the action choice remains deterministic: it depends only on the characteristics of agents at initialization such as income and education. There is no feedback between the effectiveness of previous actions taken by BN1 households or their peers and current agents' choices regarding water use. Thus, BN1 agents in Exp2 do not learn at the CA stage.

Experiment 3 is run in order explore how the learning process on precautionary measures is reinforced based on previous experiences. Here, agents employ two BN learning algorithms: BN1 for the threat appraisal and BN2 for the CA. When facing cholera risk, agents in Exp3 learn to perceive risk and subsequently learn to protect themselves by making adaptive decisions based on their own previous experience and their neighbors' experience. The epidemic curves of Exp2 and Exp3 fall within a similar range (Fig. 6b), with one important difference; namely, BN2-agents seem to be over-confident about their disease prevention choices at the epidemic's onset (approx. day 23), but quickly learn to alter strategies immediately after the peak (Fig. 8b).

Cholera begins to spread from the first few days of the simulation in both Exp2 and Exp3. The total number of infected agents during the cholera epidemic is approximately the same: on average, 14.7% of the simulation's population (5000 individuals) in both Exp2 and Exp3. However, a qualitative difference exists in the type and dynamics of preventive actions. Figure 8b demonstrates that, over time, agents driven by growing RP learn to boil water based on the previous experience, which leads to a steady increase of D3 strategy use in the BN2 agent population. Among middle and low-income household agents enhanced with BN2, no agents purchase water.

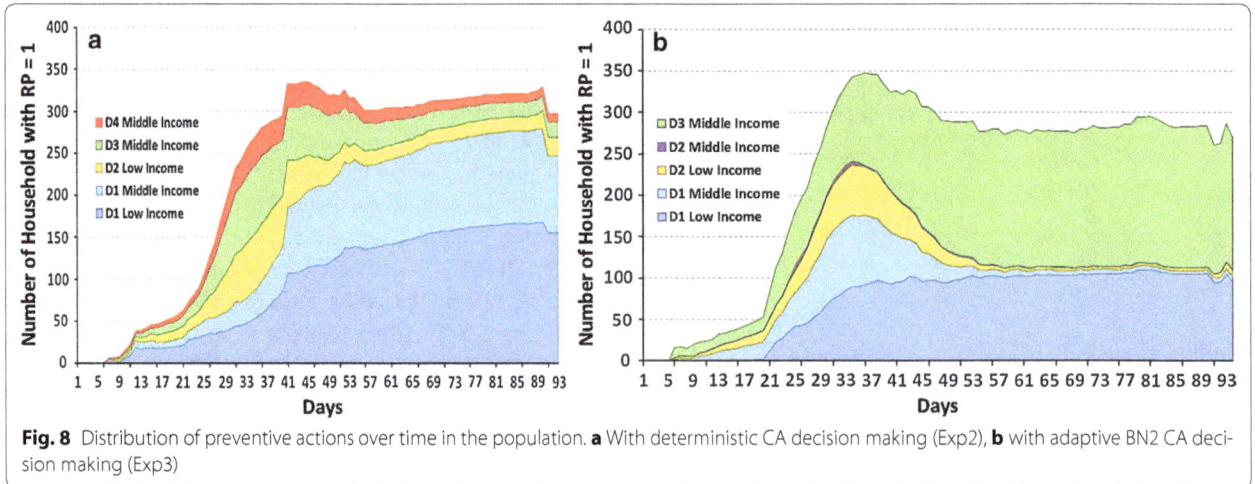

Fig. 8 Distribution of preventive actions over time in the population. **a** With deterministic CA decision making (Exp2), **b** with adaptive BN2 CA decision making (Exp3)

Instead, they switch to boiling water (see green D3 zone in Fig. 8b). Simultaneously, the number of middle-income households taking water from their usual, now suspicious-looking fetching point is nearly reduced to zero over time (see the light blue zone in Fig. 8b). BN2-agents also learn that walking to another water collection point still may result in a negative outcome.

The distribution of coping strategies between Exp2 and Exp3 also varies in space and by income class (Fig. 9). When low-income BN2-agents learn to compare efficacy and costs based on past experience in Exp3, they realize that walking to another fetching point may not be worth the effort. Instead, in Exp2, low-income agents basing their CA decision on the deterministic rule-based process continue to walk alternate fetching points (compare left-hand side maps in Fig. 9). Non-adaptive middle-income households in Exp2 continue to use a combination of the three strategies provided at initialization. Yet, intelligent BN2 individuals in Exp3 converge to using boiled water in the majority of the cases (right-hand side maps of Fig. 9), as it proved to be most rewarding alternative to D1.

Conclusions

Risk awareness and risk prevention behavior can have a major impact on the number of disease cases during an epidemic. Models ignoring these elements of human behavior may overestimate the expected number of disease cases. While a number of comprehensive disease ABMs have been developed, few explore the implications of these behavioral aspects and learning. This article introduces an innovative contribution by integrating psychological aspects of decision-making under risk into a spatial ABM using BNs learning algorithms.

We use an empirical spatial ABM of cholera diffusion [19] as a baseline model to test the impact of a multi-stage intelligent decision-making in a risk context. Two sets of BN learning algorithms are designed and coded using R, and are further integrated with the NetLogo-based Cholera ABM. Protection motivation theory from psychology lays the foundation for designing BN learning in two stages: one for RP appraisal and another for coping appraisal. We compare the results of the spatial agent-based disease model without intelligence (zero-intelligence), with an implementation of one-stage BN1 (only RP), and a two-stage BN2 (risk and coping behavior) intelligence. Learning allows a population of heterogeneous and spatially distributed agents to perceive risk and acquire and share knowledge via a social network about the effectiveness of various disease protection actions. This spatial ABM enhanced with BNs allows us to explore the emergence of disease diffusion patterns tracing both geographic, educational, and income inequalities. The implementation strategy, in which we apply both BN1 for risk awareness and BN2 for risk appraisal, seems to outperform an implementation with a single BN. As agents learn about the effectiveness of preventive measures in addition to learning to recognize risks, the society as a whole makes healthier and more cost-effective choices. The sensitivity analysis on the behavioral assumptions indicates that the model is rather robust, with minimal impact on the final outcomes.

While this research presents a step forward in ABMs of disease diffusion by integrating psychology-based intelligence the context of risk, it can be further developed in a number of directions. Firstly, in addition to spatial, hydrological, and socio-economic data, this modeling effort could benefit from disaggregated behavioral data.

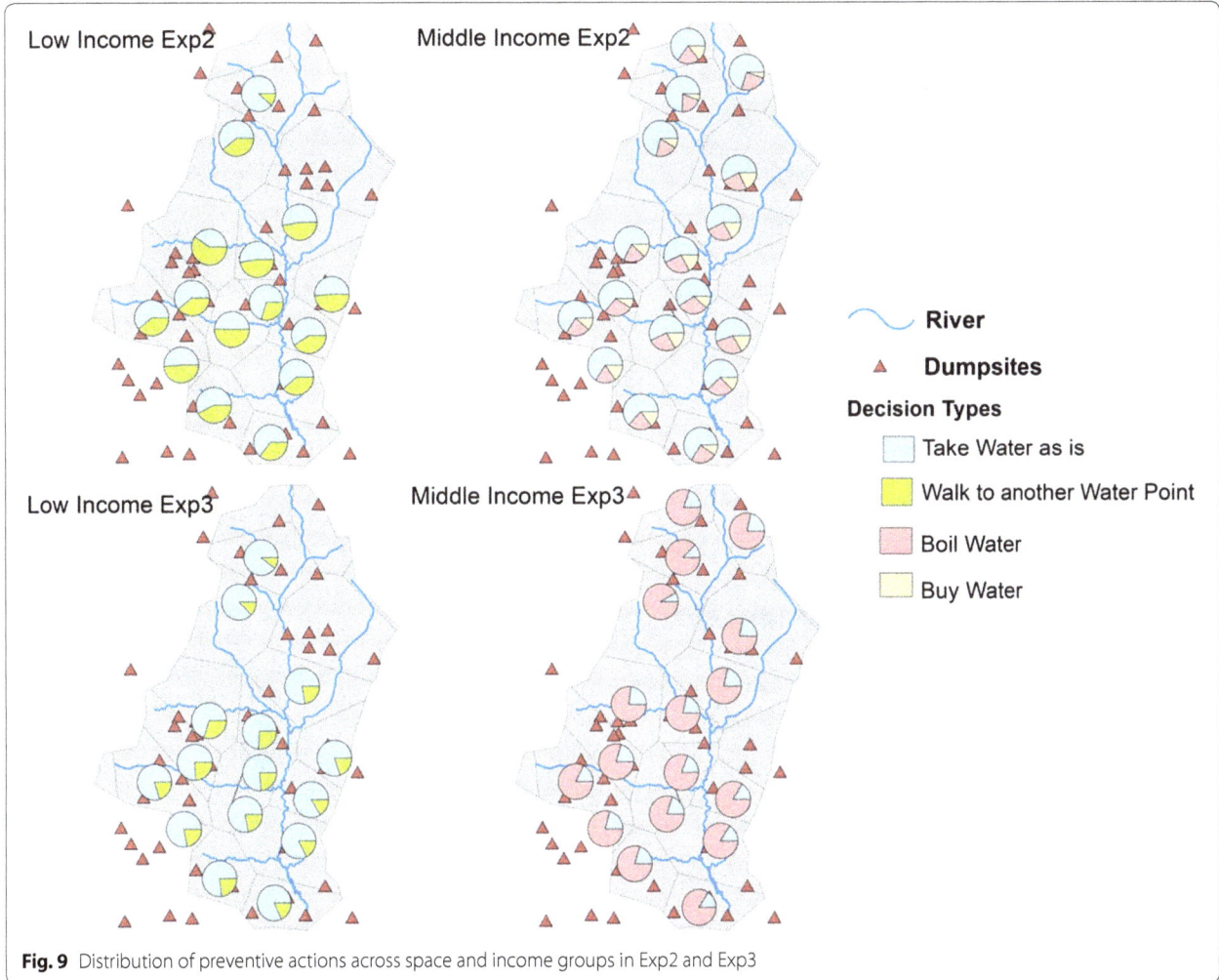

Fig. 9 Distribution of preventive actions across space and income groups in Exp2 and Exp3

Currently, our BN1–RP model is updated based on information obtained via personal communication, media, and visual observations of the environment. While we use data from the survey among students from developing countries to parameterize initial weights for RP factors, this may not be fully representative of the population in Kumasi. Disaggregated data on socio-demographic and behavioral characteristics of a target population is in demand to gain better insights on the interplay of factors influencing human behavior during a disease outbreak. This is especially true for visual perception of the environment, as a current lack of information exists on how this factor influences total RP. In addition, a survey to collect data on how media affects people would improve the simulation. Model runs with richer datasets is within the scope of our future work.

Secondly, individual RP and coping appraisal can be implemented in disease ABMs using different ML algorithms. Besides BNs, genetic algorithms or neural networks might also prove useful. Further research is needed to explore the impact of various ML algorithms within the same base ABM. In addition, a systematic study on the performance of one ML algorithm across multiple ABMs for different types of risks in various geographic environments will provide a comprehensive understanding of the implications of introducing intelligence to agent-based modeling will have.

The implementation of risk and coping appraisals in disease ABMs will ultimately aid in supporting decisions regarding the timing of media attention to societal risks, and on the information that must be communicated to the public in order to prevent as many disease cases as possible.

Authors' contribution
The authors' contribution is primarily done by the corresponding author as a part of her PhD under the supervision of the authors TF, YTM, and EWA in terms of fully guiding the process of implementing the model and been involved in drafting the manuscript and revising it critically for important intellectual content. All authors read and approved the final manuscript.

Author details
[1] Department of Governance and Technology for Sustainability (CSTM), Faculty of Behavioral, Management, and Social Sciences (BMS), University of Twente, Enschede, The Netherlands. [2] Department of Computer Science, College of Science, University of Duhok (UoD), Duhok, Kurdistan Region, Iraq. [3] Department of Geo-Information Process (GIP), Faculty of Geo-Information Science and Earth Observation (ITC), University of Twente, Enschede, The Netherlands. [4] Faculty of Science, University of Zakho (UoZ), Duhok, Kurdistan Region, Iraq. [5] School of Systems, Management and Leadership, Faculty of Engineering and Information Technology, University of Technology Sydney, Ultimo, Australia.

Competing interests
The authors declare that they have no competing interests.

Funding
The financial support of this research comes from the split-site PhD program of the Iraqi Kurdistan-region government (KRG) represented by ministry of higher education and scientific research, and the NWO DID MIRACLE project (640-006-012).

Appendix 1: Sensitivity analysis of BN1 and BN2

Each parameter (node) in the BNs is associated with a probability (weight). The initial weights for BN1 in Exp2 are estimated from a small sample of data ($N = 194$) collected within the GeoHealth MOOC in Sep, 2016. To test the impact of the initial weights on the RP in BN1 we performed a simple[1] sensitivity analysis (Table 6) changing the initial weights of one parameter at a time for VP, media and CNH.

Results show that the model behavior is rather robust. Increasing the weight of VP from 0.8 to 1 causes an increase of 10% in the risk perception. Any visual pollution observed will lead to risk awareness. A decrease in the VP weight has no effect.

Changes in the initial weights of media show a change of 8% (Table 6) occurs when the influence of media (both M1 and M2) drop by 20 and 40% correspondingly. While dropping CNH by 40% leads to decrease the number of agents perceiving risk 4%.

BN2 in Exp3 is triggered only when risk is perceived. We checked the sensitivity of the coping strategies of agents with respect to changing the initial weights for the income level in BN2. The shares of agents' disease coping decisions vary as the probabilities of belonging to a specific income group change (Table 7).

As income levels in the agent population drops (Income*1, 37% increase in the probability of agents with low income level, Table 7), we observe an increase in the uptake of strategies D1 and D2 (drinking water from the river either from the same or an alternative fetching point). If we increase the number of middle-income households, we notice that 7% of the agents start buying water (D4). This explains the decrease in D3 (compared to the original 51%).

Table 6 Sensitivity of the number of agents perceiving risk of cholera (BN1) on the initial weights (probabilities) of the decision nodes (factors)

Nodes with changed weights	Weight	N of agents with RP = 1 (outcome of BN1)	Difference from the base (%)
VP_1^a	Low = 1.0, high = 0.0	34,019	110
Base BN1 (Exp2) VP_0	Default VP: low = 0.8, high = 0.2	30,847	100
VP_2^a	Low = 0.6, high = 0.4	30,482	99
Base BN1 (Exp2) M_0	Default M no = 0.99, yes = 0.01	30,847	100
M_1^a	No = 0.79, yes = 0.21	33,174	108
M_2^a	No = 0.39, yes = 0.69	33,254	108
CNH_1^a	No = 1, yes = 0	31,341	102
Base BN1 (Exp2) CNH_0	Default CNH no = 0.8, yes = 0.2	30,847	100
CNH_2^a	No = 0.6, yes = 0.4	29,519	96

[a] Based on the mean values across 25 runs

---

[1] The full scale sensitivity analysis of Bayesian Networks is a major computational exercise [32], and is outside the scope of this paper.

Table 7 Sensitivity of the coping strategy choices made by agents with RP = 1 to the initial weights in BN2

Node	Weight	Percentage of decision types of agents with RP = 1			
		D1%	D2%	D3%	D4%
Income$_2^a$	Low = 0.17, middle = 0.83	38	6	49	7
Income	Default: low = 0.27, middle = 0.73	42	7	51	0
Income$_1^a$	Low = 0.37, middle = 0.63	57	24	19	0

[a] The results are based on the mean values from 25 Cholera ABM runs

Appendix 2: R code of BN1 and BN2

BN1: risk perception

```
#################### Loading libraries####################################
library(gRbase)
library(gRain)
library(Rgraphviz)
################# Creating BN1 ###########################################
BN1 <-function(vp,hh,Me,M,CNH){
  #constructing the BN of Threat Appraisal
  g <- list (~vpollution, ~healthS, ~Amemory, ~media, ~Contact, ~EE | media: Contact, ~Thret | vpollution: healthS
: Amemory: EE)
  threatBN<-dagList(g)
  lh <-c("low","high")
  ny <-c("no","yes")
  lmh <-c("low","mediam","high")
  VP <-cptable(~vpollution, values = c(8,2),levels = lh)
  HS <-cptable(~healthS, values = c(99,1), levels = ny)
  AM <-cptable(~Amemory, values = c(9,1), levels = ny)
  Me <-cptable(~media, values = c(9,1),levels = ny)
  CN <-cptable(~Contact, values = c(8,2),levels = ny)
  DL.MeoA <-cptable(~EE | media : Contact, values = c(85,1,05,25,45,3,3,45,25,05,1,85), levels = lmh)
  Tht.VPHSDL <- cptable(~Thret | vpollution : healthS : Amemory :EE, values =
c(85,15,55,45,25,75,15,85,55,45,35,65,25,75,25,75,55,45,35,65,25,75,2,8,45,55,35,65,25,75,15,85,4,6,2,8,4,6,2,
8,3,7,2,8,4,6,1,9),levels = ny)
  plist <- compileCPT(list(VP, HS, AM, Me, CN, DL.MeoA, Tht.VPHSDL))
  grn1 <-grain(plist)
  grn1c <- compile(grn1)
  grn1c <- propagate(grn1c)
  grn1c.ev2 <-setEvidence(grn1c, c("vpollution","healthS","Amemory","media","Contact"), c(vp,hh,Me,M,CNH))
  x<-querygrain(grn1c.ev2, nodes=c("Thret"), type="marginal")
  return(x)
}
```

BN2: coping appraisal

```
################### Loading libraries #################################
library(gRbase)
library(bnlearn)
library(Rgraphviz)
################### Creating BN2 ######################################
myBN2 <-function (inc,edu,me,ne){
  BN2 <-
model2network("[Income][Education][Myexperience][Nexperience][Decision|Income:Education:Myexperience:Ne
xperience]")
  Income.lv <- c("low","middle")
  Education.lv <- c("no","yes")
  experience.lv <- c("pos","neg")
  Decision.lv <- c("D1","D2","D3","D4")
  Income.prob <- array(c(0.73,0.27),dim=2,dimnames = list(Income=Income.lv))
  Education.prob <- array(c(0.67,0.33), dim = 2, dimnames = list(Education =Education.lv))
  Myexperience.prob <- array(c(0.7,0.3), dim = 2, dimnames = list(Myexperience = experience.lv))
  Nexperience.prob <- array(c(0.8,0.2), dim = 2, dimnames = list(Nexperience = experience.lv))
  Decision.prob <-
array(c(0.7,0.15,0.1,0.05,0.6,0.25,0.1,0.05,0.1,0.7,0.15,0.05,0.05,0.7,0.2,0.05,0.2,0.6,0.05,0.15,0.2,0.3,0.05,0.45
,0.2,0.45,0.3,0.05,0.05,0.15,0.6,0.2,0.6,0.25,0.1,0.05,0.2,0.45,0.15,0.2,0.2,0.45,0.3,0.05,0.05,0.25,0.65,0.05,0.2,
0.5,0.05,0.25,0.05,0.1,0.2,0.65,0.15,0.6,0.2,0.05,0.05,0.1,0.7,0.15),
                dim = c(4,2,2,2,2), dimnames = list(Decision=Decision.lv, Income=Income.lv,
Education=Education.lv, Myexperience=experience.lv, Nexperience=experience.lv))
  cpt <- list(Income=Income.prob, Education = Education.prob, Myexperience=Myexperience.prob,
Nexperience=Nexperience.prob, Decision=Decision.prob)
  BN22<- custom.fit(BN2,cpt)
  jglob <- compile(as.grain(BN22))
  #grn2c <- propagate(jglob)
  jcond <-setFinding(jglob, nodes = c("Income","Eductation","MyExperience","NeighborExp"), states =
c(inc,edu,me,ne))
  c.decision <- querygrain.grain(jcond,nodes=c("Decision"), type="joint")
  return(c.decision)
}
```

References

1. Pablo AL, Sitkin SB, Jemison DB. Acquisition decision-making processes: the central role of risk. J Manag. 1996;22(5):723–46.
2. Williams DJ, Noyes JM. How does our perception of risk influence decision-making? Implications for the design of risk information. Theor Issues Ergon Sci. 2007;8(1):1–35.
3. Sitkin SB, Weingart LR. Determinants of risky decision-making behavior: a test of the mediating role of risk perceptions and propensity. Acad Manag J. 1995;38(6):1573–92.
4. Bauch CT, D'Onofrio A, Manfredi P. Behavioral epidemiology of infectious diseases: an overview; 2013.
5. Manfredi P, D'Onofrio A. Modeling the interplay between human behavior and the spread of infectious diseases. Berlin: Springer; 2013.
6. Bassett RL, Ginis KAM. Risky business: the effects of an individualized health information intervention on health risk perceptions and leisure time physical activity among people with spinal cord injury. Disabil. Health J. 2011;4(3):165–76.
7. Rogers RW. Cognitive and physiological processes in fear appeals and attitute change: a revised theory of porotection motivation. IN: Social psychophysiology: a sourcebook; 1983, p. 153–177.
8. Filatova T, Parker DC, van der Veen A. The implications of skewed risk perception for a dutch coastal land market: insights from an agent based computational economics model. Agric Resour Econ Rev. 2011;40(3):405–23.
9. Haer T, Botzen WJW, de Moel H, Aerts JCJH. Integrating household risk mitigation behavior in flood risk analysis: an agent-based model approach. Risk Anal. 2017;37(10):1977–92.
10. van Duinen R, Filatova T, Jager W, van der Veen A. Going beyond perfect rationality: drought risk, economic choices and the influence of social networks. Ann Reg Sci. 2016;57(2–3):335–69.
11. Gotteland C, McFerrin BM, Zhao X, Gilot-Fromont E, Lélu M. Agricultural landscape and spatial distribution of Toxoplasma gondii in rural environment: an agent-based model. Int J Health Geogr. 2014;13(1):45.
12. Perez L, Dragicevic S. An agent-based approach for modeling dynamics of contagious disease spread. Int J Health Geogr. 2009;8(1):50.
13. Crooks AT, Hailegiorgis AB. An agent-based modeling approach applied to the spread of cholera. Environ Model Softw. 2014;62:164–77.
14. Wise S. Using social media content to inform agent based models for humanitarian crisis response; 2014.
15. Bieberstein A. "Background to Risk Perception". In An Investigation of women's and men's perceptions and meanings associated with food risks. Wiesbaden: Springer Fachmedien Wiesbaden; 2014. p. 25–62.
16. Kim DJ, Ferrin DL, Rao HR. A trust-based consumer decision-making model in electronic commerce: the role of trust, perceived risk, and their antecedents. Decis Support Syst. 2008;44(2):544–64.

17. Asgari S, Awwad R, Kandil A, Odeh I. Impact of considering need for work and risk on performance of construction contractors: an agent-based approach. Autom Constr. 2016;65:9–20.

18. Seidl R, Kuhn S, Elbers M, Ernst A, Klemm D. "Modelling risk perception and indicators of psychosocial sustainability in private households: the risk perception module in DeepHousehold". In: Regional assessment of global change impacts. Cham: Springer; 2016. p. 347–53.

19. Augustijn EW, Doldersum T, Useya J, Augustijn D. Agent-based modelling of cholera diffusion. Stoch Environ Res Risk Assess. 2016;30(8):2079–95.

20. Heckerman D. A tutorial on learning with Bayesian networks. Innovations in Bayesian networks. Berlin: Springer; 1995.

21. Zhang M, Tan Z, Zhao J, Li L. A bayesian learning model in the agent-based bilateral negotiation between the coal producers and electric power generators. In: 2008 In: Intelligent information technology application workshops. IEEE; 2008, vol 2, p. 859–862

22. Kocabas V, Dragicevic S. Bayesian networks and agent-based modeling approach for urban land-use and population density change: a BNAS model. J Geogr Syst. 2013;15(4):403–26.

23. Lei Z. Distributed modeling architecture of a multi-agent-based behavioral economic landscape (MABEL) model. Simulation. 2005;81(7):503–15.

24. Frias-Martinez V, Rubio A, Frias-Martinez E. Measuring the impact of epidemic alerts on human mobility. In: Pervasive urban applications; 2012. p. 18

25. Funk S, Gilad E, Watkins C, Jansen VAA. The spread of awareness and its impact on epidemic outbreaks. Proc Natl Acad Sci USA. 2009;106(16):6872–7.

26. Asase M, Yanful EK, Mensah M, Stanford J, Amponsah S. Comparison of municipal solid waste management systems in Canada and Ghana: a case study of the cities of London, Ontario, and Kumasi, Ghana. Waste Manag. 2009;29(10):2779–86.

27. Danquah L, Abass K, Nikoi AA. Anthropogenic pollution of inland waters: the case of the Aboabo River in Kumasi, Ghana. J Sustain Dev. 2011;4(6):103–15.

28. Melegaro A, et al. Social contact structures and time use patterns in the Manicaland Province of Zimbabwe. PLoS ONE. 2017;12(1):e0170459.

29. Mitchell TM. Machine learning. McGraw-Hill Science/Engineering/Math; 1997.

30. Ghana Statistical Service. 2010 Population and housing census. In: Ghana statistical service; 2012. p. 1–117.

31. Miezah K, Obiri-Danso K, Kadar Z, Fei-Baffoe B, Mensah MY. Municipal solid waste characterization and quantification as a measure towards effective waste management in Ghana. Waste Manag. 2015;46:15–27.

32. Jensen FV, Nielsen TD. Bayesian networks and decision graphs. New York: Springer; 2007.

16

Contextual influences affecting patterns of overweight and obesity among university students: a 50 universities population-based study in China

Tingzhong Yang[1*†], Lingwei Yu[1†], Ross Barnett[2], Shuhan Jiang[1], Sihui Peng[1], Yafeng Fan[3] and Lu Li[4]

Abstract

Background: Many studies have examined childhood and adolescent obesity, but few have examined young adults and the effect of their home and current living environments on prevalence rates. The present study explores contextual factors affecting overweight and obesity among university students in China and, in particular, focuses on how the SES–obesity relationship varies across different geographical contexts.

Methods: Participants were 11,673 students, who were identified through a multistage survey sampling process conducted in 50 universities. Individual data was obtained through a self-administered questionnaire, and contextual variables were retrieved from a national database. Multilevel logistic regression models were used to examine urban and regional variations in overweight and obesity.

Results: Overall the prevalence of overweight and obesity in the study sample was 9.5% (95% CI 7.7, 11.3%). After controlling for individual factors, both attributes of the home location (regional GDP <gross domestic product> per capita and rurality) and the current university location (city population) were found to be important, thus suggesting that the different origins of students affect current levels of obesity. At the individual level, while students with more financial resources were more likely to be obese, the extent of this relationship was highly dependent upon area income and city size.

Conclusion: The results of this study add important insights about the role of contextual factors affecting overweight and obesity among young adults and indicate a need to take into account both past as well as present environmental influences when considering the role of contextual factors in models of the nutrition transition.

Keywords: Overweight and obesity, Young adults, Context effects, China

Background

The prevalence of overweight and obesity is increasingly evident in both richer and poorer countries [1]. Although greater attention has been paid to environmental determinants of obesity in recent years [2], this research has largely occurred in western countries and focused on various neighborhood factors affecting obesity prevalence [3].

In low and middle income countries, while the impact of the nutrition revolution has been noticed for some time [4, 5], less attention has been paid to the independent effect of contextual risk factors affecting overweight and obesity and how these may differ from those of richer countries. However, the studies which have occurred have largely focused on factors affecting national variations in obesity [6] and variations in the impact of socio-economic status (SES) [6] and other contributing factors [7]. While others have explored urban and regional differences in obesity at the sub-national scale [8], many of these studies have not always adequately controlled for individual level

*Correspondence: Tingzhongyang@zju.edu.cn
†Tingzhong Yang and Lingwei Yu are co-first authors
[1] Department of Social Medicine/Center for Tobacco Control Research, Zhejiang University School of Medicine, Hangzhou 310058, China
Full list of author information is available at the end of the article

factors [9]. In some cases regional variations in obesity are largely seen as an outcome of individual level differences [10] or where independent macro-level effects have been identified, with few exceptions [11, 12], often these have been unspecified [13, 14]. Thus, in view of such trends, it is important to pay greater attention to the significance of various environmental determinants of obesity and why these may be important in countries at earlier stages in the nutrition revolution. The objective of this study, therefore, is to investigate the effects of both the home (region) and current (university city) living contexts on obesity among university students in China.

Because of their high mobility rates, studies of obesity among young adults provide an opportunity to simultaneously examine the effect of a variety of contextual effects, characteristic of their home and current locations, which may contribute to obesity [15]. Current patterns of obesity most likely reflect different cultural and behavioral norms relating to the home locations of students [16] as well as the socio-economic and other characteristics of the environments where they now reside. A frequent criticism of contextual studies of health is that they are cross-sectional in nature and do not take account of prior environmental conditions that people have been exposed to. While there have been many studies of childhood and adolescent obesity [17], there has been less focus on the importance of earlier life conditions on current levels of obesity. For example, in the United States, Zheng and Tumin [18] found that women's obesity status at older ages was influenced by early childhood conditions and place of residence, while adulthood factors seemed to be more important for males. Among the few studies of younger adults the evidence suggests that, for some groups (e.g. African Americans) neighborhood deprivation clearly plays a role in later patterns of obesity [19]. Similarly in Denmark, birthplace played a role in explaining regional differences in the prevalence of obesity. Young men currently living in provincial rural areas surrounding Copenhagen had a greater risk of obesity, especially if their birthplaces were also rural [8].

In low and middle income countries attending university may also increase the risks of obesity [20]. Since more affluent students are most likely to attend university, higher rates of obesity are likely to be found among this group [21], especially among rural dwellers migrating to more urbanised places [22]. However, the strength of the socio-economic status (SES)–obesity relationship is likely to be context dependent. As Jin and Lu [46] have noted, with the exception of cross-national studies [6], most of the existing studies on the relationship between SES and obesity have ignored spatial variations in the nature of this relationship. This has been particularly evident in studies within particular countries where the

factors producing obesogenic environments, and hence the nature and strength of the SES–obesity relationship, are likely to vary over geographic space. Thus it might be expected that more affluent students originating from higher income regions or who are currently studying in more urban and economically developed environments will be most at risk, because exposure to obesogenic factors is likely to be greater in such places [12].

While there have been numerous regional studies of obesity [10, 14, 23, 24] there have been few multi-level approaches [13, 25] which have examined the independent influence of city or regional contextual factors on obesity among young adults. The few studies which have occurred have largely focused on children and adolescents, usually at the local neighborhood level [17, 26]. While neighborhood effects are important, so too are influences which operate at other spatial scales. These may be levels of urbanization or area income differences, both of which are likely to be related to the greater availability of energy dense foods or reduced daily physical activity [11]. In addition the effects of income inequality are likely to be greater in such places and thus should strengthen the relationship between overconsumption among the rich and food insecurity among the poor [12]. Despite the importance of macro-level variables a recent review of contextual determinants of obesity paid little attention to such factors [3].

In the light of the preceding comments this paper poses two questions:

1. Independent of individual characteristics, what contextual attributes of a student's home location are important in explaining current patterns of overweight and obesity and do these remain significant when taking into account attributes of the student's current university city location?
2. Given the well-known link between individual SES and increased obesity in low and middle income countries, to what extent is this evident for university students and does the strength of this relationship vary across different geographic contexts?

To answer these questions the rest of the paper is organized as follows. First we outline the methodology of the study. This is followed by the results and a discussion of the most important findings, placing them in a wider context of international research on obesity and other Chinese studies. We conclude by emphasizing some of the wider theoretical and policy implications of our study.

Methods

Data source

This study reports data from the Global Health Professions Student Survey (GHPSS) on Tobacco Control in

China GHPSS (Extended version). The GHPSS is part of the Global Tobacco Surveillance System and is a university-based survey. The GHPSS was initially completed in 31 countries between 2005 and 2007. In China the GHPSS provided a valuable source of information on health and related health behaviours, including obesity.

The study employed a multistage sampling design and collected the sample in 2013. In Stage 1, 50 universities with medical programs were selected from 42 cities across China and differentiated by regional location (see Fig. 1). Stage 2 of the sampling strategy involved the selection of classes within each university, and all students in these classes were eligible as the sampling frame. A more detailed description of the survey and the data can be found in Yang et al. [27]. The study was approved

by the Ethics Committee at the Medical Center, Zhejiang University, and verbal consent was obtained from all participants prior to data collection.

Measures
Dependent variable
Body mass index (BMI) was calculated by dividing body weight (kg) by squared height (m^2). Overweight and obesity were defined as recommended by guidelines for the prevention and control of chronic diseases in China (Department of Disease Control and Prevention [28]): individuals with BMI scores of 24.0–27.9 kg/m^2 were categorized as overweight, and those with scores of ≥ 28.0 kg/m^2 were categorized as obese, which is the national standard [28]. As the prevalence of obesity was

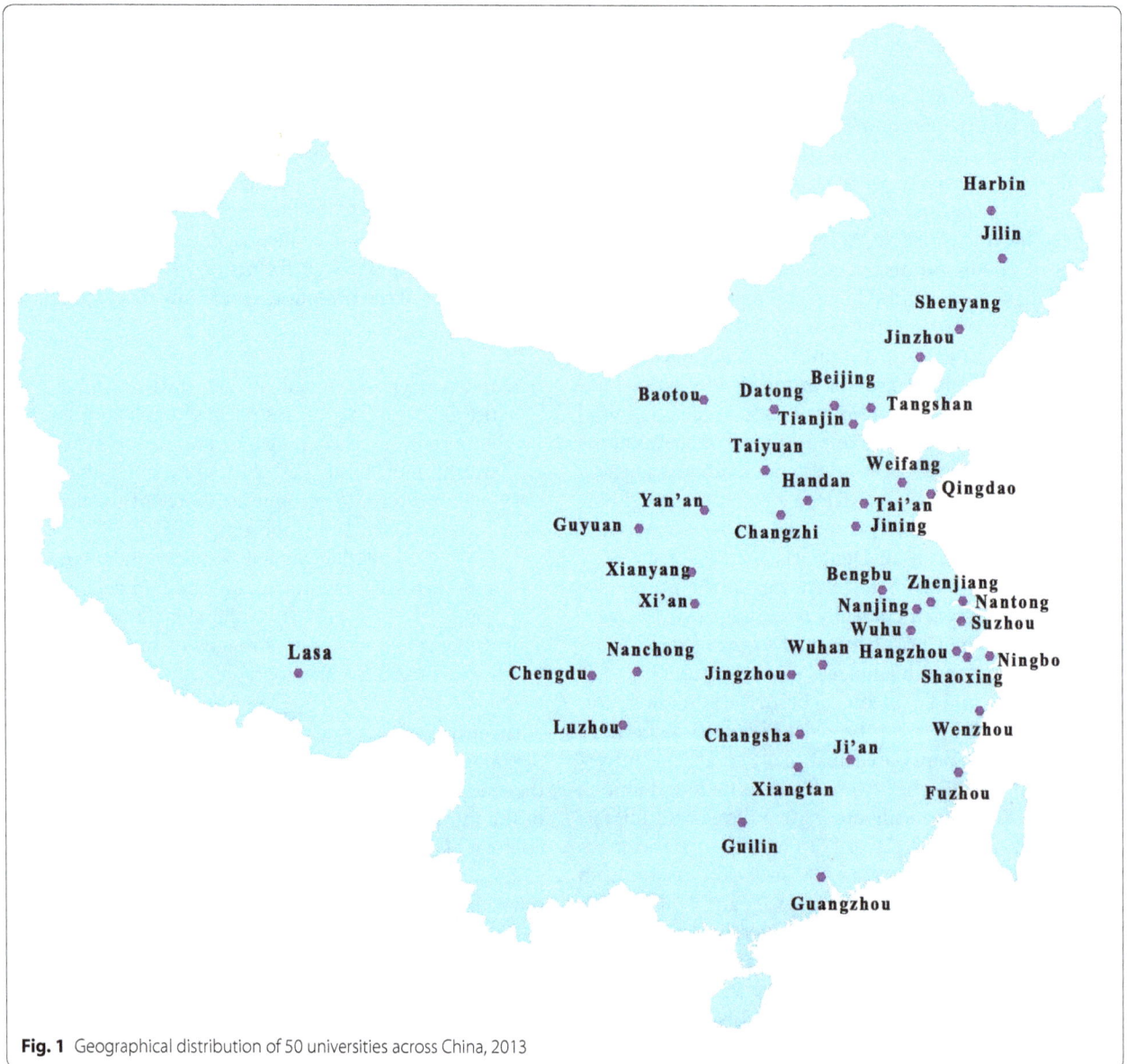

Fig. 1 Geographical distribution of 50 universities across China, 2013

low in this sample of university students, the categories of overweight and obesity were combined in the analyses.

Height and weight were measured by self-report. Given the potential problems of this measure [29], we objectively measured height and weight among 170 subjects from two universities in Hangzhou in order to validate the self-reported prevalence of overweight and obesity and for obesity alone. Concordance was 97.1% for the combined prevalence of overweight and obesity, and 98.8% for obesity.

Individual-level independent variables

In order to control for possible individual-level confounders, questions were utilized to determine age, gender, ethnicity, parents' occupation, monthly expenses and smoking. With few exceptions, most Chinese studies have shown that obesity tends to increase with age [30] and be higher for male children and adolescents [31, 32]. Given the well-established link between SES and obesity in China, three measures of SES, parents' occupation, family income and monthly student expenses, were included. Occupation was recorded in three categories: operations and commercial work (operations referring to mainly farmers and workers), staff and administration (which included mainly government jobs and company management jobs); teacher, scientific and technical work) (9, 10). Family income (in RMB Yuan) was measured through the question: "how much was the income of each person in your family over the last year?" Categories ranged from less than ¥1000, ¥1000 to ¥1999, and ¥2000 and over. We also included a variable, monthly student expenses (in RMB Yuan), which was measured though the question: "how much do you spend each month?" In addition, in view of the very high rates of smoking in China, which has been related to overweight and obesity, we also included this as a background factor [13, 33–35].

Home location and current contextual factors

Two sets of contextual variables were included, relating to characteristics of the student's family home location and of the university city where they were studying. In terms of the former, family location was defined in terms of both their home region (Northeast, North, Eastern, Centre, Southwest and Northwest) and whether students came from a city, county 'town' or rural area. In addition, gross domestic product (GDP) per capita was included to highlight differences in area income between the students' home provinces.

Given that many studies have stressed the link between the penetration of obesogenic environments and a country's level of urbanisation [11], we included urban population size and area income (GDP per capita) to describe the university cities where the students were studying.

Finally we also determined the characteristics of the universities which the students attended. Given that different universities have different social resources and some are far more prestigious than others, then it was important to include such a measure since, because of large differences in tuition fees, university type is also an indirect measure of family income. University type was determined using the China university ranking system ("high level," "middle level," and "low level") as established by the National Ministry of Education [36].

Data analysis

All data were entered into a database using Microsoft Excel. The dataset was then imported into statistical analysis system (SAS) (9.3 version) for statistical analyses. Descriptive statistics were calculated to determine the prevalence of overweight and obesity, which was also mapped at the provincial level. For the purposes of mapping prevalence rates were defined according to the home provinces of the students in the sample.

A logistic model was utilized to assess associations between the dependent and each of the independent variables. Both unadjusted and adjusted methods were considered in the data analyses and implemented to examine these associations. SAS survey logistic procedures were applied in the unadjusted analysis, using the university as the clustering unit, in order to account for a within-clustering correlation, attributable to the complex sample for unadjusted analysis. The multilevel analysis was weighted using sampling, subject-level weights, and post-stratification weights, respectively [37].

In terms of the first study objective, we applied multilevel logistic regression models using the SAS GLIMMIX procedure (Table 2). We started with the Null Model, a three -level (individual, university, and original home province) model with random intercepts. First we constructed an individual model which included variables relating to gender, monthly expenses and smoking. The second (home location) model included the above individual factors but also three variables relating to region of origin, urban–rural background and GDP per capita of the home region. Models were run both including and excluding the student's home region. The third (university city model) added three new contextual variables to the above individual characteristics, university type, university city GDP and city size. Finally, since we also wished to examine the relative importance of both home location and university city characteristics, the final (combined) model included all of the above variables.

It should be mentioned that family income is an appropriate indicator of family economic resources. However, family income was surveyed in only some universities and obtained for 4902 students due to a printing error in the questionnaire. Consequently we used an indirect measure of family income, monthly student expenses in the multilevel models. This was a valid measure because families tend to fund most students' expenses. Not surprisingly the latter was significantly associated with family income ($r = 0.30$; $p < 0.001$).

With respect to the second objective, we assessed the interaction between our measure of student income, monthly expenses, and four contextual variables: the rural–urban home location of the student, university city population and the GDP per capita of the student's home region and university city. Thus for each group we were able to assess the strength of the individual SES–obesity relationship as well as the (weighted) prevalence of overweight and obesity. We also examined the relationship between urban–rural origin and obesity by university type.

Results

A total of 12,211 questionnaires were completed. Of those who responded 11,942 students were available for general analysis. BMI was calculated for the 11,673 respondents (97.4%) who provided complete data. There were no significant differences in demographic characteristics between responders and non-responders. Of the sample, 16% were less than 20 years of age and 21% were aged 23 years and over. There were more females (64.2%) than males, most (93%) of the students were of Han ethnicity and the majority (over 75%) came from families where the parents were engaged in operations or commercial work. Almost 38% recorded high levels of monthly expenditures (over 1500 RMB). Most students came from the countryside or townships (67%) and about half attended universities in middle-size cities.

Overall the prevalence of overweight and obesity in the study sample was 9.5% (95% confidence interval (CI) 7.7, 11.3%), and obesity prevalence was 2.2% (95% CI 1.3, 3.1%) there was considerable geographic variation. A higher prevalence occurred in northeast and southwest China (Fig. 2), with the highest rates being recorded in Liaoning (34.9%), Neimenggu (18.7%), Shanxi (15.5%) and Beijing (14.9%).

The unadjusted logistic analysis showed that of the individual-level variables gender (male), higher monthly expenses and smoking were associated with being classified as overweight and obese (Table 1). Parents' occupation was not significant. However in the limited sample there was a significant relationship between family income and overweight and obesity with higher income families more likely to be overweight or obese. The unadjusted odds ratios (ORs) were 1.61** (95% CI 1.19, 2.17) (for 10,000 and over RMB vs <10,000RMB) and 1.35** (CI 1.14, 1.59) (for 20,000 and more RMB vs <10,000RMB). This relationship remained after adjusting

for other individual variables [the respective ORs were 1.61** (CI 1.10. 2.20) and 1.29** (CI 1.08, 1.55)] and all variables [1.38** (CI 1.09, 1.75) and 0.82 (CI 0.57, 1.18)]. In all models there were no significant differences between monthly expenses and overweight and obesity after considering family income.

Of the home contextual factors, students who originated from Northeast China (Fig. 2), from larger towns and cities and from provinces with higher GDP per capita were more likely to be overweight or obese. Of the three contextual factors a more urbanised family home location increased the chances of being overweight and obese to a much greater extent than region of origin or home province GDP. Contextual characteristics of the university cities were also important. Larger and wealthier destination cities were also related to overweight/obesity prevalence levels as was the type of university. Compared to high level universities, students enrolled at lower and middle level universities had a reduced risk of being overweight or obese.

We also performed unadjusted analyses for males and females separately and some gender differences occurred (table not shown). Parental occupation became significant compared to female students who had fathers engaged in operations and commercial work, those whose fathers were teachers or were employed in scientific and technical work were more than twice as likely to be overweight or obese. The effect of daily smoking increased the risk of being overweight or obese for females (unadjusted OR 7.79; 95% CI 1.82, 33.23), but was not significant for males. By contrast, home region GDP was only significant for males (unadjusted OR 1.26; CI 1.11, 1.44), while university city GDP and population size had little effect on male trends in overweight and obesity compared to females (the respective ORs 2.39; CI 1.05, 5.48 and 1.80; CI 1.76, 2.75).

In the multilevel individual and family location models being male, a regular smoker and having higher monthly expenses remained significant (Model 1) as did the student's urban–rural origin and area income of the home province (Model 2) (Table 2). However, home region became not significant, thus suggesting that regional differences in overweight and obesity were highly related to differences in urbanisation and levels of GDP. For this reason we re-ran Model 2 excluding home region and also omitted this variable in the final model. In the university city model no contextual variables were significant (Model 3). However, if controls were made just for individual factors then university type was significant, with students attending low level universities being less likely to be overweight or obese (OR 0.55; CI 0.40, 0.74). Similarly if controls were made just for individual factors then students attending university in the largest cities

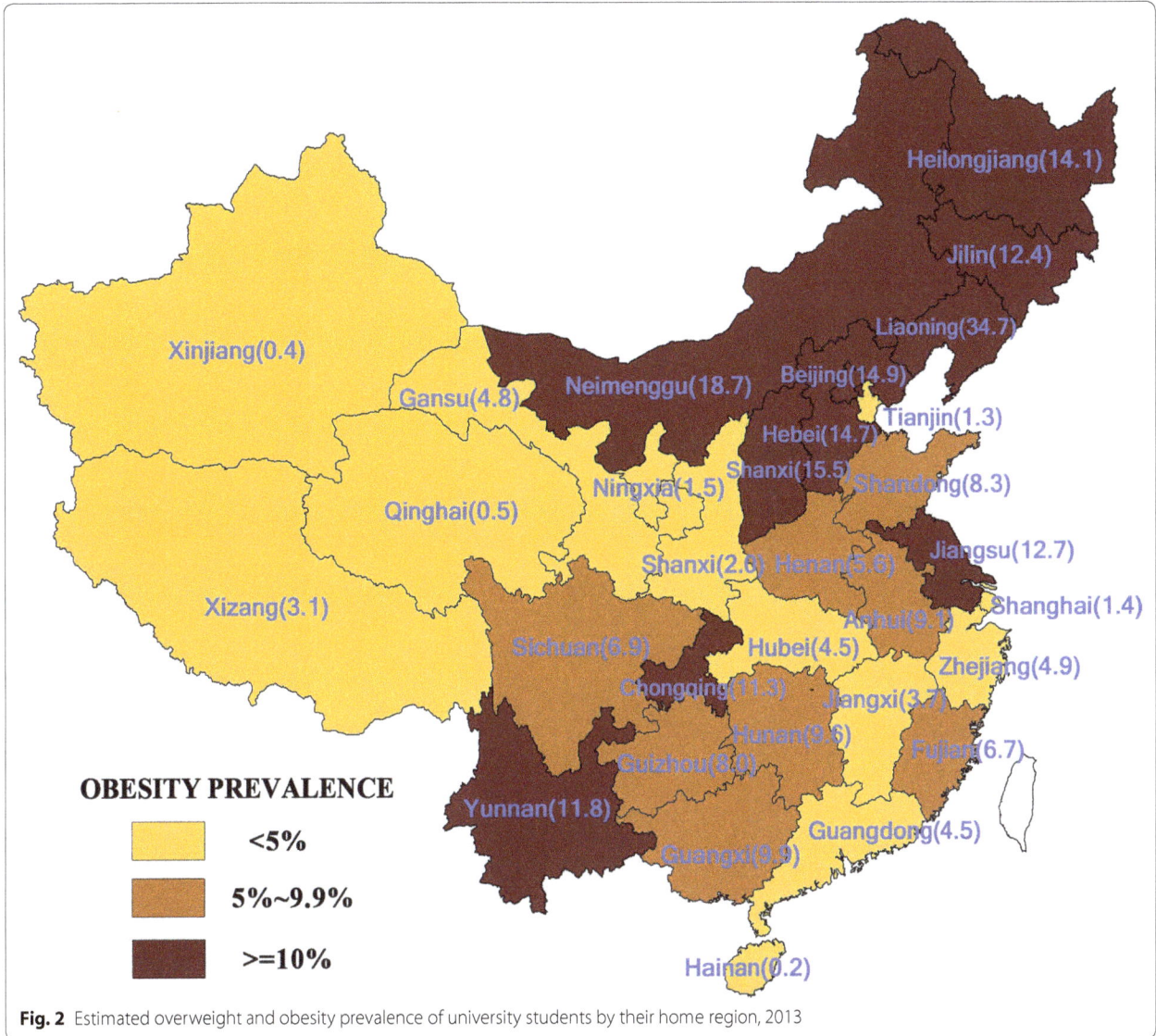

Fig. 2 Estimated overweight and obesity prevalence of university students by their home region, 2013

were more likely to be overweight or obese (OR 1.55; CI 1.02, 2.36). Finally in the combined model, incorporating both home and university city contextual factors, urban–rural origin, home provincial GDP and population size of the university city remained significant (Model 4).

Controlling for gender, monthly expenses and smoking, students who originated from cities versus rural and township areas were between 60 and 82% more likely to be overweight or obese. In addition we investigated the interaction between home location and individual level expenses since both factors have independent influences on obesity. However, analyses showed no significant interaction between these two factors (Wald Chi Square: 2.74, p: 0.0979).

In terms of the relationship between student monthly expenses and obesity and urban/area income contextual

factors the results suggest that association between individual SES and obesity was strongest for students who originated from rural areas and for those who attended universities in smaller cities (Table 3). The results are less clear for home region GDP but in the case of university city GDP higher income students were more likely to be overweight or obese in poorer cities. In terms of the actual prevalence of obesity the highest rates occurred among more affluent students originating from (28.7%) or currently living in (21.2%) larger places and among more affluent students coming from wealthier areas.

Discussion

This aim of this study was twofold; to assess the importance of home location and university contextual effects on patterns of student overweight and obesity and to

Table 1 **Demographic characteristics of sample and overweight and obesityprevalence**

Group	Unweighted N	Unweighted % of sample	Weighted % of sample	Weighted overweight and obesity prevalence	Weighted OR (95% CI)
Age (years)					
<20	1831	15.7	12.9	10.1	1.00
20	2324	19.9	31.5	6.5	0.67 (0.43, 1.07)
21	2709	23.2	30.8	7.1	0.70 (0.34, 1.41)
22	2396	20.5	14.5	8.0	0.68 (0.38, 1.21)
23 and over	2413	20.7	10.3	7.9	0.79 (0.47, 1.32)
Gender					
Male	4177	35.8	43.9	9.4	1.00
Female	7496	64.2	56.1	5.7	0.40 (0.27, 0.60)**
Ethnicity					
Han	10,884	93.2	94.6	7.6	1.00
Minority	789	6.7	5.4	6.9	0.90 (0.36, 2.26)
Father's occupation					
Operation and commercial work	9269	79.4	71.8	9.0	1.00
Staff and administration	1681	14.4	18.8	10.3	1.66 (0.79, 1.73)
Teacher, scientific and technical work	723	6.2	9.4	11.8	1.16 (0.46, 2.97)
Mother's occupation					
Operation and commercial work	9397	80.5	72.4	8.9	1.00
Staff and administration	1500	12.9	16.6	10.1	1.18 (0.79, 1.73)
Teacher, scientific and technical work	776	6.5	11.0	12.7	1.17 (0.45, 2.97)
Income of each person in family (RMB)					
<10,000	1773	36.2	34.0	6.1	1.00
10–19,999	1241	25.3	20.7	9.5	1.61 (1.19, 2.17)**
20,000 and over	1888	38.5	45.3	8.1	1.35 (1.14, 1.59)**
Monthly expenditures (RMB)					
<1000	1273	10.9	7.6	7.4	1.00
1000–1499	6048	51.8	49.0	8.8	1.21 (0.67, 2.16)
1500–1999	3406	29.2	30.2	8.5	1.18 (0.60, 2.30)
2000 and over	946	8.1	13.5	15.0	2.37 (1.39, 4.06)**
Academic major					
Medical	10,270	87.9	81.1	6.5	1.00
Other	1403	12.1	18.9	7.8	1.21 (0.93, 1.58)
Smoking status					
Non-smoker	10,735	92.0	87.3	8.9	1.00
Occasional smoker	706	6.1	8.9	10.7	1.22 (0.61, 2.43)
Daily smoker	232	2.0	3.8	20.1	2.56 (1.33, 4.92)**
Home region					
Northeast	889	7.6	5.1	21.1	1.00
North	1785	15.2	14.4	15.3	0.67 (0.33, 1.37)
Eastern	1784	15.3	17.0	11.1	0.47 (0.24, 0.93)*
Centre	4968	42.6	39.2	7.4	0.30 (0.16, 0.55)**
Southwest	959	8.2	16.3	7.7	0.31 (0.16, 0.60)**
Northwest	1288	11.0	8.0	2.4	0.09 (0.03, 0.32)**
Urban–rural home location					
Countryside or township	3276	67.0	59.6	4.3	1.00
County town	741	15.1	17.7	9.1	2.35 (1.10, 5.02)*
City	876	17.9	22.8	15.5	5.22 (1.70, 16.3)**
GDP of home province					
<50,000	5868	50.3	51.3	8.2	1.00

Table 1 continued

Group	Unweighted N	Unweighted % of sample	Weighted % of sample	Weighted overweight and obesity prevalence	Weighted OR (95% CI)
50,000–99,000	3483	29.8	26.7	9.8	1.21 (0.81, 1.82)
100,000 and over	2322	19.9	22.0	12.2	1.17 (1.05, 1.41)*
Type of university					
High level	4154	35.1	58.3	11.5	1.00
Middle level	6823	53.3	39.2	6.8	0.56 (0.43, 0.74)**
Lower level	696	6.0	2.5	5.2	0.42 (0.34, 0.53)**
University city GDP (per capita)					
<50,000	3986	34.1	16.0	7.1	1.00
50,000–99,000	6221	53.3	60.7	8.9	1.28 (0.96, 1.72)
100,000 and over	1466	12.6	23.3	12.8	1.94 (1.25, 3.00)**
University city population (m)					
<1.0	3019	25.8	12.1	6.3	1.00
1.0–3.9	5866	50.2	57.7	10.1	1.68 (1.11, 2.55)*
4 and over	2788	23.9	30.2	9.8	1.62 (1.10, 2.40)*

* p < 0.05; ** p < 0.01

investigate the extent to which the SES–obesity relationship varied depending upon the geographic context. While this is not the first Chinese study to investigate obesity among young adults [9] or university students in particular [21], it is the first Chinese research to examine these factors using a multi-level framework taking into account both past and current locations. Internationally, the research is also one of the few studies [46, 47] to consider variations in the nature of the SES–obesity relationship within a particular national context.

With respect to the first objective three main conclusions are evident. First, with respect to the student's home environment, independent of individual characteristics, levels of urbanization and provincial GDP per capita emerged as the key predictors of overweight and obesity. Students who came from county towns or larger cities were twice to almost four times more likely to be obese or overweight compared to students originating from rural areas. Similarly those who were born in more affluent regions were more likely to be overweight or obese, independent of their own individual income status. These patterns suggest the importance of lifestyle and dietary factors on overweight and obesity because students' basic lifestyles are partly formed during childhood and adolescence. These findings are similar to other research both in China [21] and elsewhere [13, 18, 26] which points to the significance of early life conditions on patterns of adult obesity.

Second, there was also evidence of contextual influences in the destination cities of the students. Students who attended university in the larger cities were more likely to be overweight or obese compared to students who lived in smaller cities and this effect remained

significant in the final model after controlling for the urban–rural home origins of students. These results are similar to the findings of Ji and Chen [38] who found that over the period 1985–2010 the rate of increase in overweight and obesity (amongst children and adolescents) was greatest in the largest cities, the authors suggesting that adult prevalence rates in such places were approaching those found in developed countries. They also support the results of other studies of students [21] and adults [39] as well as children and adolescents in China [38] where urban–rural differences in obesity, despite decreasing in recent years [40], are still very apparent.

Although in the expected direction, university city GDP was not significant. University type was significant when just individual factors were controlled for but not in the final model nor in the university model when the two other university contextual characteristics were included. This most likely reflects the fact that the most prestigious universities are located in the largest cities, places where students will be most exposed to obesogenic environments. Nevertheless the pressures of studying at China's most prestigious universities should also be taken into account. One can only speculate that sedentary behavior is more likely to be common among such students who have little time for other activities. Li et al. [21], for example, reported that obese students in Guangdong were more likely to indicate that they never exercised or engaged in daily exercise. Thus it was no surprise that, when university type was considered, the highest prevalence of overweight and obesity was typical of students with urban origins studying at China's top universities.

Table 2 Results of multiple level model (weighted)

	Null model	Model 1 (individual model)	Model 2 (home location model)	Model 3 (university city model)	Model 4 (combined model)
Group					
Gender					
Male		1.00	1.00	1.00	1.00
Female		0.38 (0.24, 0.65)**	0.40 (0.27, 0.68)**	0.41 (0.26, 0.69)**	0.40 (0.24, 0.67)**
Monthly expenses					
<1000		1.00	1.00	1.00	1.00
1000–1499		2.32 (0.70, 7.54)	2.43 (0.72, 7.61)	1.06 (0.66, 1.76)	2.41 (0.73, 7.99)
1500–1999		1.52 (0.38, 5.86)	1.47 (0.39, 5.85)	1.03 (0.62, 1.81)	1.51 (0.42, 5.49)
2000 and over		4.07 (1.27, 13.2)**	4.10 (1.29, 13.2)**	2.65 (1.54, 3.35)**	4.23 (1.33, 13.16)*
Smoking					
Non-smoker		1.00	1.00	1.00	1.00
Occasional smoker		1.15 (0.56, 2.44)	1.19 (0.55, 2.46)	0.77 (0.37, 1.58)	1.19 (0.57, 2.49)
Daily smoker		2.12 (1.12, 3.89)*	2.07 (1.14, 3.98)*	1.30 (0.61, 2.84)	2.06 (1.06, 3.99)*
Family home location					
Rural or township			1.00		1.00
County town			2.24 (1.36, 2.75)**		2.22 (1.34, 3.61)**
City			3.79 (1.20, 12.27)*		3.73 (1.15, 12.01)*
Type of university					
High level				1.00	1.00
Middle level				0.76 (0.54, 1.15)	1.51 (0.90, 2.45)
Lower level				0.79 (0.48, 1.39)	1.14 (0.95, 1.36)
GDP per capita of home region					
<50,000			1.00		1.00
50,000–99,000			1.51 (0.89, 2.51)		1.52 (0.92, 2.54)
100,00 and over			1.43 (1.05, 1.42)*		1.43 (1.04, 1.42)*
University city GDP per capita					
<50,000				1.00	1.00
50,000–				0.92 (070, 1.21)	1.12 (0.55, 2.29)
100,000–				1.21 (0.66, 1.21)	1.39 (0.55, 3.71)
City population (million)					
<1.0				1.00	1.00
1–3.9				1.28 (0.82, 1.93)	1.71 (1.10, 2.68)*
4 and over				1.41 (0.80, 2.35)	1.48 (1.04, 2.31)*
Fixed parameters	37.36 **	19.12**	17.25**	16.42**	15.75**
Random parameters between universities	4.41**	3.89**	4.25**	2.43*	2.25*
Random parameters between the original provinces	62.04**	39.87**	35.41**	37.82**	15.89**

* p < 0.05; ** p < 0.01

Third, the findings suggest that characteristics of the home locations of students are more important than those of the places to which they migrated in influencing overweight and obesity. This should not be surprising given the short length of residence of many of the students in the university cities. It would be tempting to suggest that the selective migration of more affluent students from their homes to university accounted for most of the variation in obesity amongst this student sample.

However, other studies have suggested that differences in the prevalence of obesity could not be accounted for by birthplace or later selective migration [8] and that resident children are more likely to be obese than migrant children [32]. Such findings thus point to the importance of local context effects, which are likely to become more important over time, in affecting obesity prevalence among the student population. Thus the fact that urban size remained significant in the final model suggests the

Table 3　Relationships between student monthly expenses and obesity by urban–rural home location and area income

Monthly expenses	Overweight and obesity prevalence (%)	Adjusted OR (95% CI)[a]	Overweight and obesity prevalence (%)	Adjusted OR (95% CI)[a]	Overweight and obesity prevalence (%)	Adjusted OR (95% CI)[a]	Overweight and obesity prevalence (%)	Adjusted OR (95% CI)[a]
	Home location of student		University city population		Home region GDP per capita		University city GDP per capita	
	Rural/township		< 1 million		Low		Low	
<1000	1.0	1.00	1.5	1.00	4.3	1.00	5.5	1.00
1000–1499	4.3	1.40 (0.64, 3.10)	5.9	1.73 (1.06, 2.83)*	9.2	1.34 (0.88, 2.06)	11.1	1.13 (0.69, 1.86)
1500–1999	4.3	1.42 (0.65, 3.18)	7.9	2.03 (1.49, 2.77)**	7.0	1.96 (1.34, 2.88)**	14.6	1.54 (1.03, 2.29)*
2000 and over	8.5	2.46 (1.22, 4.68)*	8.4	2.33 (1.17, 4.68)**	10.0	1.88 (1.15, 3.07)*	14.4	2.26 (1.45, 3.53)**
	Small city		1.0–3.9 million		Medium		Medium	
<1000	0.0	N/A	5.6	1.00	11.9	1.00	8.7	1.00
1000–1499	10.3	N/A	9.6	1.04 (0.71, 1.51)	8.4	0.93 (0.70, 1.24)	8.9	0.90 (0.59, 1.38)
1500–1999	11.8	N/A	10.5	1.27 (0.89, 1.78)	9.5	1.07 (0.77, 1.47)	6.0	1.05 (0.73, 2.00)
2000 and over	1.3	N/A	13.4	1.59 (1.08, 2.35)*	20.2	1.27 (0.87, 1.87)	17.7	1.35 (0.92, 2.00)
	Large city		4 million and over		High		High	
<1000	23.6	1.00	13.4	1.00	4.2	1.00	5.5	1.00
1000–1499	19.3	0.61 (0.20, 1.87)	8.1	0.61 (0.41, 0.92)*	7.6	2.67 (1.50, 4.77)**	6.3	0.62 (0.40, 1.02)
1500–1999	3.4	0.60 (0.25, 1.48)	5.9	0.75 (0.56, 1.04)	10.4	3.01 (1.83, 4.94)**	10.4	0.98 (0.62, 1.56)
2000 and over	28.6	1.51 (0.54, 4.18)	21.2	1.15 (0.76, 1.47)	18.5	1.93 (1.14, 3.28)*	10.5	1.08 (0.59, 1.81)

Adjusted odds ratios in italics are statistically significant at the * $p < 0.05$; ** $p < 0.01$

N/A = sample sizes too small

[a] Controlling for gender

importance of destination factors in modifying patterns of obesity amongst the most at-risk populations.

With respect to the second objective, the study found further evidence of the well known link between individual socio-economic status and obesity, which was evident in all the models. Unlike western countries where obesity is highest amongst the poor and certain ethnic groups [24], the pattern of higher prevalence of obesity among students from higher income families is typical of countries in the earlier stages of the nutrition transition [5, 6]. However, the fact that income differences in obesity were generally strongest for students originating from rural locations and for those who attended university in smaller cities suggests that the nutrition transition is at an earlier stage than in larger cities where, although obesity rates are higher, individual SES differences are much less pronounced (Fig. 3b). Thus the results suggest a need for more thought to be given to geographical variation in the SES–obesity relationship especially in countries as diverse as China. In other words, models of the nutrition revolution, rather than focusing just on international differences in the relationship between SES differences and obesity (Fig. 3a), need to take greater account of the forces operating within low and middle income countries. For example, at what point in the urbanization process do factors relating to obesogenic environments start to become much more important compared to individual-level determinants of obesity? Do particular thresholds exist? Such considerations are important in all low and middle income countries where the obesogenic epidemic is at an earlier stage. Answering such questions obviously has implications for population programs aiming to target the most at-risk groups.

Thus, in contrast to some other views [10] the geographic distribution of obesity cannot simply be read off from individual SES variations, but also reflects a range of context effects which will modify the individual SES–obesity relationship. Important here is the level of urbanization and regional affluence which will be highly correlated with the penetration of obesogenic environments. As He et al. [12] have suggested, these will include the greater availability of energy dense foods at a cheaper cost, the spread of obesity-related health knowledge [13] or the adoption of higher-SES groups of western cultural norms regarding body shape, all of which may narrow SES differences in obesity. On the other hand, higher rates of income inequality and increased food consumption among the rich [41, 42] or the effects of transportation infrastructure and other labour saving devices which result in reduced daily physical activity [11], are likely to increase social disparities in obesity. The above results thus suggest an urban–rural diffusion of the obesity epidemic in China. However, while the spread of the obesity epidemic to rural areas, to some extent, has already been identified [30, 38, 47] exactly how the local environment helps shape the social distribution of obesity in different places remains unclear. Thus more research which focuses on the role of contextual factors influencing obesity at smaller spatial scales, such as cities and neighbourhoods, would seem to be a high priority.

Limitations

This study has a number of limitations. First, and most important, is that our range of contextual factors was relatively limited. Although it was beyond the scope of this study greater attention to cultural factors affecting urban and regional differences in diet, the food environment and to the effects of income inequality on patterns of food consumption is necessary. More attention also needs to be paid to the nature of obesogenic environmental factors and they affect different SES groups. Second, the study was based on cross sectional design, which precludes causal inference and calls for cohort and other

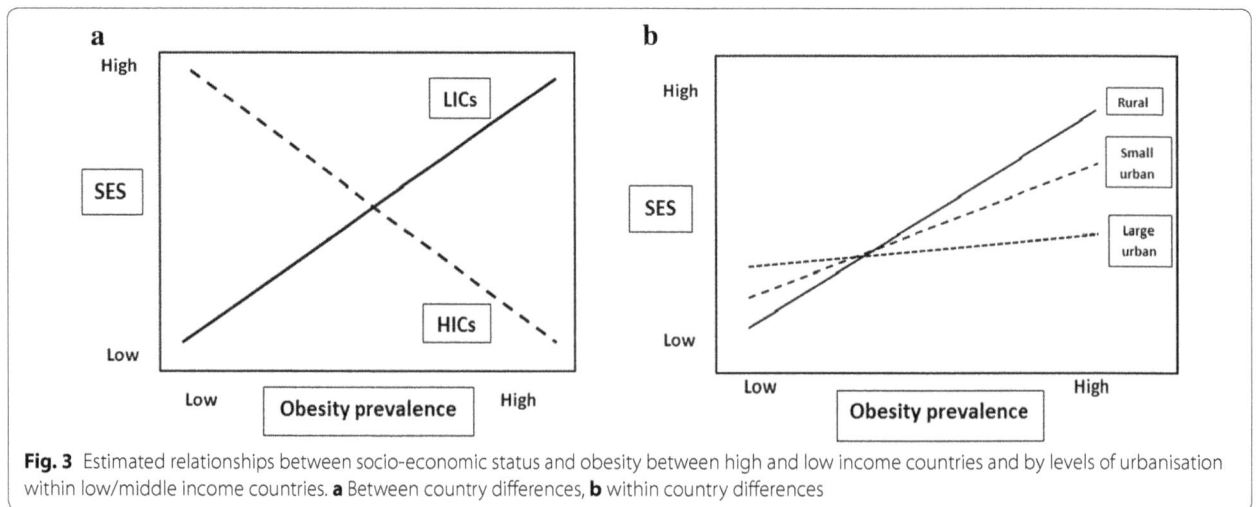

Fig. 3 Estimated relationships between socio-economic status and obesity between high and low income countries and by levels of urbanisation within low/middle income countries. **a** Between country differences, **b** within country differences

longitudinal studies on overweight and obesity in China to advance etiologic understanding, and to inform the design and evaluation of generic and tailored interventions. Third, the sampling frame was university students, most of which were medical students. Hence, the findings are not generalizable to the whole of China. Fourth, because not all universities recorded data for the urban–rural origins of the students, this was available for only 41.9% of the total sample. As a result the sample appears to under represent urban students (those who came from cities and county towns).

Conclusion

This study adds important insights about the impact of home and university environments on the prevalence of overweight and obesity among university students. By emphasizing the importance of contextual effects we suggest that more attention needs to be paid to the environmental conditions, such as urbanization and rapid economic development. These have helped change health beliefs, patterns of food consumption, health behavior and lifestyles and have contributed to the growing obesity epidemic in China and other low and middle income nations. Many of these factors have influenced the growing obesity of children and adolescents, but, as would be expected, have become particularly apparent among young adults. As Dutton and McLaren [43] have suggested modeling these population-level factors is an important avenue for future research. Given that not all places or population groups are equally affected then more attention to how local environments are changing and the effects of such changes on the diet, lifestyles, as well as the social norms and perceptions of obesityon the part of different groups is necessary.

Effective strategies that take into account contextual influences are also needed to implement policy and public health interventions to prevent overweight and obesity, especially since that there is minimal evidence that the obesity epidemic is slowing down. However, central and provincial governments in China have largely ignored food and other policies which may go some way towards slowing the growth of obesity [44] although the recent policy shift encouraging more healthy cities suggests that this view is changing [45]. This is also true among university environments and thus this study provides preliminary evidence for public health policymakers and educators and suggests the need for an approach for intervening to avert or reduce overweight and obesity among college students. Such an approach needs to take account of the diverse origins of students, since such differences will be important in affecting the social distribution of obesity and the attitudes of students to any policy interventions. Thus we recommend that there is a need for strategies which address both environmental and individual factors as such a multi-faceted approach is essential to help curb the growing obesity epidemic.

Abbreviations
GDP: gross domestic product; SES: socio-economic status; GHPSS: Global Health Professions Student Survey; BMI: body mass index; SAS: statistical analysis system.

Authors' contributions
TY conceived the study design, conceptualized the ideas, and supervised the data management and analyses. YL, SJ, SP and YF organized the data collection. TY wrote the initial manuscript. RB and LL provided the revision of the manuscript. All authors reviewed previous drafts. All authors read and approved the final manuscript.

Author details
[1] Department of Social Medicine/Center for Tobacco Control Research, Zhejiang University School of Medicine, Hangzhou 310058, China. [2] Department of Geography, University of Canterbury, Private Bag 4800, Christchurch, New Zealand. [3] Department of Nursing, Hangzhou Normal University, Hangzhou 310036, China. [4] Institute of Family and Social Medicine, Zhejiang University School of Medicine, Hangzhou 310058, China.

Acknowledgements
We thank local teams from the "Building advocacy capacity for tobacco control in medical universities in China (Bloomberg global control project)" project organizing the data collection.

Competing interests
The authors declare that they have no competing interests.

Funding
This study was partly funded by the National Nature Science Foundation of China (Major Project, 71490733), the National Nature Science Foundation of China (71473221), Center for Tobacco Control Research, Zhejiang University School of Medicine. This project universities, local government and Center for Disease Control and Prevention also partly fund this survey. These funding was used for the design of the study and collection, analysis, and interpretation of data and in writing the manuscript.

References
1. Ng M, Fleming T, Robinson M, Thomson B, Graetz N, Margono C, Mullany EC. Global, regional, and national prevalence of overweight and obesity in children and adults during 1980–2013: a systematic analysis for the Global Burden of Disease Study 2013. Lancet. 2014;384:766–81.
2. Pearce J, Witten K, editors. Geographies of obesity: environmental understandings of the obesity epidemic. Burlinton: Ashgate Publishing Ltd; 2010.
3. Kim D, Kawachi I. Contextual determinants of obesity: an overview. In: Pearce J, Witten K, editors. Geographies of obesity: environmental understandings of the obesity epidemic. Burlinton: Ashgate Publishing Ltd; 2010. p. 39–54.
4. Popkin BM. The nutrition transition and obesity in the developing world. J Nutr. 2001;131:871S–3S.
5. Popkin BM, Adair LS, Ng SW. Global nutrition transition and the pandemic of obesity in developing countries. Nutr Rev. 2012;70:3–21.

6. Monteiro CA, Moura EC, Conde WL, Popkin BM. Socioeconomic status and obesity in adult populations of developing countries: a review. Bull World Health Organ. 2004;82:940–6.

7. Peltzer K, Pengpid S, Samuels T, Özcan NK, Mantilla C, Rahamefy OH, et al. Prevalence of overweight/obesity and its associated factors among university students from 22 countries. Int J Environ Res Public Health. 2014;11:7425–41.

8. Halkjaer J, Sørenson TI. Psychosocial and demographic determinants of regional differences in the prevalence of obesity. J Biosoc Sci. 2004;36:141–52.

9. Wan Y, Jiang X, He Y, Zhang Y, Liang Y, Pan F, Xu Y, Shang L. Body mass index of young men in China: results from four national surveys conducted between 1955 and 2012. Medicine. 2016;95:e2829.

10. Ji CY, Cheng TO. Prevalence and geographic distribution of childhood obesity in China in 2005. Int J Cardiol. 2008;131:1–8.

11. Monda KL, Gordon-Larsen P, Stevens J, Popkin BM. China's transition: the effect of rapid urbanization on adult occupational physical activity. Soc Sci Med. 2007;64:858–70.

12. He W, James SA, Merli MG, Zheng H. An increasing socioeconomic gap in childhood overweight and obesity in China. Am J Public Health. 2014;104:e14–22.

13. Siddiqui MZ, Donato R. Overweight and obesity in India: policy issues from an exploratory multi-level analysis. Health Policy Plan. 2016;31:582–91.

14. Willms JD, Tremblay MS, Katzmarzyk PT. Geographic and demographic variation in the prevalence of overweight Canadian children. Obes Res. 2003;11:668–73.

15. Poobalan A, Aucott L. Obesity among young adults in developing countries: a systematic overview. Curr Obes Rep. 2016;5:2–13.

16. Kumanyika SK. Environmental influences on childhood obesity: ethnic and cultural influences in context. Physiol Behav. 2008;94:61–70.

17. Alvarado SE. Neighborhood disadvantage and obesity across childhood and adolescence: evidence from the NLSY children and young adults cohort (1986–2010). Soc Sci Res. 2016;57:80–98.

18. Zheng H, Tumin D. Variation in the effects of family background and birth region on adult obesity: results of a prospective cohort study of a Great Depression-era American cohort. BMC Public Health. 2015;15:1.

19. Curtis DS, Fuller-Rowell TE, Doan SN, Zgierska AE, Ryff CD. Racial and socioeconomic disparities in body mass index among college students: understanding the role of early life adversity. J Behav Med. 2016;39:866–75.

20. Pengpid S, Peltzer K. Prevalence of overweight/obesity and central obesity and its associated factors among a sample of university students in India. Obes Res Clin Pract. 2014;8:e558–70.

21. Li Y-q, Li J, Ze W-x, Li X-y, Bin L, Zo H-q. Investigation of obesity in undergraduate students of an university in Guangdong province and its influence factors. J Southeast Univ (Med Sci Edit). 2013;4:012.

22. Antiporta DA, Smeeth L, Gilman RH, Miranda JJ. Length of urban residence and obesity among within-country rural-to-urban Andean migrants. Public Health Nutr. 2016;19:1270–8.

23. Li R, Wang D, Chen J, Chai J, Tang M. Regional differences in smoking, drinking, and physical activities of Chinese residents. Asia Pac J Public Health. 2015;27:NP230–9.

24. Myers CA, Slack T, Martin CK, Broyles ST, Heymsfield SB. Change in obesity prevalence across the United States is influenced by recreational and healthcare contexts, food environments, and Hispanic populations. PLoS ONE. 2016;11:e0148394.

25. Matozinhos FP, Gomes CS, de Souza Andrade AC, Mendes LL, Pessoa MC, de Lima Friche AA. Neighbourhood environments and obesity among adults: a multilevel analysis of an urban Brazilian context. Prev Med Rep. 2015;2:337–41.

26. Nau C, Schwartz BS, Bandeen-Roche K, Liu A, Pollak J, Hirsch A. Community socioeconomic deprivation and obesity trajectories in children using electronic health records. Obesity. 2015;23:207–12.

27. Yang T, Yu L, Bottorff JL, Wu D, Jiang S, Peng S, Young KJ. Global Health Professions Student Survey (GHPSS) in tobacco control in China. Am J Health Behav. 2015;39:732–41.

28. Department of Disease Control and Prevention, National Ministry of Health. Guidelines for the prevention and control of overweight and obesity in China. Beijing: National Ministry of Health; 2003.

29. Le A, Judd SE, Allison DB, Oza-Frank R, Affuso O, Safford MM, Howard VJ, Howard G. The geographic distribution of obesity in the US and the potential regional differences in misreporting of obesity. Obesity. 2014;22:300–6.

30. Lao XQ, Ma WJ, Sobko T, Zhang YH, Xu YJ, Xu XJ, Yu DM, Nie SP, Cai QM, Xia L, Thomas GN, Griffiths SM. Overall obesity is leveling-off while abdominal obesity continues to rise in a Chinese population experiencing rapid economic development: analysis of serial cross-sectional health survey data 2002–2010. Int J Obes. 2015;39:288–94.

31. Andegiorgish AK, Wang J, Zhang X, Liu X, Zhu H. Prevalence of overweight, obesity, and associated risk factors among school children and adolescents in Tianjin, China. Eur J Pediatr. 2012;171:697–703.

32. Liu W, Lin R, Li B, Pallan M, Cheng KK, Adab P. Socioeconomic determinants of childhood obesity among primary school children in Guangzhou, China. BMC Public Health. 2016;16:1.

33. Lv J, Chen W, Sun D, Li S, Millwood IY, Smith M, Guo Y, Bian Z, Yu C, Zhou H, Tan Y, Chen C, Chen Z, Li L. Gender-specific association between tobacco smoking and central obesity among 0.5 million Chinese people: the China Kadoorie Biobank Study. PLoS ONE. 2015;10:e0124586.

34. Pei L, Cheng Y, Kang Y, Yuan S, Yan H. Association of obesity with socioeconomic status among adults of ages 18 to 80 years in rural Northwest China. BMC Public Health. 2015;15:1.

35. John U, Hanke M, Rumpf HJ, Thyrian JR. Smoking status, cigarettes per day, and their relationship to overweight and obesity among former and current smokers in a national adult general population sample. Int J Obes. 2005;29:1289–94.

36. National Ministry of Education. Annual report on university graduates' employment in 2015. Beijing: National Ministry of Education; 2016.

37. Grilli L, Pratesi M. Weighted estimation in multilevel ordinal and binary models in the presence of informative sampling designs. Surv Methodol. 2004;30:93–104.

38. Ji CY, Chen TJ, Working Group on Obesity in China (WGOC). Empirical changes in the prevalence of overweight and obesity among Chinese students from 1985 to 2010 and corresponding preventive strategies. Biomed Environ Sci. 2013;26:1–2.

39. Zou Y, Zhang R, Zhou B, Huang L, Chen J, Gu F, Zhang H, Fang Y, Ding G. A comparison study on the prevalence of obesity and its associated factors among city, township and rural area adults in China. BMJ Open. 2015;5:e008417.

40. Song Y, Ma J, Wang HJ, Wang Z, Hu P, Zhang B, Agard A. Secular trends of obesity prevalence in Chinese children from 1985 to 2010: urban–rural disparity. Obesity. 2015;23:448–53.

41. Jones-Smith JC, Gordon-Larsen P, Siddiqi A, Popkin BM. Cross-national comparisons of time trends in overweight inequality by socioeconomic status among women using repeated cross-sectional surveys from 37 developing countries, 1989–2007. Am J Epidemiol. 2011;173:667–75.

42. Subramanian SV, Perkins JM, Khan KT. Do burdens of underweight and overweight coexist among lower socioeconomic groups in India? Am J Clin Nutr. 2009;90:369–76.

43. Dutton DJ, McLaren L. How important are determinants of obesity measured at the individual level for explaining geographic variation in body mass index distributions? Observational evidence from Canada using quantile regression and Blinder–Oaxaca decomposition. J Epidemiol Commun Health. 2016;70:367–73.

44. Wang H, Zhai F. Programme and policy options for preventing obesity in China. Obes Rev. 2013;14:134–40.

45. Xu B, Yang J, Zhang Y, Gong P. Healthy cities in China: a Lancet Commission. Lancet. 2016;388:1863–4.

46. Jin H, Lu Y. The relationship between obesity and socioeconomic status among Texas school children and its spatial variation. Appl Geogr. 2017;79:143–52.

47. Gao Y, Huang Y, Song F, Dai D, Wang P, Li H, Zheng H, et al. Urban-rural disparity of overweight/obesity distribution and its potential trend with breast cancer among Chinese women. Oncotarget. 2016;7:56608–18.

Permissions

All chapters in this book were first published in IJHG, by BioMed Central; hereby published with permission under the Creative Commons Attribution License or equivalent. Every chapter published in this book has been scrutinized by our experts. Their significance has been extensively debated. The topics covered herein carry significant findings which will fuel the growth of the discipline. They may even be implemented as practical applications or may be referred to as a beginning point for another development.

The contributors of this book come from diverse backgrounds, making this book a truly international effort. This book will bring forth new frontiers with its revolutionizing research information and detailed analysis of the nascent developments around the world.

We would like to thank all the contributing authors for lending their expertise to make the book truly unique. They have played a crucial role in the development of this book. Without their invaluable contributions this book wouldn't have been possible. They have made vital efforts to compile up to date information on the varied aspects of this subject to make this book a valuable addition to the collection of many professionals and students.

This book was conceptualized with the vision of imparting up-to-date information and advanced data in this field. To ensure the same, a matchless editorial board was set up. Every individual on the board went through rigorous rounds of assessment to prove their worth. After which they invested a large part of their time researching and compiling the most relevant data for our readers.

The editorial board has been involved in producing this book since its inception. They have spent rigorous hours researching and exploring the diverse topics which have resulted in the successful publishing of this book. They have passed on their knowledge of decades through this book. To expedite this challenging task, the publisher supported the team at every step. A small team of assistant editors was also appointed to further simplify the editing procedure and attain best results for the readers.

Apart from the editorial board, the designing team has also invested a significant amount of their time in understanding the subject and creating the most relevant covers. They scrutinized every image to scout for the most suitable representation of the subject and create an appropriate cover for the book.

The publishing team has been an ardent support to the editorial, designing and production team. Their endless efforts to recruit the best for this project, has resulted in the accomplishment of this book. They are a veteran in the field of academics and their pool of knowledge is as vast as their experience in printing. Their expertise and guidance has proved useful at every step. Their uncompromising quality standards have made this book an exceptional effort. Their encouragement from time to time has been an inspiration for everyone.

The publisher and the editorial board hope that this book will prove to be a valuable piece of knowledge for researchers, students, practitioners and scholars across the globe.

List of Contributors

Yanchao Cheng, Nils Benjamin Tjaden, Anja Jaeschke, Stephanie Margarete Thomas and Carl Beierkuhnlein
Department of Biogeography, University of Bayreuth, Universitätsstr. 30, 95447 Bayreuth, Germany

Renke Lühken
Bernhard Nocht Institute for Tropical Medicine, World Health Organization Collaborating Centre for Arbovirus and Hemorrhagic Fever Reference and Research, Hamburg, Germany

Ute Ziegler
Friedrich-Loeffler-Institut, Institute of Novel and Emerging Infectious Diseases, Südufer 10, 17493 Greifswald – Insel Riems, Germany

Carl Beierkuhnlein
BayCEER, Bayreuth Center for Ecology and Environmental Research, Bayreuth, Germany

Winfred Dotse-Gborgbortsi
Kibi Government Hospital, Ghana Health Service, Accra, Ghana

Winfred Dotse-Gborgbortsi, Nicola Wardrop, Ademola Adewole, Mair L. H. Thomas and Jim Wright
Geography and Environment, University of Southampton, Highfield, Southampton SO17 1BJ, UK

Wahida Kihal-Talantikite
LIVE UMR 7362 CNRS (Laboratoire Image Ville Environnement), University of Strasbourg, Strasbourg 6700, Strasbourg, France

Christiane Weber
UMR Tetis (Territoires, environnement, télédétection et information spatiale), Montpelier, France

Gaelle Pedrono
The French National Public Health agency, Saint-Maurice, France

Claire Segala
SEPIA-Santé, Baud, France

Dominique Arveiler
Department of Epidemiology and Public Health, EA 3430, FMTS, Strasbourg University, Strasbourg, France

Clive E. Sabel
School of Geographical Sciences, University of Bristol, Bristol BS8 1SS, UK

Séverine Deguen
Department of Environmental and Occupational Health, School of Public Health (EHESP), Sorbonne Paris Cité, Rennes, France
Department of Social Epidemiology, Sorbonne Universités, UPMC Univ Paris 06, INSERM, Institut Pierre Louis d'Epidémiologie et de Santé Publique (UMRS 1136), Paris, France

Denis Bard
Department of Quantitative Methods in Public Health, School of Public Health (EHESP), Sorbonne Paris Cité, Rennes, Paris, France

Eva R. Maguire, Thomas Burgoine, Tarra L. Penney and Pablo Monsivais
UKCRC Centre for Diet and Activity Research (CEDAR), MRC Epidemiology Unit, University of Cambridge School of Clinical Medicine, Institute of Metabolic Science, Cambridge Biomedical Campus, Cambridge CB2 0QQ, UK

Nita G. Forouhi
MRC Epidemiology Unit, University of Cambridge School of Clinical Medicine, Institute of Metabolic Science, Cambridge Biomedical Campus Cambridge CB2 0QQ, UK

Pablo Monsivais
Department of Nutrition and Exercise Physiology, Washington State University Elson S Floyd College of Medicine, Spokane WA 99210, USA

Irene Garcia-Marti and Raúl Zurita-Milla
Department of Geo-Information Processing (GIP), Faculty of Geo-Information and Earth Observation (ITC), University of Twente, Enschede, The Netherlands

Arnold J. H. van Vliet
Department of Environmental Sciences, Wageningen University, Wageningen, The Netherlands

Willem Takken
Department of Plant Sciences, Wageningen University, Wageningen, The Netherlands

Boris Kauhl, Jürgen Schweikart, Andrea Keste and Marita Moskwyn
Department of Medical Care, AOK Nordost – Die Gesundheitskasse, Berlin, Germany

Boris Kauhl and Jürgen Schweikart
Department III, Civil Engineering and Geoinformatics, Beuth University of Applied Sciences, Berlin, Germany

Thomas Krafft
Department of Health, Ethics and Society, School of Public Health and Primary Care (CAPHRI), Faculty of Health, Medicine and Life Sciences, Maastricht University, Maastricht, The Netherlands

Hannah Verhoeven, Linde Van Hecke, Benedicte Deforche and Jelle Van Cauwenberg
Department of Public Health, Faculty of Medicine and Health Sciences,Ghent University, Corneel Heymanslaan 10, 9000 Ghent, Belgium

Hannah Verhoeven, Linde Van Hecke, Peter Clarys and Benedicte Deforche
Physical Activity, Nutrition and Health Research Unit, Faculty of Physical Education and Physical Therapy, Vrije Universiteit Brussel, Pleinlaan 2, 1050 Brussels, Belgium

Hannah Verhoeven, Linde Van Hecke, Delfien Van Dyck
Research Foundation - Flanders (FWO), Brussels, Belgium

Delfien Van Dyck
Department of Movement and Sport Sciences, Faculty of Medicine and Health Sciences, Ghent University, Watersportlaan 2, 9000 Ghent, Belgium

Tim Baert and Nico Van de Weghe
Department of Geography – CartoGIS, Faculty of Sciences, Ghent University, Krijgslaan 281, 9000 Ghent, Belgium

Enrique Gracia, Miriam Marco and Marisol Lila
Department of Social Psychology, University of Valencia, Av. Blasco Ibáñez, 21, 46010 Valencia, Spain

Antonio López-Quílez
Department of Statistics and Operations Research, University of Valencia, C/Doctor Moliner, 50, 46100 Burjassot, Valencia, Spain

Eun-Hye Yoo and Youngseob Eum
Department of Geography, University at Buffalo, Buffalo, NY, USA

Patrick Brown
Department of Statistical Sciences, University of Toronto, Toronto, Canada

Man Sing Wongs, Hung Chak Ho, Wenzhong Shi and Jinxin Yang
Department of Land Surveying and Geo-informatics, Hong Kong Polytechnic University, Kowloon, Hong Kong

Lin Yang
School of Nursing, Hong Kong Polytechnic University, Kowloon, Hong Kong

Ta-Chien Chan
Research Center for Humanity and Social Sciences, Academia Sinica, Taipei, Taiwan

Melanie Tomintz
GeoHealth Laboratory, Department of Geography, University of Canterbury, Private Bag 4800, Christchurch 8140, New Zealand

Bernhard Kosar
Geoinformation and Environmental Technologies, Carinthia University of Applied Sciences, Europastrasse 4, 9524 Villach, Austria

Graham Clarke
School of Geography, University of Leeds, Leeds LS2 9JT, UK

Juliano André Boquett, Marcelo Zagonel-Oliveira, Luiz Gonzaga Jr., Maurício Roberto Veronez Nelson Jurandi Rosa Fagundess and Lavínia Schüler-Faccini
Instituto Nacional de Genética Médica Populacional (INaGeMP), Porto Alegre, Brazil

Juliano André Boquett and Nelson Jurandi Rosa Fagundes
Post-Graduate Program in Genetics and Molecular Biology, Departamento de Genética, Universidade Federal do Rio Grande do Sul, Agencia Campus UFRGS, Caixa Postal 15053, Porto Alegre, RS CEP 91501-970, Brazil

Marcelo Zagonel-Oliveiras, Luiz Gonzaga Jr. and Maurício Roberto Veronez
Advanced Visualization and Geoinformatics Laboratory (VIZLab), Applied Computing Graduate Program, Universidade do Vale do Rio dos Sinos, São Leopoldo, RS, Brazil

Luis Fernando Jobim and Mariana Jobims
Department of Immunology, Hospital de Clínicas de Porto Alegre, Porto Alegre, Brazil

Claire A. Quiner and Yoshinori Nakazawa
Poxvirus and Rabies Branch, Division of High-Consequence Pathogens and Pathology (DHCPP), National Center for Emerging and Zoonotic Infectious Diseases (NCEZID), US Centers for Disease Control and Prevention, Atlanta, GA, USA

Imelda K. Moise and Jaclyn F. Verity
Department of Geography and Regional Studies, University of Miami, 1300 Campo Sano Ave, Coral Gables, FL 33124, USA

Joseph Kangmennaang
University of Waterloo, Waterloo, ON N2L 3G1, Canada

Shaheen A. Abdulkareem
Department of Governance and Technology for Sustainability (CSTM), Faculty of Behavioral, Management, and Social Sciences (BMS), University of Twente, Enschede, The Netherlands
Department of Computer Science, College of Science, University of Duhok (UoD), Duhok, Kurdistan Region, Iraq

Ellen-Wien Augustijn
Department of Geo-Information Process (GIP), Faculty of Geo-Information Science and Earth Observation (ITC), University of Twente, Enschede, The Netherlands

Yaseen T. Mustafa
Faculty of Science, University of Zakho (UoZ), Duhok, Kurdistan Region, Iraq

Tatiana Filatova
School of Systems, Management and Leadership, Faculty of Engineering and Information Technology, University of Technology Sydney, Ultimo, Australia

Tingzhong Yang, Lingwei Yu, Shuhan Jiang and Sihui Peng
Department of Social Medicine/Center for Tobacco Control Research, Zhejiang University School of Medicine, Hangzhou 310058, China

Ross Barnett
Department of Geography, University of Canterbury, Private Bag 4800, Christchurch, New Zealand

Yafeng Fan
Department of Nursing, Hangzhou Normal University, Hangzhou 310036, China

Lu Li
Institute of Family and Social Medicine, Zhejiang University School of Medicine, Hangzhou 310058, China

Index

www.ingramcontent.com/pod-product-compliance
Lightning Source LLC
Chambersburg PA
CBHW061253190326
41458CB00011B/3657